Crossing Over

Crossing Over

Narratives of Palliative Care

Revised Edition

DAVID BARNARD, PHD, JD
Department of Medicine
Section of Palliative Care and Medical Ethics
Center for Bioethics and Health Law
University of Pittsburgh
Pittsburgh, Pennsylvania

ANNA TOWERS, MD
Supportive and Palliative Care Services
McGill University Health Centre
Montreal, Canada

PATRICIA BOSTON, PHD
Department of Family Practice
Faculty of Medicine
University of British Columbia
Vancouver, Canada

YANNA LAMBRINIDOU, PHD
Department of Science, Technology, and Society
Virginia Polytechnic Institute and State University
Blacksburg, Virginia

OXFORD
UNIVERSITY PRESS

OXFORD
UNIVERSITY PRESS

Oxford University Press is a department of the University of Oxford. It furthers
the University's objective of excellence in research, scholarship, and education
by publishing worldwide. Oxford is a registered trade mark of Oxford University
Press in the UK and certain other countries.

Published in the United States of America by Oxford University Press
198 Madison Avenue, New York, NY 10016, United States of America.

Library of Congress Cataloging-in-Publication Data
Names: Barnard, David, 1948- editor. | Towers, Anna, 1953- editor. |
Boston, Patricia, editor. | Lambrinidou, Yanna, editor.
Title: Crossing over : narratives of palliative care / [edited by] David Barnard,
Anna Towers, Patricia Boston, and Yanna Lambrinidou.
Other titles: Crossing over (Barnard) Description: Revised edition. |
New York, NY : Oxford University Press, [2023] |
Preceded by Crossing over : narratives of palliative care / David Barnard ... [et al.]. 2000. |
Includes bibliographical references and index.
Identifiers: LCCN 2022028805 (print) | LCCN 2022028806 (ebook) |
ISBN 9780197602270 (paperback) | ISBN 9780197602294 (epub) | ISBN 9780197602300
Subjects: MESH: Palliative Care | Terminal Care |
Terminally Ill—psychology | Personal Narrative
Classification: LCC RT87.T45 (print) | LCC RT87.T45 (ebook) |
NLM WB 310 | DDC 616.02/9—dc23/eng/20220803
LC record available at https://lccn.loc.gov/2022028805
LC ebook record available at https://lccn.loc.gov/2022028806

DOI: 10.1093/med/9780197602270.001.0001

1 3 5 7 9 8 6 4 2

Printed by Sheridan Books, Inc., United States of America

Praise for the 2000 Edition

The text would be an excellent addition to any collection on death and dying. In a non-judgmental manner the authors have examined the individualism of dying while maintaining the clinical aspects.
—*Bibliotheca Medica Canadian*, 2000 Winter

All the narratives are engrossing. They are also instructive, illustrating how the issues that arise in palliative care can be addressed through a team process.
—*JAMC*, March 20, 2001

The affective void of traditional medical writing gives way to the richly varied texture of lived existential experience. The narrator's voice is also clear. Qualitative research posits that the researcher is a dynamic, interactive element in the human equation.
—*Annals*, March 2001

This text is an excellent reminder that when we die, we will be able to decide what is right for us. For clinicians and lay people, and a must for the library of any clinician who deals with end-of-life issues.
—*ChoiceMiddletown*, Connecticut, May 2001

A welcome addition to the fast-growing literature in this field of human need and response.
—Dr. Derek Doyle

Too many times clinicians and caregivers alike want to decide what is good and what is bad about a death experience. This text is an excellent reminder that when we die, we will be able to decide what is right for us. While others may make suggestions or offer information, they must allow the patient to decide how this event should proceed. (Weighted Numerical Score: 100–5 Stars!)

—*Doody's*

Crossing Over is an impressive collection of 20 "narratives" of people facing the ends of their lives alongside their professional and informal careers. What makes this book quite outstanding is the wealth of clinical experience contained within its pages—covering the physical, psychosocial, and spiritual issues of dying. This book emphasizes all aspects of holistic care with equal importance in the day-to-day work of end-of-life care. Because the text is about the actuality of "crossing over," it is not surprising that spirituality and religious ritual play an important part in the text. This book will be extremely helpful for all disciplines working within the field of special palliative care. The emotional energy that many of the narratives must have consumed just to work with, let alone write down, is enormous. The authors need to be congratulated for bringing together an extremely coherent masterpiece in an easy-to-read style.

—*Progress in Palliative Care*, 2000

Crossing Over is written with the education and training of physicians, nurses, chaplains, therapists, and social workers in mind. The author-investigators have taken pains to capture and convey the perspectives of patients and their families. This is cinema-verite projected in written word: the experience of illness, dying, and caregiving photographed with available light, through clinical lenses. *Crossing Over* reads as biography, ethnography, comparative sociology, and medical anthropology. However, true to its intention, it remains a clinical report. The book ultimately succeeds in conveying the essence of palliative care.

—Ira Byock, *Hastings Center Report*, Nov.–Dec. 2000

This work is a collection of narratives that each provide a glimpse into the later stages of a terminal illness. The narratives cover a wide range of concerns, touching on the emotions of both patients and caregivers, physical symptoms, spiritual concerns, stress on family relationships, and the challenge of providing adequate hospice and palliative care. At the end of the book, the authors of each narrative provide commentary and raise questions for discussion. Additionally, the book is complete with an index of themes and an extensive list of further reading.

—*Journal of Social Work Education*, Winter 2001

[A]n insightful and challenging attempt to document the gap that exists between the theories of palliative care and the realities of its day-to-day practice . . . this book is refreshing in its avoidance of false hope and tidy resolutions.

—*Journal of Palliative Care*

[P]rovides an extraordinary portrait of the processes of giving and receiving palliative care . . . ideal for practitioners and trainees in medicine, nursing, gerontology, ministry, counseling psychology, allied health, and social work.

—End-of-Life Physician Education
Resource Center (EPERC), January 2001

[P]rovides a much-needed service by supplying us with rich tales of dying in North America and, in doing so, they have given more realistic and contemporary alternatives to Ivan Ilych . . . fascinating, important additions to palliative studies.

—*Theoretical Medicine*, 2001

[U]ndoubtedly moving, and provide some real insights into the experience of those dealing with dying and death.

—*Social Sciences & Medicine*, 2002

This book is about the human side of palliative care, viewed in depth and from a variety of perspectives. For students of palliative care and their teachers, this is a wonderful resource, complete with lists of questions and discussion topics in the final chapter. For those who work in palliative care, this book will stimulate professional self-reflection and challenge such basic tenets as to whether or not all the things we do and regard as "good" are really beneficial to the patients and their families. Highly recommended.

—IAHC website, November 2002

To
Balfour Mount,
Mentor, Colleague, Friend
and
To all who are striving to make systems of care more equitable and more just

Contents

Foreword from the Previous Edition

In a famous 1906 lecture to medical students, entitled "Science and Immortality," Sir William Osler referred to his records of 500 death-bed cases. These were studied through the nurses at the Johns Hopkins Hospital, Baltimore, and showed that the actual sensations of dying in the great majority of patients were "like their birth—a sleep and a forgetting."[1] The cards on which patient details are recorded are kept in the Osler Library at McGill University and, so far as I know, are the first attempt at such a study. It is moving to see and handle them, but it also arouses questions about the illnesses that preceded this peaceful dying.

Nearly a century later, this book describes in perceptive detail the sometimes tortuous journeys toward such final moments. It concentrates on personal and family struggles with inexorable illness rather than on the details of the medical treatments, nursing, and other support that palliative care teams aim to offer.

The authors do not idealize these very real people; rather, like so many patients I recall after 50 years in this field, these people teach us what it means to be human. There are many lessons in living to be learned from the dying, and some of these are described here with quiet objectivity.

Many of us in palliative care spend much of our time helping people face crises and have to assess and analyze a situation with speed as well as sensitivity. We may have only a small part in a whole continuity of care and family dynamics. It is, however, often from the rarer situation when we can follow a patient alone or with a family through weeks or months that we may learn to meet more urgent needs. One of our patients at St. Christopher's Hospice, London, who had amyotrophic lateral sclerosis, was such a person. A lonely musician (a flautist), he challenged all our skills, understanding, and patience. Near the end of his year-long saga with us he dictated the following during a poetry workshop:

[1] Osler W. *Science and Immortality*. New York: Arno Press; 1906/1977: 17.

Smoke Rings
I can't blow smoke rings any more
My tongue, it will not budge,
But other people's various powers
I never would begrudge.

It's not for me to jealous be
And make a silly fuss.
If everybody were like me
Then who'd look after us?

The more I lose my little skills
The more I see God's plan,
I see what really counts with Him:
The essence of a man.
—James Haylock-Eyre[2]

It is "the essence of a man" that we meet in this book, and I believe we will be wiser and more confident in both our service and living because of what we have learned here.

—Dame Cicely Saunders, OM, DBE, FRCP
Chairman, St. Christopher's Hospice, London

[2] Heylock-Eyre J. Smoke rings. In: Saunders C, ed. *Beyond the Horizon* London: Darton, Longman & Todd; 1992: 11.

Preface to the Revised Edition

The first edition of *Crossing Over* appeared in 2000. It was the fruit of three years of research that we conducted between 1995 and 1998. At that time, the specialty of palliative medicine—as distinct from hospice care, which had emerged in its modern form some three decades earlier—was just beginning to come into its own.* A growing number of textbooks and scholarly journals were making the scientific and clinical aspects of palliative care more widely known than ever before. Yet, despite this profusion of publications, which continues today, there was—and is—a gap. As two reviewers of several of those early textbooks put it, "Most palliative care textbooks, including the *Oxford Textbook*, do not speak to the heart, nor do they give an adequate sense of the range of psychological, spiritual, social, and existential suffering or the opportunities for personal growth and healing that dying presents."[1]

This was our aim: to speak to the heart by telling as vividly as possible stories of giving and receiving palliative care—with particular emphasis on the inner life or subjective experience of patients, families, and caregivers. We still believe this to be a valid aim, and we are grateful to Oxford University Press for reaching out to us to prepare a revised and updated edition for a new generation of readers. We particularly thank Tiffany Lu, Marta Moldvai, and Emily Hu at Oxford University Press for their steady interest and support.

To be sure, since *Crossing Over* first appeared, many other books have "spoken to the heart" by telling stories from the world of palliative care. Here, too, *Crossing Over* was—and is—different. The great majority of these books are written by a single author—usually a palliative care clinician—and from the single point of view of that author. We admire many of these books for their passion and their advocacy of an empathic, holistic approach. Yet these very characteristics—advocacy and close personal involvement—limit these books in important respects. As advocates who selected their narratives retrospectively to illustrate the merits of a particular style of end-of-life care,

---

* In this book, we use "palliative care" as an umbrella term for comprehensive, supportive care for people with life-threatening illness, within which are the various clinical disciplines such as palliative medicine and nursing and particular forms for delivering palliative care such as hospice.

the authors are apt to minimize some of the inadequacies or ambiguities of their philosophies when applied to particular patients. More important is their singular narrative point of view, especially in the many prominent books written in the first-person voice of a physician. For all the authors' evident empathy for the experiences of patients and families, their approach inevitably privileges the physician's point of view. This is what we sought to avoid. We actively sought out the experiences and perceptions of the widest possible range of participants in each of our narratives, which include voices of patients, families, doctors, nurses, social workers, chaplains, volunteers, friends, and neighbors. And we adopted third-person narration when describing the events in our book precisely to allow voices to emerge in a way that reflected the actors' actual role and importance. Very often, the important roles were not that of the physician.

The narratives in this book describe events that took place nearly a quarter-century ago. Why republish them now? In the first place, the thoughts, actions, and feelings of the individuals who lived, died, and provided care in these narratives are profoundly human. They occurred in the past, but they will be immediately recognizable today by anyone who has been touched by life-threatening illness as sufferer, caregiver, or companion. The people in this book still have much to teach us about dying and caring for the dying—lessons that feel more urgent in a world ravaged by COVID-19. We have opened this edition of *Crossing Over* with Anna Towers's narrative of living and working as a palliative care physician in the midst of the COVID-19 pandemic, which, as this is written, has yet to abate. Anna's narrative is a bridge between the world in which the narratives in this book took place and the world we live in today.

As Anna remarks in the Afterword to her narrative, all of us today are living with a newly heightened awareness of personal vulnerability, the fragility of our institutions, and the gaping inequalities in our societies that the pandemic has made starkly visible. We have endured ruptures in every facet of our everyday lives. We have observed and lived through cruel separations from loved ones as people's lives have ended. And we have watched health systems buckle before the pandemic's sweep. Yet, we have also borne daily witness to the resilience, courage, even heroism, of friends, neighbors, and colleagues—not least in the practice of palliative care. These themes—vulnerability, fragility, inequality, resilience, courage, heroism—are all present in the narratives in this book. We believe they will resonate even more strongly for readers who encounter them today.

We have therefore kept the narratives essentially intact, though we have edited them lightly to tighten and streamline the text. At the same time, we appreciate that there have been many changes in palliative care and in society, in both Canada and the United States, since our book first appeared. To account for these, we have made major changes in this edition, in addition to the pandemic narrative by Anna Towers. The most important changes are in the General Introduction and the Authors' Comments that follow each individual narrative. Just as we situated the narratives originally in the context of our understanding of palliative care in North America in the 1990s, for this revised edition we have situated them in the context of the 2020s. The General Introduction provides an initial, broad overview of the contemporary context. In the Authors' Comments, we look more closely at the specific life choices and clinical decisions made by the individuals involved. There, we emphasize the changes in society—which as we write this Preface include a profound racial reckoning—and in professional practices that might lead certain aspects of these individuals' experiences to be approached differently today. We also comment where the narratives illustrate enduring problems in caring for the dying and their families that persist despite the evolution of the field.

At a more personal level, this revised edition gives us as authors an opportunity to look at our narratives through new eyes. We are 20 years older! Just as the field of palliative care has evolved in the past 20 years, so have our individual understandings of death and dying, the nature of caring relationships, ethics and professionalism, and the relations of science, medicine, and society. We have drawn on these perspectives in writing new or thoroughly revised commentaries for each narrative. Our goal is to produce an edition of *Crossing Over* that is as reflective of its authors today as it is of its new readers.

—D. B., A. T., P. B., Y. L.
November 2021

Reference

1. Quill TE, Billings JA. Palliative care textbooks come of age. *Ann Intern Med.* 1998:129(7):590–594.

Preface to the First Edition

The preface usually gets written last, which seems especially fitting for a book on palliative care. For the preface is as much an opportunity to look back, take stock, and give thanks as it is to alert readers to what lies ahead. In our case, we have much to acknowledge in the way of colleagueship (among the four of us), collaboration (with patients, families, and caregivers), and support (from our sponsors and home institutions).

For the authors, this book grew out of shared interests and experience in care for the dying and dissatisfaction with currently available stories of what that experience is like. Two of us (Anna Towers and Patricia Boston) are clinicians who are working or have worked directly with the dying. One of us (David Barnard) teaches medical humanities and palliative care to health professionals who care for the dying and is involved administratively with palliative care programs. And one of us (Yanna Lambrinidou) combines interest in the subject of end-of-life care with a broader interest in the ethnographic study, and faithful rendering, of human experience with illness and health. As we worked together, the four of us came to enjoy a form of collaboration, interdependence, and mutual respect that, we all agree, has been unique in our professional lives.

Almost exactly three decades ago, Paul Ramsey published one of the pioneering works in the young field of medical ethics, *The Patient as Person*. The care of the dying figures very prominently in Ramsey's seminal book. In a chapter entitled "On (Only) Caring for the Dying," Ramsey made an observation that could easily serve to summarize the subject matter of our book.

> Upon ceasing to try to rescue the perishing, one is then free to care for the dying, Act of caring for the dying are deeds done bodily for them which serve solely to manifest that they are not lost from human attention, that they are not alone, that mankind generally and their loved ones take note of their dying and mean to company with them in accepting this unique instance of the acceptable death of all flesh.[1]

What is it like, we wanted to know, to "company with" the dying? This book is our effort to answer that question from the points of view of family members, hospice workers, palliative care staff, friends and loved ones, and—to the extent possible—from the point of view of the dying themselves.

To state this goal is to proclaim immediately the enormous debt we owe to the patients and families who accepted us into their living and dying, so that we might tell others of their experiences. In a sense, they are the true authors of this work, and we but the transcribers and editors.

We are also indebted to the staff of the Palliative Care Service at the Royal Victoria Hospital, Montreal, and at the Hospice of Lancaster County, Lancaster, Pennsylvania. These superb and generous clinicians and volunteers were willing to open themselves to our view in the midst of the day-to-day routines and emergencies of end-of-life care, with no time to rehearse—and no protection in the thought that if a case didn't turn out well we would exclude it from the book. We admire these people for their professionalism and for their commitment to improving hospice and palliative care through research and honest self-reflection.

None of these people can receive acknowledgment by name, in keeping with our promise of confidentiality. Several other people, however, can be acknowledged publicly for their crucial contributions to our project.

Eileen Lavery provided essential administrative and clerical support in Montreal. June Watson, Administrative Assistant in the Department of Humanities at the Pennsylvania State University College of Medicine, prepared the final draft of the entire manuscript (as well as several almost-final ones) and supervised all of the complicated administrative aspects of an interinstitutional and binational collaboration. During the writing of this book David Barnard was University Professor and Chair of the Department of Humanities at the Penn State College of Medicine.

Angela Martin, who at the time was a medical student at Penn State, helped lay the foundation for the Lancaster County fieldwork. Gina Tuncil transcribed the Lancaster County interviews. Dr. Cathy Jarvis assisted with some of the data collection and medical editing in Montreal. Elizabeth C. Hechtman, at the Philadelphia Center for Social Therapy, provided clinical supervision that was invaluable to Yanna Lambrinidou during the Lancaster County fieldwork. Lauren Enck was our skilled and supportive editor at Oxford University Press.

Finally we are pleased to acknowledge a major research grant from the Open Society Institute's Project on Death in America. Essential additional support was generously provided by the Greenwall Foundation, the Social Sciences and Humanities Research Council of Canada, the T. R. Meighen Foundation, and the Walter J. Blackburn Foundation.

—D. B., A. T., P. B., Y. L.
October 1999

Reference

1. Ramsey P. *The Patient as Person*. New Haven: Yale University Press; 1970: 153.

1

Prelude—Palliative Care in the Time of Pandemic

"I Am a soldier, a Different Person . . . a Ghost"

Anna Towers

As humans we meet through shared narratives. There will be as many COVID-19 narratives as there are humans. I am, by nature, a note-taker. At the start of the pandemic, I decided to take more detailed notes from the viewpoint of a palliative care physician, as I sensed that interesting times were coming. This narrative is based on my experience during the first year of the crisis in Quebec, up to March 2021. Although the situation is still evolving, I feel that the topics and themes most relevant to palliative care and to me as a person had emerged by then.

I hesitated often as I wrote because I am one of the lucky ones. I live in a peaceful country, not one at war. In Canada, we have a government-funded healthcare system where no one need fear healthcare costs when faced with sudden illness—or a pandemic. I am 68 years old, but healthy. I have a loving family and friends. I am a well-off physician and have had a privileged life. Many essential workers were, and are, exposed to far more COVID risk than I was—in crowded, poorly ventilated environments, without adequate protection. Too many in the world do not yet have access to the vaccine. I therefore present this first-person account in all humility.

Like many physician providers, I work in several clinical contexts and areas: on a palliative care service in a main McGill University hospital, including an inpatient unit, a consultation service, and a supportive care clinic for cancer patients; on a palliative home care program, and—for a few hours per week—on a ward in a chronic care facility.

In some ways, this has been an ordinary year for physicians. We did not lose our jobs! We are used to dealing with death and dying, with persons in distress, and with emergencies of all sorts. But in those ordinary contexts we work and problem-solve over a period of hours or days before taking a mental break in normal surroundings. In the first year of the pandemic, COVID-19 never let up. It was a unique experience for all and distressing to many.

A New Reality

March 5, 2020

Every winter a good friend and I try to get away from the Canadian cold, snow, and ice for two weeks. I am recently back in town, well-rested after a Caribbean holiday. We had irregular internet access and were cut off from daily news. We heard intermittently about the coronavirus outbreaks in China, Europe, and the USA. The first confirmed case in Quebec was in Montreal, last week—a woman returning from Iran.

Back home, I turn on my computer and face a new reality of emails and bulletins full of calls to action. Those of us in palliative care—like all health professionals—are suddenly preparing late into the evening, reading and interpreting Ministry of Health and hospital directives.

Hospital nurses come to train our team on personal protective equipment (PPE). I double-check our clinic's PPE kits: masks, visors or face shields, gowns, as well as the constantly updated emergency directive sheet on how to deal with patients with respiratory symptoms who may turn up at the clinic.

My palliative care colleagues are involved in shifting patients so the hospital can create designated wards for those infected, who are expected to arrive within the next few weeks. Our role as palliative care providers is twofold: to prepare to deal with ill and dying coronavirus patients and to help inform non-specialists on basic end-of-life care. Team members are adapting pharmaceutical protocols and other guidance that will be useful to non-palliative physicians and nurses who will be dealing with those dying in respiratory distress. We email this information to medical teams across the region, trying to minimize the risk of opioid and sedative dosage errors. The key message to our colleagues was twofold: (1) appropriate medication for comfort will not hasten death. (2) As far as dosages go, start low, go slow, but GO.

There is a general sense of dread. We know from Europe that the death rate will be high. We review the antibiotic and other protocols, knowing full well that there is no specific treatment for this novel virus.

I prepare my own PPE. The hospitals provide surgical scrubs, but they don't fit me properly. I buy a dozen sets of scrubs online: purely for aesthetics, I choose white, beige, or turquoise for spring and summer; gray for winter. I imagine that this is all that I will be wearing for the foreseeable future.

March 18, 2020
The World Health Organization declared coronavirus (now known as COVID-19) a pandemic on March 11. The tally of cases is growing in Canada, with many now linked to the United States. (New York State is only 60 miles south of here.) Two days from now, the 8,891-kilometre-long US–Canada border will close to non-essential travel.

I feel a sense of foreboding, like we are entering a war situation. The COVID peak in our region is predicted by mid-April. The urgent videoconference and telephone calls continue. Outbreaks have started in chronic care hospitals, also known as long-term care (LTC) facilities. The provincial Ministry of Health declares that, as of now, families and private care assistants can no longer visit their loved ones in hospitals, LTCs, or in private residences for seniors. At one of my side jobs in an LTC, the nurses, my physician colleagues, and I are now spending a lot of time every day speaking on the phone with distraught family members. Luckily, COVID cases are still few.

Because they come in various sizes, we get fitted for the N95 respirator masks in case we need to work in particularly high-risk COVID situations. I mentally prepare the exercise of managing the PPE, as I go from an uninfected hospital area to a COVID-positive zone: remove the old procedural mask, wash hands, don gown, don a new procedural mask, don face shield, don gloves, enter the COVID ward. Then doff gloves, doff gown, wash hands, doff mask and visor, wash hands, don new mask, don gloves, sanitize and store face shield, doff gloves.

I feel a split between my professional self and my personal self. On the professional side, I still work full-time in a hospital environment. I have a job to do. I take orders from above and interpret orders for those under my supervision. On the personal side, I wonder: Will I myself get very sick? Will my 32-year-old son, Daniel, a student who still lives with me, get sick? What about my older friends, my elderly mother who is now isolated, my co-workers? But there are practical matters to be seen to. Like everyone else, I stock up on frozen food and essentials. I make an appointment with the bank to ensure that Daniel has power-of-attorney on my accounts, and I brief him on finances.

Then I get back into physician mode. I remind myself once more that I am experienced in dealing with emergencies and leading team members in new and changing situations. I am in perfect health. I have a very good immune system. I seldom even get colds. I can do this!

April 9, 2020

There are now hundreds of cases in Quebec. Non-essential businesses were shut down on March 23. My services are required in an LTC hospital in which there are already 30 COVID patients. I see in the daily public health bulletins that most LTCs in the region are similarly affected. COVID beds in the acute care hospitals are rapidly filling. We are asked to minimize transfers from LTC settings to emergency rooms. That directive causes me some distress. In "peacetime," we can automatically send very ill yet appropriate LTC patients to an acute care hospital. I will now have to justify every transfer to a hospital colleague who is the on-duty "gatekeeper." They may refuse the transfer. And it somehow feels like all these discussions happen at 2 A.M.

After my morning at an MUHC supportive care clinic, I round on an LTC hospital ward for those with stroke or advanced dementia. I am relieved that there is no COVID on this ward! However, family members need to be alerted regarding the likelihood that their loved one will not be transferred to an acute care hospital should they contract COVID. I need to urgently update dozens of level-of-care or medical directive forms. These patients are not competent to sign advance directives, so I need to find the relative who is their legal representative. Only a physician can have this discussion, normally face to face. So how does one speak about COVID, advance directives, and levels of care over the telephone, while wearing a face mask, to someone whose first language may be neither English nor French and who may also be elderly and partially deaf?

My rounds are over for the day. I sit at home with telephone call list in front of me. At least at home I don't need to wear PPE in order to work. On the downside, these are calls concerning patients whom I might have just seen briefly; their full medical and nursing records are not available to me. Almost invariably, the family member I am speaking with is distraught and has very specific questions about the immediate status of their loved one—questions that I cannot answer. The ward nurse does not have a cellphone and will be busy dealing with ill patients. She cannot be answering my every landline call.

I pass on the same information, over and over, to family members—and try to deal with their emotional reactions. Someone with advanced dementia and other comorbidities such as heart or lung disease who is bedbound, I tell them, would likely not survive a cardiac arrest nor its aftermath. Should they develop respiratory failure and be intubated, they would likely not be successfully weaned off a ventilator, and—in the minuscule chance that they would survive—they would not have much brain function left. Transfer to an acute medical ward would not change the outcome, I say. Some family members fear that a do-not-resuscitate (DNR) or a "do not transfer" order means that their spouse, mother, or father will be abandoned and not receive any care. I have to explain, again and again, about appropriate level of care: that we can still provide physician coverage and intravenous medication, oxygen, blood tests, and X-rays where indicated; that we will transfer their parent to the acute care hospital if it would change the outcome or improve their comfort. Some family members require long discussions, and some say that they need to consult with siblings before authorizing changes in level of care. The discussions continue late into the evening and into the night.

In the larger world, many national borders have now closed, as well as some provincial borders. My trip to the UK this week is cancelled, and so is a European conference next month. In Quebec, professional bodies are asking retired healthcare personnel to help. Government officials tell us that more support is coming. But how long will it take? Non-healthcare workers such as teachers and librarians are asked to volunteer in hospitals. I wonder: How will outside helpers be kept safe from infection if they are not used to hospital protocols?

Once more, I feel like I am preparing for a war front. It is my duty to go, but I am afraid. Do I have the right skills to protect the life of COVID patients who are not ICU candidates, just with basic medical and proper supportive care? At short notice, health authorities have not had a chance to acquire all the supplies that we will need. We are told that there are shortages of PPE, that we will need to reutilize masks and face visors. In a touching gesture, a friend who is not in healthcare offers to donate the few surgical masks that she has been able to acquire for her personal use. The more protective "blue" overall gowns are in short supply, as are the specialized respirator masks. Some mask sizes are not available. But we just have to get on with it.

April 12, 2020

As I round on the LTC ward, a nurse comes up to me with a personal problem: she has a sore throat and asks me to have a look. Normally I might oblige but now I tell her to call the hospital employee COVID line. They tell us that COVID tests are not widely available, that testing capacity will improve soon, but for now indications are limited. The screening staff are abiding by strict checklists of "significant" symptoms. If you have just one symptom, such as fever or sore throat, you don't get tested. The employee COVID service tells the nurse to stay home until she has been symptom-free for 24 hours and then come back to work.

I head an outpatient supportive care team that is based outside the main hospital. I need to brief the team members who are under my supervision. I am up late at night or early in the morning, scanning emails and public health sites so I can interpret guidelines for our staff and plan procedures in minute detail, adapted to our specific clinic. We need to go through all our patient appointments that have been scheduled a year in advance. How do we screen these outpatients? Who do we see in-person and who do we see virtually? Where do we direct patients who are ill? We telephone patients the day before their appointment to tell them not to come to their clinic if they are unwell. What do we do in an emergency with a person who might arrive at our door feeling ill and in respiratory distress, despite our telephone pre-screening procedure? What do we do if one or more team members become ill, or if we are recruited at short notice to work elsewhere?

All physicians in my department are asked to do COVID ward duty unless we have a medical condition or (based on what we know at this time about risk to life) are age 70 or over. At the LTC hospital especially, it truly feels like we are at war. Our virtual team meetings are called "war rounds."

I am leaving most parts of myself behind. I am a soldier, a different person . . . a ghost.

April 17, 2020

Today I am doing an eight-hour shift on the COVID ward in the acute care hospital. There are now three "step-down" COVID isolation wards here, units housing patients who are recently off ventilators or those who may not (yet) require a ventilator. I will do a couple of shifts here, and then I have been released to spend more time in the LTC setting where the need is greater. In marked contrast to the LTC, these three COVID wards are in a recently built pavilion, with state-of-the-art ventilation systems. In the antechamber,

I change into PPE in the well-equipped staff room. I notice staff levels are good here. There are two nurses to orient me. The COVID patients have been put into single, negative-pressure rooms to limit virus-contaminated air from escaping. The physicians can view the patient through glass and speak to them through a monitor. Only the primary nurse and nursing assistant in best available PPE go into the patient rooms. Although there is some air exchange, it feels pretty safe for the MDs. Nevertheless, I notice that my physician colleague is using a clear plastic bag to house his cellular phone, and he is taking notes through the bag. I wonder how I will protect my own phone when I go to the LTC.

Back home I continue my telephone calls to the families of the LTC ward patients that I know. Spouses, daughters, sons are anxious and have many questions. Whereas ordinarily they might have visited daily, they have not been able to see their loved one for the past month. Many ask for daily updates. Social workers and ancillary staff working from home have been recruited to place calls after briefings from nurses. Understandably, the relatives wish to speak with a nurse or a doctor who has actually seen their loved one that day. Do they have a fever? How is their breathing? I do what I can with the briefing information that I have. I am still trying to update some level-of-care directives. How can I get through all this? From lack of personnel and communication channels there seems to be chaos as to how information is transmitted. One son is angry with me because I am reporting that his COVID-positive father is stable when in fact he died earlier today.

April 19, 2020
I have been putting in up to sixteen-hour days. This was supposed to be my only day off in two weeks, but they called for LTC COVID work because they are short of MDs. Two of our younger physician colleagues tell us that they have hardly been going home. They have not seen their children. In between their medical tasks they have been helping to feed and wash the patients, and late into the evening they are facilitating phone and video calls between the patients and their anxious family members. I hear on the news that over one thousand personnel from the Canadian Armed Forces will be coming to twenty of the hardest-hit LTCs to help with staffing and infection control.

April 20, 2020
Our charitably funded MUHC Supportive Care Program now has financial concerns. The fund manager tells me that there are, and will be, fewer

charitable donations during COVID. One of my hospital programs is threat-ened. I speak to the Ministry of Health about it. They cannot help: the hos-pital must take care of it within existing budgets. I am forced to cut staff temporarily.

COVID tests are still not widely available. We don't really know who among us might be asymptomatic and yet contagious. Three more patients on my supposedly COVID-free, "cold" LTC ward test positive for COVID. I go in to see one of them, a bedbound woman with advanced dementia and chronic lung disease. She looks very unwell. I call her daughter, the desig-nated decision-maker. Luckily, she understands the futility of aggressive measures and does not insist on acute hospital transfer. As I am writing a note on this case, a nurse next to me comments that she has conjunctivitis. I tell her that could be a sign of COVID. She seemed not to be aware. I suggest she call about getting tested. As I say that, I again realize that she might be refused testing because she does not have two or more of the current specific significant symptoms. In this crisis, the authorities' definition of "significant" symptoms is changing according to the testing resources available. This we must accept.

The LTC hospital pharmacist emails us to advise that we may face shortages of some basic injectable palliative care drugs. We now have limited supplies of methotrimeprazine and midazolam—our most used sedatives. We discuss alternatives. As far as PPE is concerned, I notice that we are short of the wall-mounted hand sanitizer gel. Most of the pumps are empty. An infection con-trol coordinator brings us a few small bottles. This is not adequate, I say to myself. I email my supervisors about the insufficient protection.

I drive home at the end of another long day. Even having reached home, I cannot disengage from this crisis. In the driveway, I perform the daily rou-tine. I disinfect the inside of the car with wipes—the steering wheel, shift control, and doorknobs. I walk up to the front door, strip off my clothing. I keep to the top floor of our three-floor dwelling, while my son stays in a basement suite. We share a kitchen. I run up to get showered and wash my hair. I disinfect the faucet taps, my phone, my keys. I come down and do more laundry. I worry about my son becoming infected in addition to myself. I wonder if I should be cooking, given the chance that I might be a positive carrier. However, I do not want to put all the burden of cooking onto my son. I decide that I will cook. I start to prepare some soup but first I wash my hands again, perhaps for the fiftieth time today.

Cases Rising

April 24, 2020

Across the province, the LTC statistics are alarming. There are now over 100 infected in the LTC hospital where I am helping out. Today I start on what was my "cold" ward. Thirteen out of 29 patients are positive. One week ago there were none. They have now been transferred to the "hot" unit across the way, where all the patients are COVID-positive. At the PPE station there are no gloves my size. I must go to another ward to find some. Many of the hand gel dispensers are empty. I will disinfect and reuse my face shield until I can no longer see through it.

Compared to the acute-care COVID ward where I worked last week, there are no isolated private rooms here. Most patients are in two- or three-bed rooms, but the unit is basically being run as an open ward. There are no barriers between staff and patients beyond our PPE.

I start by rounding on the sickest COVID patients. One of these is Mrs. G, aged 75. I have known her for years. She survived a stroke but now has dementia and diabetes. She has been on the COVID ward for a week. She was stable yesterday, but today, like several others here, she has turned "bad"— breathing fast, more sleepy, less conscious. Oxygen saturation levels are dropping. The nurse calls her brother, asking if he wants to come see her, stressing the risks and outlining the PPE procedure. On compassionate grounds, the government decree does allow for limited visiting at the end of life, by one family member only. The brother is older, at risk and vulnerable, but he soon arrives. Staff help him with PPE. I see him, in gown, mask, visor. "I'm sorry, I say." "Thank you for everything," he says. I want to touch his shoulder, comfort him somehow. I keep 6 feet apart.

When these older, frail patients do go "bad," I note that death is fairly swift and merciful. They require minimal doses of morphine and midazolam for respiratory distress. They rapidly become comatose. They have minimal lung secretions. They need hardly any scopolamine for terminal rales, probably because they are kept in a "dry" state to try to maximize lung function.

I continue to walk around the ward. I note that the patients who are in their second week of infection and look like they will survive have had few symptoms. One is happily eating her dinner. Another is sitting in a chair outside the nursing station, wearing a pretty flowered hat. She smiles at me. My eyes above the mask and behind the visor smile back. "One day at a time,"

I say. "Yes, and we pray," she says. Back at the nursing station, I sign one death certificate after another.

April 26, 2020

I am on in the LTC hospital for the next seven days straight, in addition to my regular job at MUHC. Today is Sunday. We are three physicians covering over 300 patients, of whom 120 are COVID-positive. Acute care emergency rooms in the city are overwhelmed. We must keep the patients here, but we are desperately short of nurses. On the COVID ward today we have one nurse for 38 patients, many of whom are very ill. It's the same situation in LTC facilities across the city.

Some of our PPE is inadequate. Each new batch seems to come from a different manufacturer. The masks dispensed today are too small and the elastic breaks easily. This morning there are no gloves my size, and none covers my wrists properly. We were trained that we should have a buddy who ensures that we are properly protected and who double-checks our technique. But there is no one here. By myself, I gown up, gear up, and go through the plastic sheet barrier that separates "cold" from "hot" zones. It is dark on the ward. For some reason they have turned the lights down low. I feel alone.

I start my rounds. Mr. B, a stroke survivor on COVID day 12, has managed to avoid respiratory problems. But he is refusing to eat. He hides under the covers. Next, two female patients who seemed well yesterday are now actively dying. I go to the nursing station to update their orders. The nurse gives me messages to return calls. Some family members want to speak with a doctor every day. "How is she? Does she have fever? Is she still on oxygen? What is her oxygen level?" And, "How much is he eating and drinking? Does he have an IV? What about his spirits? Is he agitated? Is he upset? Could I please speak with him on video?" We have family members crying out for a chance to connect with their loved ones through virtual calls but not enough staff to fulfill that need. There is only one computer tablet for 38 patients that staff can use for video calls with each other and with family members.

We are having to rely on our personal cell phones to make the connections. When I get the chance, I facilitate contact between families and their loved ones. I worry about my cell phone continually being near the patients' mouths or faces. I experiment with various commercial plastic casings. But the casings interfere with the video and audio of my phone. Finally, I give up and resign to using the bare phone, despite any risk. I see patients light up, spouses, children expressing their love. It is worth every minute, I think. I stand by the bedside, witnessing tears, expressions of love. "Look we are all here! We are praying for you! We love you!" The time is never enough. The most touching are the exchanges between spouses when one is clearly dying. "*Chéri* [darling], you'll be fine! Look, I'm here. Remember to drink! And you must eat! I love you so much! I will see you soon, don't worry!"

It is dark by the time I get home. Disinfect, doff layers, disinfect. I take my third shower today. My skin is dry, and my hands are sore. I don a fresh T-shirt and loose pants and get ready to make more phone calls to families. I have not had time to cook or shop. A friend has offered to have meals delivered in a few days. I am very grateful for that.

April 27, 2020
I am on the COVID unit for twelve hours straight. They have locked the staff toilets on the ward to try to minimize viral transmission amongst the staff. Alternative facilities are in other parts of the building, which involve removing and redonning all PPE. In any case, we are discouraged from circulating in COVID-free areas of the hospital. Since I can't easily take toilet breaks, I have taken to wearing diapers, just in case. Common eating areas are also closed. After five hours, I slip away to eat a packed lunch in my car.

In the whole chronic care sector of the city, exponentially more patients, personal attendants, and nurses are becoming infected. We get detailed daily statistics on the COVID-positive patients, but no one tells us how many staff are ill or have tested positive. We don't ask, and we don't discuss it amongst ourselves. Privately, I am upset that LTCs are expected to look after the COVID-positive patients as if we were in an acute care setting, minus the staff to carry out our medical orders in a timely fashion. This afternoon there is still only one nurse for every 38 patients, and two auxiliary nurses. Our managers tell us that reinforcements are coming soon.

At 8 P.M. I go home to continue to call families and communicate with the other MDs.

Before I deal with calls, emails, and team reports I go through the routine: peel off layers outside, go up for a shower, launder work clothes from the day, disinfect doorknobs and light switches. I don't want to get too near my son.

In the evening I notice that I have a sore throat . . . but no fever or other symptom considered "essential" to trigger self-isolation or COVID testing at this time.

April 28, 2020

I go to work on the COVID ward, but I have a strange malaise. I manage to finish morning rounds. At noon, a manager tells me that local funeral homes are overwhelmed and that our own facility's morgue is now full.

"We have to put bodies one of top of the other," he says.

I look at him. He looks at me.

"Don't worry," he says. "We will separate the men and the women."

Later he tells me that they called for a refrigerated van that is now parked behind the building. In a sister LTC institution, the carpenters have had time to install shelves in the van, so the bodies are separated. The manager says that the carpenters here may be too busy. I see them at work on the wards, creating more wood-framed plastic sheet barriers to separate those infected from those who are not.

After lunch I still have malaise, so I go home early. In the evening I have a few chills but again, no fever.

I Have Become Ill

May 1, 2020

For the past three days I have been working from home because I have had low-grade fever, "brain fog," sore throat, nausea, fatigue. Daniel says that I am mixing my words. Then, two hours later, I feel normal again. My drive-through polymerase chain reaction (PCR) test comes back negative. I am relieved, but I don't feel right at all. Is this a false-negative? Was I tested too early? Colleagues message me to find out how I am doing. One tells me that the false-negative rate for the PCR is around 30%.

In the evening, I email my team leader to tell him that I still have symptoms and that I worry about being on call overnight in a few days for 320 patients, half of whom are COVID-positive. I ask for a buddy to be on backup call in case my judgment is affected.

I feel badly about this. I have a brief cry. I feel that I am letting down my colleagues who are still putting in 12- to 16-hour days, every day, as the COVID caseload mounts.

I am self-isolating as long as I have symptoms, and I am trying to protect my son. I am not shopping or cooking. I only leave the house to walk our dog when there is no one around in the streets.

May 4, 2020
A second PCR test from yesterday was negative. A relief, but I am still un-well, working from home. I now have unusual GI symptoms: colitis-like, with bleeding, which I have never had in my life. I call the occupational health nurse again. She says this can happen with COVID. I am to wait until symptom-free for 24 hours before going back to the hospital.

I reach out to my sister for support. She is a health professional herself. Her husband is a physician on a hospital ward where they have had positive cases. He has been unwell for the past few days, sleeping all the time. We share stories. I am grateful to have her there.

May 15, 2020
I am now physically back on an LTC COVID ward. What a different atmos-phere compared to two weeks ago! The ward seems physically brighter. We have more staff now, which is such a relief. One of the new nurses here today has been relocated from a family medicine clinic. She happily chats as she prepares the long list of injections and pills. Another nurse is from a neo-natal care unit. She is also cheerful, despite being in this environment. It must be a change from caring for newborn babies! There are several volunteers and more patient attendants. I see two of the nurses who have been here for weeks, some working double shifts, with very little time off. "All is good!" they respond to my greeting. They carry on, so focused, so calm.

Patients are recovering—those who are not among the 28% who have died over the past five weeks. The nearby emergency rooms have been less busy and have been accepting LTC transfers. I note that, of the patients that we had transferred at the request of families, most have not returned but have died in the acute care hospital. Transfer seems to have made no difference.

My team leader gives me some good news: as there are fewer newly infected cases, I will no longer be needed on the "hot" unit. I can devote more time to my full-time palliative care duties at my base hospital and in home care. Not being on a COVID ward decreases risk significantly. I feel like I have been given my personal life back. I can now ease into becoming an uncontami-nated person—one less likely to make family members and friends ill just by carrying the virus in or on my person or in my car. I wonder how the LTC nurses and patient attendants cope, though—the ones who have been on the COVID wards for weeks and weeks, in rooms with multiple patients, with no special ventilation systems, in full protective gear all day. What about *their* families? My team leader talks about how, for the past two months, he has been sleeping in the basement of their house, away from his family, apart from his wife. How and when do we get back together with spouses or partners? We get no guidance on this.

May 22, 2020

I read that across the province there are many thousands of cases in our chronic care institutions. Many sites have over one-third of patients affected, and, of those, the death rate is 30–35%. In some sites the death rate is close to 60%. At our LTC, the infection rate so far is 53%, and, among those, 29% have died directly from COVID. A colleague tells me that for COVID-positive home care patients, the reported mortality rate is 25%. I think to myself: the home care population is younger, with fewer comorbid conditions.

My original LTC ward held those with the most advanced dementias. I count. Half of them have died. Mrs. M., my oldest at age 106, has survived. I see her in her room, dozing placidly after breakfast, a half-smile on her face.

June 24, 2020

Montreal's public health authority reports that, by mid-June, 75% of the city's LTC facilities had COVID cases and of the 3,200 people who have died of COVID-19, 85% were in chronic care facilities or in seniors' centers.

I read in various reports that the overall COVID case-fatality rate is around 4–5% in Canada (8–9% in New York City) and about 30% in hospitalized patients and in those over age 80. However, the impact of this virus will be larger than the reported figures, it seems to me. Some of my LTC hospital patients who survived were permanently weakened by the illness and died a few months later, before their time. They were COVID-free at the time of death but having had the virus contributed to their decline. Is COVID being indicated as "contributory" on death certificates? How are these deaths being counted in official statistics?

What about staff? At the LTC hospital where I am helping, they report that 100 staff members out of 300 were symptomatic and tested positive for COVID. I note that some staff who got ill two months ago have not yet come back. We do not yet have routine COVID screen-testing. So, I think to myself: What about asymptomatic staff, who were not tested? What about the false-negatives, of which I might have been one?

This wave of the pandemic seems to be almost over, for this LTC hospital anyway. Many have died without family near. Relatives have had to grieve alone. I have learned that the symptom control aspect of end-of-life care for non-ICU COVID patients is straightforward. They require only small doses of the usual medications for comfort care. Those who die of COVID tend to have underlying illnesses; nevertheless, they die prematurely.

Summer Respite

August 15, 2020

The summer brings some relief. In our private lives, we can see friends again. Although limited by government rule to masked and distanced groups of ten, we bask in the sun, appreciate our small outside gatherings. My widowed Italian 93-year-old mother, a social soul who lives in a seniors' complex, is glad that she can see her children and grandchildren again, even though she cannot hug and kiss them. She lived through World War II in a village in Italy where there were bombing raids, various armies coming through. I ask her how this experience compares.

"This pandemic and the quarantines are worse," she says.

I express surprise.

She explains: "At least, during the war, we were all together, all the time. We hid from the bombs, but then we could come out, gather vegetables from our gardens, prepare a chicken to cook, put on the pasta and share food, wine, and stories with our *paesani* (fellow villagers)."

I go to a friend's home for tea. She is a microbiologist and is considered a national COVID expert. We can visit without masks, she says, because she has had COVID. After hearing about my illness, she tells me that the false-negative test rate can be up to 50%, that from my clinical picture I had COVID. I felt reassured to have an explanation for the symptoms that I had experienced—me, who is never ill.

I am getting ready to do palliative care home visits again, with protective gown, mask, visor, shoe covers. For the last six months I have been working virtually, while our nurse has gone into the homes in full PPE gear. But now my nurse sends me a message to say that she has tested positive for COVID! I phone her. She feels unwell but not bad enough to get any special medical attention. She is off for two weeks. I work on my own.

Second Wave

November 15, 2020

After a relatively quiet summer, our region is experiencing a second COVID-19 wave. Once more, physicians and other staff are getting daily calls to serve. I start looking after COVID-positive patients again. Two of the MDs in my LTC team have just contracted the virus. Back in the acute care hospital, two colleagues also become ill and test positive. A third becomes ill but tests negative. When will this end?

December 14, 2020

One of the COVID-19 vaccines is becoming available next week. LTC patients and staff will be the first to be immunized, and I have been invited to do so, too. I am relieved, but then I think: this vaccine will protect me from becoming ill, but it will not necessarily protect others. I could still transmit the virus. We are told, of course, to continue to wear protective equipment.

Acute care hospital wards and ICUs are getting full. The nurse manager at the LTC tells me today that most of her nurses are now COVID-positive. One nurse who is there this evening has been working up to 16-hour days without a break, and her young family is complaining that she is not home this Christmas holiday.

Going into the holiday period, no social gatherings are allowed, except with members of the same household. People are asked not to leave home unless it is essential, except for those living alone who may visit one other home. Christmas has been essentially cancelled. I will not be seeing my mother or my sisters.

As I walk along the streets in our neighborhood, I see that families hunkered inside have put out many more holiday lights than usual. "Ça va bien aller" (It's going to be OK), declare the rainbow banners on the streets and walls.

We hope things will be better in a year's time.

January 7, 2021

With new and more virulent strains in the community, this is beginning to feel like a long-term siege. Hospitalizations are rising rapidly. Public health experts predict that our next peak in hospitalizations will occur in mid-January.

We are facing a novel ethical dilemma—new for peacetime. Hospital staff in the region are now doing online training for the "advanced triage protocol" to prepare for the possibility that we may soon be forced to rate and categorize critically ill patients. This is part of a centralized healthcare system response, once all ICUs in Quebec are overcapacity. In Ontario as well, patients will be scored on a short-term mortality risk assessment that assigns a percentage to the odds they will live a year. Those with the best chance for survival will get access to scarce resources, such as ventilators or the less-invasive helmet-based ventilation systems. Those refused ICU care will receive treatment in other parts of the hospital. Mortality rates will be very high.

This is a serious and historic move for the provinces. Essentially, we are bracing for the possibility that a panel of physicians would decide the fate of persons using anonymous case descriptions. At our weekly hospital-wide COVID video conference, our director discusses the details of the process. Rather than involving the treating ICU physician, who might find making such decisions untenable, a committee of three people—consisting of two other physicians along with a third person, such as a medical ethicist— would receive de-identified clinical and prognostic data. They would then prioritize patients and inform the teams who is next to be taken off life support to make room for a patient who has a better prognosis. It is a triage system, but the briefs do not use that word. Addressing the media, our ICU chief expresses distress that they could soon have to remove people from respirators who will die because other patients need the beds. "I'm told this happens on the battlefield all the time, but I never saw our medical system as a battlefield," he says. "And I guess that's what some of us need to change our perspective on."

What would be the role of palliative care staff? We would have to counsel and deal with the distress of the families whose loved ones have been taken off life support to make way for others who have a better chance of survival. And these dealings would likely happen over the telephone, days, evenings, nights. It's a horrific thought, bringing back memories of what we went through last spring, having to discuss life and death with families at a distance. But we would have to do our part.

I am supervising a palliative care resident today. We are discussing MAID (Medical Aid in Dying, or physician-administered active voluntary euthanasia) which has been legal in Quebec for the last five years. She is worried about what she might do if she is consulted for a COVID patient in the emergency room who is in distress with respiratory symptoms and who has been triaged to the "no ICU" group. The resident imagines that this patient might then request MAID for that reason (a possible scenario, since there is a high

MAID rate in Quebec compared to other provinces). I have no answer for her distress other than to acknowledge it. I share it.

"Montreal Hospitals Nearing Critical Triage Point, When Doctors Must 'Kill People' to Save Others," reads the headline in the evening paper.

January 28, 2021
Are we halfway through this pandemic yet? There are now new, more infectious variants of the virus in circulation. The vaccine supply from Europe on which we were relying has dried up. I have not had my second vaccine dose, due three weeks ago. As per new government guidelines, I will have to wait three months. This feels like a limbo or purgatory, the daily virus threat on one side, crumbling life on the other, while we wait.

Ripples

February 6, 2021
Today's *Globe and Mail* newspaper: The City of Toronto has revealed that 79% of Torontonians suffering from COVID-19 are people from visible minority groups. These are the people in service jobs, keeping supplies flowing. It now strikes me that, although forming 34% of the Montreal population, almost 100% of those who work at the LTC are people of color. Those who deliver my groceries, and my online purchases, are people of color.

I also worry about lack of access to the vaccine in low- and middle-income countries. They might have to wait a year or more while their population is ravaged. Many places do not even have adequate running water. The head of the WHO warned last week that the world is on the brink of a "catastrophic moral failure" if wealthier nations don't ensure the equitable distribution of vaccines. We are one world family. The virus is demonstrating that to us, if we were not aware before.

March 3, 2021
The US has surpassed 500,000 deaths. In 2020, COVID was the third leading cause of death in Canada. In Quebec, 15% of cases are now of the more contagious UK variant, and the statistic might reach 30–40% by the end of March. The variant is now in workplaces and schools. We will have a third wave. Is this like a war, where we don't know where the enemy might be hiding and in what shape or form? In our region, hospitalization rates are

leveling off, for the moment. We have not yet had to invoke the emergency algorithm.

In the meantime, my virtual personal life goes on. My sons, friends, mother, sisters, colleagues go through illness, accidents, small-scale and distanced weddings, childbirth—worries, joys, and tribulations. I try to participate as much as I can. But COVID, and wariness of what might happen next, takes up a sizeable portion of my consciousness. I long for soul-space, for a respite, to reconnect with my creative self, my inner life.

March 11, 2021
The WHO declared the pandemic one year ago today. Across Canada, provinces and municipalities are arranging memorial services and lowering flags at half-mast. At 11 A.M., we will observe a province-wide minute of silence. For that I am grateful: ritual and remembrance will help us heal and move on.

Quebec province has chosen a white rose as the emblem for the day. "In addition to evoking both strength and delicacy, the flower is associated with honor and reverence," the government says. On their website, they provide a poster with an image of a white rose and invite citizens to download and use the image. I print it out and place it before me. "On March 11th," the poster reads, "I remember the victims of COVID-19, for myself, my family, and their loved ones." My eyes well up. This is part of healing, for the strength and wisdom to carry on, to do the right thing, for ourselves and for everyone.

At some point, we will all have to reckon with our experiences. How do we deal with grief when we cannot mourn face to face, in the company of loved ones? What will be the impact of COVID on grief counseling? What will be the extent of posttraumatic stress disorder (PTSD) after this pandemic, especially for nurses who have worked with COVID patients for months and months, nonstop? I know several who are on extended leave, but we don't talk about it. Staff have witnessed many deaths within a very short period, in a context where there may have been lack of personnel or facilities and inadequate protective equipment. Although the institutions are sending us emails regarding psychological services for employees who are tired or burnt out, I wonder how many are taking advantage of such services. We are not used to looking after ourselves and seeking help.

Even within palliative care teams, where there is a strong tradition of debriefing and in-person staff support—either individually or in groups—the present culture around our workplace is such that we do not speak with each other about our experiences. We hide staff illness. If we become ill, we feel somehow ashamed, that we are letting our teammates down. We do not grieve for our fellows. We feel that we just need to carry on, for as long as we are needed.

Afterword, September 2021

I offer this narrative of the first year of the pandemic to feature the role, the dilemmas, and the impact on myself as a palliative care physician and a person, as well as to express sympathy for those who have suffered the most all over the world. My co-authors and I also offer it as a Prelude to this Revised Edition of Crossing Over. *Of the myriad ways the world has changed since this book first appeared in 2000, perhaps none has been so radical as the changes in consciousness and self-understanding forced upon us by the pandemic. As clinicians we have had to reckon with the fragility of our systems of care in the face of surging demand. We have had to question the capabilities of our institutions, our governments, and our leaders to respond equitably and efficiently to a fast-moving but entirely predictable global threat. And, while we celebrate the resilience and courage of our colleagues and the unprecedented achievements in vaccine development, we are shaken and humbled by these failures.*

Our world also looks different today because the pandemic laid bare the wide inequalities within and between our nations. As COVID pierced whatever illusions of invulnerability we might have cherished for our modern, technologically advanced society, it also demonstrated unmistakably that some of us are much more vulnerable than others to adversity and risks. As we turn, then, in the shadow of this pandemic, to the narratives of palliative care in this book, I wonder: How shall we reckon and process our collective and personal griefs and nurture together the emerging seeds of hope and of new, more just visions of the future? Will we learn to be better citizens of this planet?

2

General Introduction

The goals of palliative care are easy to state. Realizing them is not so easy. The Center to Advance Palliative Care defines palliative care as "specialized medical care for people living with a serious illness. This type of care is focused on providing relief from the symptoms and stress of the illness. The goal is to improve quality of life for both the patient and the family."[1] More briefly, the American Academy of Hospice and Palliative Medicine states, "Palliative care focuses on improving a patient's quality of life by managing pain and other distressing symptoms of a serious illness."[2]

When one tries to achieve these goals in the real world, one is brought face-to-face with limits of knowledge, institutional limitations, human foibles, problems giving care in teams, and challenges of cultural diversity, among other things. Dying, even with the best possible care, can be messy and difficult. Yet much can be done to make the time of a person's dying more comfortable and meaningful, and much is done, every day, by patients, family members, and dedicated hospice and palliative care workers. That is the theme of this book.

A Book of Stories

This is a book of stories—narratives of giving and receiving palliative care in the context of end of life. This is not a textbook that portrays ideal palliative care or that prescribes specific management techniques. Instead, we present stories of actual patients and families who have experienced terminal illness with the support of hospice or palliative care teams. The narratives are derived from a three-year, qualitative, ethnographic study of the experiences of patients, families, and caregivers. To protect people's privacy, all names have been changed, as have many dates, physical features, occupations, and other potentially identifying characteristics.

The cases we narrate were followed prospectively. We did not select them after the fact to illustrate ideal or exemplary care. They are meant to illustrate certain realities of what it was like to die in North America under the palliative care umbrella, in the contexts described, when we conducted our research. This book helps us compare palliative care ideals with depictions of the actual practice of the discipline. Often, the care was exemplary—at times, ennobling and inspiring. In other situations, many would criticize certain aspects of care. In some cases, there were intractable problems or symptoms that the caregivers could not help. Sometimes, personal, institutional, or social care was, frankly, inadequate. The narratives are meant to elicit empathy, understanding, and reflection.

Our narratives portray the application of scientific and technical knowledge, to be sure, but they always situate particular clinical judgments or interventions in the context of people's overall experience, including its emotional, existential, and spiritual dimensions. We have actively sought out the experiences and perceptions of the widest possible range of participants in each case. The narratives include the voices and points of view of patients, families, doctors, nurses, social workers, chaplains, volunteers, friends, and neighbors as they interact with each other and form their often-conflicting judgments over the course of the patient's illness and, in most of the cases, up to one year after the patient's death. We have attempted in each narrative to capture something of the patient's inner life or subjective experience, as well as caregivers' inner experience of giving care.

We thus offer this collection of narratives as a complement to the technically oriented textbooks such as the *Oxford Textbook of Palliative Medicine*, the *Oxford Textbook of Palliative Nursing*, or *Palliative Medicine: A Case-Based Manual*.[3-5] We recommend that professionally interested readers consult these and other textbooks to deepen their appreciation of the problems of clinical management depicted in *Crossing Over*. At the same time, we believe the narratives in *Crossing Over* will remind students and clinicians of the complex human contexts within which they must apply their knowledge. Illness always occurs in a particular family, social, and cultural context and always unfolds over time. It is a *biographical* and not merely *biological* process. And the feelings, perspectives, and motivations of the caregivers (both families and professionals) are inevitably part of the story.

We have written this book with two types of reader in mind. First, we hope it will interest a general reader who is curious about how some people have died with the support of excellent palliative care services. Such a reader will find poignant, provocative, and sometimes inspiring scenes in these narratives. It is possible to approach the book simply as a collection of stories of people who are face-to-face with some of life's most profound challenges.

We have also designed the book for healthcare professionals, students, and trainees in the health professions. For them we have included features intended to make the book useful for teaching and learning about palliative care. The most important of these are the Authors' Comments that follow each narrative. These commentaries have three purposes. First, we note changes in the field of palliative care and in society since *Crossing Over* first appeared that might lead certain aspects of the cases to be approached differently today. Later in this General Introduction, we discuss the most significant changes in the contemporary landscape of palliative care, focusing on developments in North America. In the Authors' Comments, we pinpoint specific decisions and choices of patients, families, and clinicians where today's changed context may be particularly relevant. Second, the Authors' Comments give us the opportunity to speak in our own voices—as teachers and practitioners of palliative care, bioethics, and science and society—about clinical and ethical aspects of the cases that we find praiseworthy or, in some instances, problematic. We express these judgments with humility, for we have the luxury of hindsight and are far from the fast-moving intensity of the clinical moments that were experienced by our colleagues. Finally, we highlight in the commentaries themes related to the experience of dying, or to the care of the dying, that we believe deserve special emphasis as we look again at our narratives from our vantage point in the present.

A second feature is an Index of Themes. While every narrative raises a wide range of issues related to giving or receiving palliative care, each brings out some themes more prominently than others. The index provides an inventory of these themes and, for each one, lists the cases in which that theme plays an especially important role. A student or teacher can use the index to quickly identify which cases best bring out particular themes of interest, such as, for example, difficult pain management, requests for assisted death, or the impact of preexisting family conflict on end-of-life care.

The index is a rough-and-ready guide to the narratives rather than an exhaustive content analysis. One entry does deserve comment, however: "Socioeconomic status, race, ethnicity, and culture." Everyone is shaped, of course, by cultural norms; everyone occupies a particular socioeconomic status; and everyone embodies one or more ethnicities. In selecting only a few narratives as especially pertinent illustrations of this fact, we are not trying to limit the reach of these categories to people who are outside the dominant sector—middle-class, European-American, Christian—in US and Canadian society. Nevertheless, precisely because most health-care institutions and practitioners in those societies reflect that sector, they are more likely to view culture, socioeconomic status, and ethnicity as "differences," "challenges," or "problems" in patients who are low-wealth, non-Christian, and/or people of color. That is the phenomenon we have in mind in connection with this theme.

For this edition, we have changed our approach to the Bibliography, which in the first edition included up-to-date references from the clinical literature for a range of palliative care topics. Today's practitioners are far more likely to rely on electronic resources for this type of information, which in a printed book would soon be out of date in any case. And most general readers will probably not have use for such information. We also reiterate that this is not a textbook designed to teach specific techniques of palliative care, nor are the clinical interventions we describe, including the selection and dosages of medications, intended as recommendations for practice. What we have provided instead, in our Suggestions for Further Reading, is a compendium of books and articles—some very recent, some "classics" from the past—that to our minds offer illuminating, thought-provoking perspectives on many of the salient themes in end-of-life care.

"What Is in Your Mind and in Your Heart"

A hallmark of palliative care since Dame Cicely Saunders founded the modern hospice movement has been the combination of scientific rigor with personal concern. As Dame Cicely herself frequently recalled, one of her ear-liest inspirations was a relationship she had in 1947, as a recently qualified medical social worker and former nurse, with a cancer patient named David Tasma. This 40-year-old Jewish man, who had survived World War II and the Warsaw Ghetto, spoke often with Dame Cicely about his life, his sufferings, and what he wanted from his caregivers. "I only want what is in your mind and in your heart," he told her one day, in an oft-quoted remark that addresses both the cognitive and interpersonal aspects of palliative care.[6] Accordingly, palliative care and palliative care education have embraced three broad areas: the science and techniques of pain management and symptom con-trol; knowledge of psychological, social, and spiritual aspects of dying and grieving, and self-knowledge on the part of caregivers, especially regarding personal attitudes toward death and loss.

Palliative care is "whole-person care,"[7,8] not only in the sense that the whole person of the patient (body, mind, spirit) is the object of care, but also because palliative care brings the whole person of the caregiver into play. Palliative care is, *par excellence,* care that is given through the medium of human relationships. And education for palliative care is not only education in science and clinical techniques, but also in the art of building and sustaining relationships—using *oneself* as a primary diagnostic and therapeutic instrument. This involves a level of psychological risk-taking that may be unique in the health field, a process that is demonstrated in several of the narratives in this book. One of our aims is to provide students and caregivers with material that will encourage self-reflection and discussion of these emotional issues.

Extended, richly detailed, multiperspectival case narratives are well suited to portray the physical, psychological, spiritual, ethical, and social dimensions of terminal illness, the dynamics of the caring relationship and its impact on the caregiver—even to the point of what has been called "compassion fatigue" or burnout—and how all these are interwoven and interact with each other. By going beyond conventional case reports in clinical medicine with their narrow concentration on signs, symptoms, and treatment, narratives can attend to the processes by which patients, families, and healthcare providers find personal meaning in illness and how personal meanings influence the experience, quality, and outcome of care.

Narratives can also bring into focus the often unspoken, unnoticed, and yet deeply consequential values that guide healthcare provider decision-making. Consider these common challenges, for example: assessing whether a patient who outlives their prognosis ought to remain in hospice or be discharged, determining whether an intervention requested by a patient ought to be labeled "palliative" or "active" treatment, judging whether a persistent symptom that a patient reports has been optimally or inadequately controlled, or ascertaining whether a patient's desire to die at home ought to be honored or denied. These are only a few of many dilemmas whose resolution involves value-laden judgments. Narratives have the capacity to shed light on the values behind these judgments. Especially when healthcare provider decision-making unfolds in ambiguous contexts—those that lack clear definitions, guidelines, codes of conduct, or legal requirements—narratives can help us recognize most clearly the operation of structural, implicit, or subconscious values and biases that all of us have.

Like microscopes, narratives have the capacity to magnify institutional forces at play that are normally invisible and unaccountable but that can replicate prevailing social orders and perpetuate individual, family, and community harm. As such, narratives can help us see that decisions that might be cogently rationalized or legally backed may, in fact, raise urgent questions about institutional inequities in end-of-life care and challenge us to recognize structural racism, classism, and other forms of discrimination at the very close of a human life—as the COVID pandemic has also forced us to do.[9] In the end, narratives can bring us face to face with systemic misalignments between professionals' assessments of the effectiveness of their interventions and the assessments of the people they aim to serve. The narratives' promise, therefore, is their ability to help us see weaknesses and failures as clearly as strengths and successes and to encourage us to make the improvements necessary to ensure that all people have access to palliative care that they experience as effective, desirable, and just.

Vivid and detailed cases are also a valuable contribution to societal awareness on topics related to end-of-life care. We believe this book can be an important part of the current public debate regarding optimum care for the dying, what options ought to be legally available at the end of life, and the wisest allocation of society's resources. The last issue has emerged with particular urgency, with the COVID pandemic stretching intensive care resources nearly to the breaking point, as Anna Towers describes in her opening narrative.

We are also aware, however, that the style of palliative care depicted in these narratives will not be relevant for many low- and middle-income countries. This brand of palliative care may be too expensive and technologically complex to serve the needs of the world at large. Palliative care leaders in wealthy countries have a responsibility, we believe, to ensure that research in the immediate future focuses on interventions that are adaptable to areas where costly or high-tech solutions are unavailable while also advocating for increased access, over time, to the full range of care.

Our Project: Case Narratives in Palliative Care

We constructed our narratives by employing a variety of qualitative research methods. Many procedural, philosophical, and ethical issues arise in the use of qualitative methods in medical and social research, which we explore in some depth in Chapter 23. Here we describe just enough of our methodology to help readers understand the context and construction of the narratives.

For a fuller treatment of the details, rationale, strengths, and limitations of our approach, readers should consult Chapter 23.

We carried out our research between 1995 and 1998, in two settings. In the United States, we followed cases from the Hospice of Lancaster County, Lancaster, Pennsylvania, at that time a large, free-standing community-based hospice program with an active home care service and a 12-bed in-patient facility for acute symptom management, respite care, and terminal care. In Canada, we followed cases from the Palliative Care Service at the Royal Victoria Hospital, Montreal, a large, academically based palliative care service at a major teaching hospital, with a 16-bed inpatient unit, consultation service, and—at the time of our research—a fully integrated home care service.

It is crucial to note two major differences between these settings that existed at the time of our research. The first was the difference in healthcare financing. Canadian patients were participants in the Canadian Medicare System, which meant that, except for private-duty nurses in the home and some medications, patients and families had no out-of-pocket costs for the care they received. Patients in Lancaster County were subject to the confusing and limited coverage for hospice care in the United States. People aged 65 and older could elect the package of services provided under Medicare Part B, but only after being certified by their doctor to be within six months of death and by agreeing to receive no further coverage for active treatment of their disease. Patients younger than 65, unless eligible for Medicaid by virtue of their meager financial means, were subject to the varying limits in coverage for hospice care provided by private insurance. As a result, economic hardship and financial uncertainty played a significant role in the cases from Lancaster County; these concerns were almost entirely absent in the Canadian cases.

The second difference is in the extent of physician involvement in patient care. The Palliative Care Service at the Royal Victoria Hospital was staffed with several full-time palliative care specialists who were actively involved in patient care whether the patient was in an acute care ward of the hospital, in the Palliative Care Unit, or at home. (Since this project was completed, home care has been shifted to local community health agencies, and the role of the Palliative Care Service in the home has decreased.) At the time of our research, Hospice of Lancaster County had no full-time medical staff but was served by a group of part-time physicians from the community. Especially when at home, patients had very little direct contact with physicians; most physician involvement in symptom management took place via telephone contact with a hospice nurse. As a result, nurses and social workers played a much greater role, proportionally, in Lancaster than in Montreal, though in each setting the burden of care was distributed across the team.

Since we conducted our research, Hospice of Lancaster County has grown to become the largest hospice provider in the state of Pennsylvania, changing its name in 2012 to Hospice and Community Care. Today, it has an inpatient facility with 24 beds, an outpatient palliative care clinic, and a staff that numbers ten palliative medicine physicians and twelve palliative care nurse practitioners. This growth has paralleled the field as a whole. Since palliative medicine's formal recognition as a medical subspecialty in 2008, the number of board-certified palliative care physicians in the United States had grown to 7,618 by 2019. By this date, there were more than 18,000 palliative care–certified nurses.[10] Hospice and Community Care is also among 140 US hospice agencies that were selected to participate in the Medicare Care Choices Model, a demonstration project sponsored by the US Centers for Medicare and Medicaid Services.[11] In this pilot program, initially planned for five years but extended for an additional year in 2021, hospice patients may continue to receive curative or life-prolonging treatment, under the Medicare benefit, for their underlying terminal condition. Taken together, the increased presence of palliative medicine specialist physicians and nurses and greater flexibility to integrate palliative care with ongoing treatment of the underlying disease substantially reduce the differences between the two sites that existed at the time of our research.

We followed our cases from the time a patient was admitted to the hospice or palliative care program, or when a member of the team suggested that a patient or family may be of interest to our project (which may have been later than the time of admission). Because the grief and bereavement of surviving family and friends were part of our focus, we continued our work with most of the cases until approximately one year after the patient's death, though in a few instances this was not feasible.

The main criteria for selection of cases were the willingness of the patient and family to participate and their physical and mental capacity to respond to interview questions. Where relevant, and always with the patient's permission, we invited others in the patient's circle (e.g., friends, neighbors, co-workers) to participate in the research. Healthcare providers included all members of the palliative care or hospice team who were involved in the patient's care and who were willing to participate (e.g., physicians, nurses, social workers, aides, psychologists, music and occupational therapists, chaplains, volunteers). We gave full explanations of the nature, purposes, and methods of our project to all potential participants in order to obtain their cooperation and informed consent. The project was approved by the review boards and ethics committees of the participating healthcare institutions.

We relied on four types of data to construct our narratives: (1) the patient's medical history and significant aspects of the patient's biography (e.g., their cultural background, family history, employment, important and meaningful life events, and outlook on life, whether expressed in religious or spiritual terms or otherwise); (2) the clinical course of the patient's illness, through and including the patient's death and the family's bereavement; (3) the patient's and family's perceptions and interpretations of the patient's illness and care; and (4) the caregivers' perceptions and interpretations of the patient's illness and care, as well as significant aspects of the caregivers' own biographies and value systems, as these influenced their attitudes or behaviors toward the patient.

We employed the following research methods:

- *Medical and biographical background*: Review of the medical chart and interviews with the patient and family
- *Clinical course of the illness*: Ongoing chart review, direct observation of patient and caregiver interactions, interviews at regular intervals with the patient, family, and hospice or palliative care staff, and attendance at team meetings and ward rounds
- *Patient and family perceptions*: Interviews with the patient and family at regular intervals, the actual frequency determined by the course of a particular case and the interviewees' comfort level as the cases unfolded
- *Healthcare providers' perceptions*: Providers in Montreal kept a journal to record their perceptions, reactions, and interpretations of their involvement with the care of the patient; researchers in both settings regularly interviewed the providers and also attended staff support meetings

Tape-recorded interviews of patients, families, and caregivers; chart reviews; and participant-observation were carried out by the authors. In Montreal, several of the patients were primary speakers of French. In those cases, the interviews were conducted in French or in a combination of French and English. We have translated quotations in French from those interviews into English.

While interview questions were not specified in advance, certain broad areas of inquiry were felt to be central to the project, and we were alert for opportunities to pursue them as people told their stories. (For details of our interview guides, see Chapter 23.) A first draft of each case was written by the primary researcher, who is also identified as the narrator of that case (Patricia Boston or Anna Towers in Montreal, and Yanna Lambrinidou in Lancaster County). The drafts were circulated among all the authors for critical comments and questions, and a second draft was written. David Barnard, who formulated the original plan for the project and recruited the other three authors to join him, edited the final draft of each case, which, after the primary researcher's approval, is the version printed in this book. Thus, while the initial selection of data and the narrative stance are the responsibility of the researcher who was closest to the events, the final version of each narrative is a collaborative work, growing out of collegial criticism and revisiting the raw data with new or refined ideas about salient themes in the case.

In order not to interrupt the narrative flow, we avoided explicitly injecting into the narratives our own opinions and interpretations of many of the salient issues raised by the cases, reserving those for the Authors' Comments, although, of course, these opinions and interpretations do enter *implicitly*, through our selection of incidents to recount and the language with which we describe them.

We offer the fruits of this process in all humility, mindful of these words by the critic Craig Brown, from an essay on the difficult art of biography that appeared in the *Times Literary Supplement* as this chapter was being written:

> Everyone who has ever written non-fiction will know that, from paragraph to paragraph, perhaps even from sentence to sentence, one is always obliged to pick a version of the truth: every available source has a slightly different tale to tell. It would be tedious to present each different version of each event, or the finished book would be impossibly long and impossibly boring. So which to choose? And how do you know if it is the right one?[12]

The narrative that results from the process we have described here is not *the* story of the patient's experience of dying, as if there could ever be such a thing. It is *a* story—*our* story, or perhaps *a co-created* story composed in partnership with the participants in our research—with the limitations of point of view and narrative selectivity that are inherent in our method.

Changed Landscapes in Palliative Care and Society:
From the 1990s to the 2020s

The growth and change at Hospice of Lancaster County described above are part of a bigger picture. Over the past twenty-five years, in both Canada and the United States, changes have occurred in healthcare and in society at large that have altered the environment in which people give and receive palliative care. In this section, we highlight the changes that seem to us to be most significant for the North American practice of palliative care in general and for specific points in our narratives where clinicians' decision-making, or patients' choices, might be different in today's environment.

COVID-19

Our book opened with a chronicle of the COVID-19 pandemic—the cause of the most radical and pervasive changes in our current lives. Beyond the sweeping alterations in our daily routines and our planning for the future, the pandemic has forced a remodeling of our collective mental picture of the world we live in. Even for people whose privilege or good fortune has shielded them from much of life's adversity and hurt, that picture has a darker hue now, with more prominent suggestions of fragility and vulnerability.

Embedded in Anna Towers's narrative of the pandemic are poignant scenes of family members trying to comfort loved ones through thick barriers of protective gear or on the tiny screen of a cell phone. Herein may lie one of the pandemic's gravest impacts on palliative care: the new, reflexive association that has taken hold in our minds between intimacy and danger. Perhaps not since the early years of AIDS—but with more justification now—have people throughout society felt as inhibited, if not expressly prohibited, from expressing care and comfort through closeness and physical contact. (Recent outbreaks of Ebola may provide other, more localized, examples.) And yet, the very essence of palliative care is *accompaniment*, the rich panoply of words and gestures through which we try to alleviate what the German sociologist Norbert Elias called the loneliness of the dying. In our modern civilization, Elias lamented,

> those close to the dying often lack the ability to give them support and comfort by proof of their affection and tenderness. They find it difficult to press

dying people's hands or to caress them, to give them a feeling of undiminished protection and belonging. Civilization's overgrown taboo on the expression of strong, spontaneous feelings ties their tongues and hands. And living people may half unconsciously feel death to be something contagious and threatening; they involuntarily draw back from the dying. But, as with every parting of people who are intimate, a gesture of undiminished affection is, for the one taking final leave, perhaps the greatest help, apart from the relief of physical pain, that those left behind can give.[13]

What is our self-protective response to COVID, whether by reflex or protocol, if not the literal enactment of Elias's half-unconscious fear of death's contagion? How long will it take, as we come out on the other side of this pandemic, to feel again the confidence to express comforting intimacy without fear?

The Opioid Crisis

If the COVID-19 pandemic has inhibited one of the signature features of palliative care—accompaniment through close physical presence—society's efforts to contain a different sort of epidemic has inhibited another: the use of opioids for pain management. In October 2017, the US government declared the opioid epidemic a public health emergency. In the prior year, 64,000 people had died from drug overdoses, of whom more than 42,000 had died from opioids.[14] Already between 1999 and 2008, opioid-associated deaths had increased four-fold in the US, and they kept on rising.[15] In the year April 2020 to April 2021, there were 100,000 such deaths, a nearly 30% increase over the prior year, as the social disruptions of the COVID-19 pandemic exacerbated the crisis.[16] A host of measures have been put in place to reverse this trend, whose salutary effects have been accompanied by significant negative ones, as physicians' reluctance to continue prescribing opioids forced many sufferers from cancer pain, especially, to endure inadequate treatment.

The rise of the opioid crisis in the years since we carried out our research is a story in which the hospice and palliative care communities are deeply implicated. Campaigns to combat "opiophobia" and the undertreatment of pain in advanced illness included the designation of pain as "the fifth vital sign"; dissemination of the "consensus" that opioid addiction among patients with cancer pain is a negligible problem, despite the thin body of scientific evidence; guidelines from the Joint Commission on Accreditation of Healthcare Organizations (JCAHO) mandating adequate pain control; and even the promulgation of "opioids prescribed per million inhabitants" as a national quality measure.[17] These largely well-intentioned efforts were turbocharged by pharmaceutical companies' aggressive and misleading marketing campaigns, especially for supposedly low-risk time-release opioid formulations such as OxyContin. They coalesced in an avalanche of opioid prescriptions. In 1997, there were 670,000 prescriptions for Oxycontin. In 2002, there were 6.2 million.[14] Overall opioid consumption in the United States rose from 46,946 kg in 2000 to 165,525 kg in 2012—the exact proportion of the increase in opioid-associated deaths in the same period.[15] In Canada, a study of beneficiaries of the Ontario Drug Benefit (ODB) from 2003 to 2014 found that, among opioid users, the prevalence of high-dose prescribing doubled (from 4.2% to 8.7%) over the study period. By 2014, 40.9% of recipients of long-acting opioids exceeded daily doses of 200 mg morphine or equivalent, including 55.8% of long-acting oxycodone users and 76.3% of transdermal fentanyl users. Moreover, in the last period, 18.7% of long-acting opioid users exceeded daily doses of 400 mg morphine or equivalent. Rates of opioid-related emergency department visits and hospital admissions increased from 9.0 to 14.0 per 10,000 ODB beneficiaries (55%) from 2003 to 2013.[18]

The new, profession- and industry-manufactured "opiophilia" dangerously conflated malignant and non-malignant pain, with woefully inadequate evaluation or monitoring of patients' susceptibility to opioid abuse or the risk of drug diversion. And the upward pressures on opioid prescribing coincided with lagging clinician education in opioid use and the relaxation of regulatory scrutiny by state medical boards and drug enforcement agencies.

Against this backdrop, the opioid pendulum swung back in the 2010s. Regulatory scrutiny of physicians' prescribing behavior increased; the large prescription drug plans initiated complicated, time-consuming opioid-prescribing rules that included strict limits to dosages and quantities; and many physicians concluded that the risks and stresses of continuing to prescribe opioids had become too high. In the words of a *New England Journal of Medicine* editorial,

> In our opinion . . . the most important contributor to a desire to stop prescribing opioids is the effect of opioid prescribing on clinicians' emotional

well-being. We worry about the potential unintended consequences of these medications even if they're used appropriately.[19]

As opioid prescriptions have begun to fall again, worries about undertreatment of cancer pain have resurfaced. At Houston's M. D. Anderson Cancer, for example, the median morphine-equivalent opioid dose for patients referred to the Supportive Care Center fell from 78 to 40 mg per day between 2010 and 2015.[20] The challenge to society now is to stabilize the opioid pendulum at a point that protects against rampant abuse while assuring pain sufferers the relief they need. The narratives of Miriam Lambert, Leonard Patterson, and Shamira Cook that follow illustrate this delicate balancing of goals and concerns. At present, intensive clinician education, more widespread screening to identify patients who are at risk for excessive or illicit opioid use, and a greater emphasis on multimodal approaches to pain management that incorporate nonpharmacological methods are becoming the new gold standard.[15,20]

Social Welfare Policy

If the COVID-19 pandemic and the opioid crisis have inhibited and complicated the provision of palliative care in recent years, other social trends have been more positive. Relative to the 1990s, people in Canada and the United States have more financial security in times of sickness, access to more health information, greater ability to integrate palliative care with active treatment of their underlying disease, and more options for expressing and documenting their preferences for the level of care they wish to receive.

The most dramatic change relative to financial security in sickness has occurred in the United States, which, at the time of our research, unlike Canada, did not, and still does not, have a program of universal health insurance coverage. Until the passage in 2010 of the Affordable Care Act (ACA), many millions of Americans were uninsured, underinsured, or at risk of losing their employment-based coverage if they lost or changed their jobs. Though the ACA has not eliminated these problems, it has drastically reduced the number of un- or precariously insured people in the United States.

The social safety net for family caregivers has also been strengthened in both Canada and the US, with Canada continuing to have the more generous provisions. The US Family Medical Leave Act (FMLA) of 1993 mandated that private-sector employers with more than 50 employees, and public agencies and schools regardless of the number of employees, provide eligible workers with up to twelve weeks per year of unpaid leave to care for an ill family member at home. Paid leave is much rarer in the United States. While almost 90% of American workers have some provision for un-paid medical leave through federal or state programs, only 20% receive any amount of paid leave under programs enacted by a few states.[21] Moreover, some states classify maternity leave as an FMLA claim, which can cause a problem for those having a baby in the same year they need to take time to care for a sick relative. As of 2016, Canada began to provide financial benefits to family caregivers who had to leave work to care for an ill relative. Compassionate Care benefits allow claims for up to 26 weeks. In September 2020, due to the COVID-19 pandemic, these benefits were extended to up to 52 weeks.[22] There remain few opportunities for financial support, how-ever, for family caregivers who do not work or who are not actively pursuing work outside the home.

Among our narratives, those of Klara Bergman, Sadie Fineman, and Victor Sloski in Montreal, and those of Shamira Cook, Leonard Patterson, and Joey Court in Lancaster County, portray patients and family members struggling under the weight, variously, of economic hardship, financial anxiety, and personal exhaustion—on top of the daily physical and psycho-logical burdens of the illness itself. Would the more recent social welfare pol-icies in both countries have reduced their struggles? The picture is mixed. Rachel Fineman and Ellen Bergman might have qualified for Compassionate Care benefits; Shirley Sloski, however, would not, as she was not employed. Amanda Court's anxiety about losing health insurance if she were to lose her job because of the demands of caring for Joey would very likely be alleviated with a health insurance plan obtained through the ACA. As the Pattersons discovered, however, the social safety net in the United States has many gaps, confusing eligibility criteria, and geographical variation in levels of support, circumstances that remain true today. Moreover, the most recent estimates of out-of-pocket and time costs (value of time spent receiving care) for indi-viduals with cancer in the United States in 2019, while varying according to cancer type, averaged $2,700 for people aged 65 and older and $5,900 for younger patients. These figures, the study authors note, ought to be com-pared to the resources of the 40% of American families who report being unable to afford an unexpected expense of $400.[23]

The Internet

Consider these three vignettes from our narratives:

Frances Legendre: She and her husband pressed on with their determined search for a cure, only now they felt that they were alone in their mission for her doctors were offering no more treatments. Mrs. Legendre interpreted this as a loss of interest in her and a withdrawal of support. "We had to take matters into our own hands and think up answers on our own," Mr. Legendre said. They did their own research, pored over New Age type journals, and sent away for literature described in the advertisements. They sought out unpublished information by word of mouth. At times during their quest, they felt they were being taken advantage of, Mr. Legendre said, by people who were "probably making a lot of money by giving out 'recipes' to cure cancer."

Jenny Doyle: To educate herself about her disease, Mrs. Doyle joined a support group. She liked these meetings because they gave her the opportunity to learn and help at the same time. She exchanged information and advice. She cried and laughed. The third time she went, a woman announced that her cancer had metastasized to her liver. Six weeks later, she died. Mrs. Doyle was shocked. For the first time, she had come face-to-face with the deadliness of her disease.

Susan Mulroney: Sometimes when her friend Jack visited her, Susan appeared to be preoccupied with medical books, especially gynecological books. He thought that was odd, but Susan had a curious mind and loved to read. Then she began to frequent medical bookstores and health clinics where she could get the latest information on gynecological illnesses. By then, Jack felt "something wasn't right" because she seemed so single-minded about this kind of information. But she did not go to see a doctor. Looking back, Jack thought that Susan must have had a clear idea that "something was very wrong."

Such were the strategies people employed to obtain health information in the analog world of the 1990s. In only one of our narratives—that of Richard Johnson, trained as an engineer—is there any reference to the Internet. The Johnsons must have been early adopters of that revolutionary technology.

Today, digital technologies have totally supplanted old ways of producing, communicating, and using health information, whether it be a clinician looking up a treatment algorithm or a patient worried about the possible meanings of an unfamiliar bodily sensation. In Canada, for example, the Canadian Virtual Hospice is the leading web-based resource. This organization provides information and support to more than 1.2 million people each year, 40% of whom identify themselves as healthcare providers.[24]

The Internet has democratized access to expert knowledge. The norm of automatic deference to professional authority—already subject to question and critique as part of the civil rights, consumer, and women's health movements of the 1960s and 1970s—is now thoroughly discredited among large segments of an increasingly tech-savvy, online-dwelling population. As has been apparent in the COVID-19 pandemic, however, the potential for anxious or desperate people to be taken in and harmed by quack remedies and scams is now, if anything, greater than when the Legendres were grasping at "recipes" for curing cancer. The need for trust and *trustworthiness* in professional–patient relationships has never been higher than in our digital age.

The Internet has also enabled forms of networking and social support that go far beyond what was available to people in our narratives. There are online communities for connecting with fellow sufferers or survivors of a disease, with other people burdened by family caregiving, and with the bereaved. Even our emphasis in this book on the power of narrative has found a fertile environment online. Bloggers document every phase of their experiences of illness, sometimes reaching loyal and supportive audiences in the millions. Though living (or dying) online is not for everyone, the Internet has perhaps become for many people a very modern antidote to the loneliness of the dying.

The Evolution of Palliative Care as a Field

We turn now to developments in the field of palliative care and to social policies that have specifically addressed the options people have for end-of-life care. We will be selective. Rather than a comprehensive survey of the evolution of palliative care over the past two decades (such as can be found in comprehensive textbooks or histories of the field), we call attention to aspects of the contemporary context of palliative care that put in perspective some of the clinical decisions and patient or family choices that we describe in the narratives. In this General Introduction, we paint that context with a broad brush. In the commentaries that follow the individual narratives we focus on those specific decisions and choices in more detail.

In assessing the evolution of palliative care since we conducted our research in the 1990s, we have concluded that the overall picture has remained very much the same in Canada, as it has in the United States. While there has been a significant increase in the trained workforce and dramatic growth of individual organizations, such as the transformation of Hospice of Lancaster County into Hospice and Community Care, overall access to palliative care at the national level is still patchy in both countries. Resources remain limited relative to need and are distributed unevenly. As was the case in 2000, the likelihood of receiving timely, expert palliative care today depends on who you are, where you live, what disease you have, and to what extent your local institutions have prioritized palliative care. Official policies and visions for quality palliative care have proliferated robustly over the past twenty years.[25,26] Actual practices, however, very often fall short of stated policies or standards, primarily due to resource constraints, but also due to lack of education and awareness among healthcare practitioners, policymakers, and the general public.

A national survey by the Canadian Society of Palliative Care Physicians in 2014 identified 1,114 physicians who said they provided palliative care. Of these, only 51 (5%) were specialists. Another 12% identified as family physicians with a focused practice in palliative care. The remaining 83% represented a broad range of specialties and practice areas, none of which included palliative care. The majority of respondents reported that fewer than 20% of their patients had non-cancer diagnoses, despite the fact that deaths from non-cancer causes in acute care settings outnumber those from cancer. And while 79% of respondents from urban areas worked with a specialized palliative care team, this number fell to 35% in rural or remote areas.[27]

In the United States, in addition to the increase in specialist physicians and nurses noted above, the number of Medicare-certified hospice organizations had reached 4,639 by 2018. They served 1.55 million Medicare beneficiaries that year. As in Canada, cancer is by far the most common diagnosis among Medicare recipients of hospice care, at 30%, followed by cardiovascular disease (17.4%) and dementia (15.6%).[28] Also similar to Canada is the great regional variation in availability of palliative care in the United States. While 72% of all US hospitals with 50 or more beds report having a palliative care team, only 17% of rural hospitals of that size do so. Between 2015 and 2019, palliative care availability grew the most in New England and in the

Mid-Atlantic regions of the country; in the south-central regions it grew the least.[10] Hospice enrollment also varied considerably by state in 2018, from Utah's 60.5% of Medicare decedents to Alaska's 22.8%. For Pennsylvania, where we carried out our project, the figure was 49.3%.[28]

Two additional pieces of data from the United States point to the distance yet to be traveled to ensure timely, effective palliative care across the population. First, from 2000 to 2018, the median length of stay in hospice has stayed flat at 17 or 18 days, with nearly 30% of patients in care for a week or less.[29] Second, 82% of hospice patients in 2018 were Caucasian, compared to 8.2% who were African American, 6.7% who were Hispanic, 1.8% Asian/Pacific Islander, and 0.4% Native American.[28] African American decedents, especially, continue to receive more high-intensity care at the end of life and fewer hospice services than Caucasians.[30] The multiple reasons for the enduring patterns of late referral and racial disparities in hospice care are beyond full exploration here. They undoubtedly include factors such as prognostic uncertainty, especially in diseases other than cancer; physicians' reluctance to deliver bad news; and, especially in the case of African Americans, mistrust of a medical system that has historically been a site of structural racism, discrimination, inequitable access to care, and exploitation.

Several initiatives to reduce racial disparities emerged in the years following our research. The most substantial were spearheaded by the late Richard Payne, a pain and palliative medicine specialist whose career included leadership posts at Memorial Sloan Kettering Cancer Center in New York, the M. D. Anderson Cancer Center of the University of Texas, and the Duke University Institute on Care at the End of Life. It was at Duke that Dr. Payne and colleagues created a new curriculum to teach essential clinical competencies and practical skills for culturally appropriate palliative and end-of-life care to African Americans. The national curriculum, called A Progressive Palliative Care Educational Curriculum for the Care of African Americans at Life's End (APPEAL), was funded by the Robert Wood Johnson Foundation from 2002 to 2004.[31]

A synthesis of scholarship in this area was presented at a national conference in 2004—Last Miles of the Way Home: National Conference to Improve End-of-Life Care for African Americans—and published by Duke University in 2006 as *Key Topics on End-of-Life Care for African Americans*.[32] Further compelling, in-depth analyses of racial and cultural factors affecting the quality of end-of-life care for African Americans are also to be found in the work of LaVera Crawley[33,34] and Alan Elbaum.[35]

Several of our narratives illustrate one further explanation for many patients' delay in utilizing hospice or palliative care until the very last days or even hours of life: the association of such care with giving up, of simply being left alone to die. The almost indelible taint of hopelessness and death attached to palliative care and hospice in the minds of patients and families influences many physicians as well. In the case of Jenny Doyle, at a time when she was suffering intensely not only from her advanced disease but also from the side effects of treatment, one of her oncologists told her, "When I see someone functioning as well as you are—they are looking to get back to driving and things like this—this does not spell 'hospice patient' to me."

In the United States, policy reinforces prejudice. Medicare rules strictly limit payment for active treatment of a patient's underlying disease once they elect the Medicare hospice benefit. Lancaster County patients in our narratives, such as Jenny Doyle, Shamira Cook, and Albert Hoffer, faced a stark either-or dilemma: They could pursue possibly curative or life-prolonging treatment of their disease, or they could enjoy comprehensive pain and symptom management and psychological and social support for themselves and their families. Under the rules, they could not do both.

In what promises to be the most consequential change in US social welfare policy specific to palliative care, both the Centers for Medicare and Medicaid Services (CMS) and private philanthropy are supporting pilot programs designed to bridge the hitherto nearly impassable bureaucratic chasm between hospice and palliative care and continued active treatment. One of these is the Medicare Choices Model mentioned above, in which Hospice and Community Care in Lancaster County is participating. Had such a program been in effect at the time of our research, Jenny Doyle, Shamira Cook, and Albert Hoffer may well have had more options for combining palliative care with their determination to pursue the cure or remission of their disease. CMS is also proposing a Kidney Care Choices Model, which would allow patients with end-stage renal disease to elect the hospice benefit without foregoing their dialysis treatments, as existing Medicare rules typically require them to do.[36] A version of this "concurrent care" model for dialysis patients is being tested at the University of Washington under a grant from a private foundation.[37]

Two further innovations aim to expand the reach of palliative care. One is the development of outpatient palliative care clinics, where patients with a range of non-cancer diagnoses—such as cardiovascular or pulmonary disease, or neurological diseases such as amyotrophic lateral sclerosis

(ALS)—have access to consultation and ongoing follow-up from a palliative care specialist as part of the regular management of their primary condition. The second innovation is for hospice agencies to establish contracts to provide palliative care within nursing homes and other long-term care facilities. Our narrative of Leonard Patterson describes tense relations and poor communication between hospice personnel and nursing home staff and a serious medication error by an inexperienced nursing home nurse. Such problems are greatly reduced when there is a consistent, collaborative relationship between the nursing home and a hospice agency under contract to provide care at the facility.

The vision of policymakers in Canada and the United States is of the seamless integration of expert palliative care for any life-threatening illness, regardless of the stage of the disease or the setting where care is needed. The innovations mentioned above are promising steps toward that vision. At present, however, they exist only as pilot projects or at the relatively few organizations with the human and financial resources to sustain them.

The changes in the field of palliative care that we have discussed so far have primarily been at the structural and organizational levels. Have there also been significant developments in therapeutics? Surprisingly few. Most of the symptom management approaches described in our narratives would be the same today, with one or two important exceptions. One of these is a trend toward greater use of interventions involving chemotherapy, radiation, and surgery to manage symptoms very late in the course of a patient's disease. Another is the use of methadone and anesthetic or interventional neurosurgical procedures for treatment of neuropathic pain. As described in several of our narratives, the standard treatment of neuropathic pain with a cocktail of anticonvulsant and tricyclic antidepressant medications often achieved only partial success. Many of those situations today would be managed with methadone or with newer interventions such as intrathecal injections, neurolytic procedures, or vertebroplasty.

During the past decade, several new psychotherapeutic approaches have been introduced to enhance quality of life and help people with anxiety and existential distress near the end of life. For several of these approaches, including "meaning-centered therapy" and cognitive-behavioral therapy, there is an emerging evidence base. "Dignity therapy," a form of short-term psychotherapy developed by Harvey Max Chochinov that aims to relieve psychological and existential distress has been shown to be beneficial in terms of reducing patients' and families' anxiety and lessening sadness and depression.[38–40] In our narratives, Klara Bergman might have benefitted from Dignity Therapy to help with her anxiety and fears of persecution that seemed to have roots in her past as a Holocaust survivor. One further approach to existential distress at the end of life that is only very recently gaining attention is the use of psychedelic agents such as psilocybin and MDMA.

Advance Care Planning

One central feature of palliative care today barely registered in our research: the use of advance directives to anticipate and document preferences for treatment at the end of life. Although the right to limit or refuse life-sustaining treatment had been recognized in the United States since the 1970s, only in the 1990s did advance care planning seriously begin to enter the national conversation, much less conversations between patients and their physicians. Since 1990, healthcare facilities in the United States have been required to ask every patient upon admission if they have an advance directive or if they would like information on the subject. In many institutions today, a notation about the patient's advance directive occupies a conspicuous position at the head of the medical record.

Advance directives come in three main forms. One, often referred to as a "living will," records a person's goals and priorities for medical treatment at the end of life, a statement that may or may not be accompanied by an indication of the type of treatments they would either accept or refuse under various clinical conditions. With the second form, frequently combined with the first and often called a "durable power of attorney for healthcare" or "healthcare proxy," a person authorizes someone to make healthcare treatment decisions on their behalf if they have lost decision-making capacity when decisions have to be made. The third form translates the treatment preferences expressed in the first into actual medical orders, to be followed as any other medical orders would be, by clinicians in a hospital or nursing home, or—crucially—by emergency medical personnel in the field. This type of document is usually called Physician Orders for Life-Sustaining Treatment (POLST) in the United States and Medical Orders for Scope of Treatment (MOST) in Canadian provinces where it has been adopted.

This third form of advance directive is designed to endow a person's treatment preferences with the authority of actionable medical orders, as well as to give clinicians greater certainty and confidence in their decision-making than is often provided by vague or ambiguous language in a living will. A convincing piece of evidence of the effectiveness of advance care planning in helping people realize their end-of-life care goals comes from a large study from Oregon. The study compared the location of death of almost 58,000 people with the presence or absence of a POLST form in a statewide registry, and, for the 18,000 with a POLST form, with the level of care specified on the form. The study found that only 6.4% of patients who specified "Comfort Measures Only" on their POLST form died in the hospital, compared with 44.2% whose form called for "Full Treatment," and 34.2% who had no POLST form in the registry.[41] On the reasonable assumption that a non-hospital death is more consistent with the prioritization of comfort over aggressive interventions, this result appears to support this type of advance care planning.

In both Canada and the United States, campaigns to encourage advance care planning have targeted health professionals and the general public over the past twenty years. Examples include The Conversation Project and Respecting Choices in the United States, and Advance Care Planning Canada, spearheaded since 2008 by the Canadian Hospice and Palliative Care Association. Training in communications skills related to end-of-life care conversations with patients now features prominently in health professions education at all levels. An early example, OncoTalk, was directed at oncologists. It is now part of a broader curriculum tailored to various subspecialties under the rubric Vitaltalk.[42] In addition, Medicare now reimburses physicians in the United States for one patient visit per year to review or revise a patient's preferences for care near the end of life.

Still, the use of advance directives in both countries remains relatively low. An online survey of 2,948 Canadians 18 years of age or older, conducted in February 2019, found that eight in ten have given end-of-life care some thought, but fewer than one in five has an advance care plan,[43] though this may understate the prevalence of advance care planning among particular subgroups. For example, a population-based mortality follow-back survey conducted in Nova Scotia found that 56.3% of decedents had a documented advanced directive, while 67.6% had power of attorney for healthcare. Significant predictors of decedents having an advance directive included the decedent's age, where they received most of their end-of-life care, whether they received specialized palliative care, whether they were aware they were dying, and the age of the informant.[44] Researchers in the United States carried out a systematic review of 150 studies published in the period 2011–2016 to determine the proportion of adults with a completed living will, health care power of attorney, or both. Among the 795,909 people in the studies, 36.7% had completed an advance directive, including 29.3% with living wills, proportions that were similar across the years of the review.[45]

In terms of our narratives, the absence of discussion of advance directives is not surprising, given our point of entry into people's experiences of care. In most cases, they had already made the choices that are typically specified in advance directives. On the other hand, in several narratives, patients describe conversations with physicians or hospice staff about their diagnosis or the probability of their imminent death that clearly demonstrate the importance of the communications skills training that has lately become more widely available. As we point out in our commentaries, some of these interactions are breathtakingly blunt, heavy-handed, or even harsh. We invite readers to assess for themselves what improvement has occurred in recent years.

Medical Aid in Dying

Four of the twenty patients whose experiences we describe in this book asked their caregivers to administer medication that would end their lives: Klara Bergman and Frances Legendre in Montreal, and Leonard Patterson and Jenny Doyle in Lancaster County. At the time of our research, the palliative care team could truthfully respond that, whatever their own professional or personal views on the matter, to comply with such a request would be against the law. In Canada, this is no longer the case. In Quebec, since December 15, 2015, and in the rest of Canada since June 17, 2016, a physician or nurse practitioner is legally allowed to provide Medical Aid in Dying (MAID)—at a person's request and with certain procedural safeguards—either by directly administering a medication to cause the person's death or prescribing a medication for that purpose that the person takes themselves.[46,47] In the United States, where active euthanasia is still illegal, between 1997 and 2021 nine states and the District of Columbia (though not Pennsylvania) have adopted laws permitting physician-assisted suicide (PAS).[48] Physicians in those states—as well as in Montana under a ruling by the state's Supreme Court—may provide a terminally ill person with a prescription for a lethal dose of medication for the purpose of assisting that person in ending their own life.

At the outset, all the laws in both countries incorporated the procedural safeguards in Oregon's pioneering law, which was first adopted by voter referendum in 1994 and came into effect, after court challenges and a second referendum, in 1997. Chief among these safeguards were requirements that the person requesting MAID or PAS must be terminally ill and mentally competent, and repeats the request after a 15-day waiting period. Here, too, things are beginning to change. Since March 12, 2020, in Quebec, a court has had the authority to waive the law's requirement that an otherwise qualifying patient's natural death be reasonably foreseeable.[49] To drive home the point, the Government of Canada's official website for MAID emphasizes that "you do *not* need to have a fatal or terminal condition to be eligible for medical assistance in dying."[50] As of March 17, 2023, in all of Canada, Canadians whose only medical condition is a mental illness, and who otherwise meet all eligibility criteria, will also be eligible for MAID.[51] Even Oregon has waived the 15-day waiting period for people whose life expectancy is reasonably expected to be shorter—as short, in fact, as two days.[52]

Between 2016 and 2020, more than 21,000 Canadians ended their lives under the MAID law. The 7595 people who used MAID in 2020 represented a 34.2% increase over the prior year. MAID accounted for 2.5% of all Canadian deaths in 2020; 4% on Quebec, and 3.1% in British Columbia.[53] The best long-term data from the United States come from Oregon and Washington, where 2,588 people died with PAS between 1998 and 2017—between three and four of every 1,000 deaths in the two states during the period. In Oregon, in 2020, 6.5 of every 1,000 deaths were the result of PAS.[54,55]

In both countries, the great majority of people utilizing a form of MAID were receiving hospice or palliative care at the time: in 2020, 82.8% of the people in Canada; 95% of the people in Oregon. The most common reasons people give for choosing MAID or PAS are also broadly similar. Canadians most often mention the loss of the ability to engage in meaningful activities or to perform activities of daily living. People in Oregon and Washington mention the loss of autonomy, decreasing ability to participate in pleasurable activities, impaired quality of life, and the loss of dignity.[53, 54]

Would the narratives of Klara Bergman and Frances Legendre have had different outcomes had the Canadian legal environment concerning MAID been what it is today? What of Miriam Lambert and Rose Picard, also in Montreal, whom the palliative care team maintained in states of prolonged sedation in the last days of their lives, taking pains to distinguish this approach from euthanasia? And what if Leonard Patterson and Jenny Doyle had been living under the type of law governing PAS that is now in effect in several states in the United States? Although such counterfactual questions are almost by definition unanswerable, in the Authors' Comments we explore specific aspects of these cases with the evolving legal climate in mind. We want to conclude this section with more general observations about how the practice of palliative care is being affected as it comes to terms with this changed environment. Issues are emerging in three areas: clinicians' relationships with patients and the public, relationships among palliative care colleagues, and palliative care practitioners' professional identity.

Where MAID or PAS are now legal, palliative care practitioners must be more explicit about their own position in their conversations with patients. The cloak of illegality having been stripped away, practitioners now have no choice—when a patient requests MAID or PAS—but to declare openly whether they are prepared to comply, after appropriate investigations of the patient's reasons and mental state, or whether, as the laws provide, they will conscientiously refuse and refer the patient to another physician—quite possibly a stranger—who is prepared to proceed. In Canada, offers of palliative sedation (as in our narratives of Frances Legendre, Miriam Lambert, and Rose Picard) now open the physician to questions why, once embarked on that path, the patient's dying must be prolonged rather than brought to an immediate conclusion. These questions, too, require more complicated, nuanced answers than in the past, as we discuss in our commentary on the narrative of Frances Legendre.

Among some patients, the fact that palliative care physicians are legally authorized to perform MAID or PAS may reinforce the stigma attached to palliative care, that it is "where they send you to die." For other patients, a physician's willingness to provide MAID or PAS may be a litmus test that inverts the traditional foundations of trust in the physician–patient relationship. The physician's traditional question—consistent with the prohibition of euthanasia in medical ethics since Hippocrates—has been, "can my patient trust me, amid the profound vulnerability and dependency of very advanced illness, if I might end their life?" The physician may now have to wonder, "Can my patient trust me if I *refuse* to end their life?"

As early as the mid-1990s, as state-level initiatives to allow PAS began to gain traction, the Ethics Committee of the Academy of Hospice Physicians (AHP), a predecessor of today's American Academy of Hospice and Palliative Medicine (AAHPM), promulgated a statement in opposition to the practice as the official position of the organization. Rancorous dissent within the membership revealed wide divergences of views. In due course, the AHP backtracked to an official position that is characterized on the AAHPM's website today as "studied neutrality" on the legalization of PAS.[56] Within particular hospice or palliative care teams, such conflicts now play out as serious philosophical disagreements or resentment at the amount of time and emotional resources required to carry out even one patient's request for MAID.[57,58]

Regarding professional identity, our physician colleague Talia Abecassis has commented,

> One key unwritten, yet strongly held belief among palliative care providers is that they can relieve most patients' suffering. This belief may be the key to their ability to continue to work long-term in this emotionally charged and thus challenging field. To help patients and families and to gain their trust, do they need to believe that they will not fail to provide them comfort? If palliative care physicians were to allow themselves to think that there is prevalent suffering that they fail to address, might it be too difficult for some physicians to continue in palliative care practice?[59]

The growth of public support for MAID and PAS since we conducted our research raises, in a specific, intensified form, one of our principal findings: the frequent discrepancy between professionals' assessments of the effectiveness of their interventions and the assessments of the patients and families themselves. Our narratives do describe significant suffering that palliative care failed to address. They do describe patients' unmet needs for relief. Sometimes this was due to inherent limits to what could be done. Sometimes the team was aware of the failures and worked tirelessly, if not always successfully, to make things better. Sometimes, however, the team appears to have overlooked or failed to acknowledge the continuation of a patient's distress. Today, even when pain and symptom management has been exemplary, some patients insist that this is not enough. The data on people's reasons for choosing MAID or PAS show that it is more likely a loss of meaning or satisfaction with one's *very existence*, rather than inadequate relief of physical symptoms, that determines their choice. There are thus uncomfortable questions for the palliative care professional that the new environment for MAID and PAS is bringing to light: Am I doing harm when I think I am doing good? Even when I've done my best, do some of my patients think that I am prolonging rather than relieving their suffering?

What Did We Learn?

The primary value of the narratives in this book lies in their particularity. Our project was not designed to test hypotheses and so achieve generalizable knowledge. Nevertheless, it is possible to stand back from the details and pick out some overarching themes, some larger stories being told collectively by the individual stories in the narratives.

1. We have just discussed the discrepancies that can arise between professionals' and patients' or families' assessments of the effectiveness of care. We need say no more about it here, except to note that overall definitions of a "good death" are variable, too. Among these narratives are stories of patients whose final hours were marked by astounding moments of calm, reconciliation, even humor. There are other patients who died in pain, surrounded by frantic and exhausted relatives. Yet it is impossible on the basis of these moments alone to declare that one death was "good," another "bad." Few deaths can be simply characterized one way or the other, and the family's judgment may turn out to be quite different from that of the professionals.

2. There is no hard distinction between active treatment and palliative care. Forcing patients to choose between them—either through payment mechanisms or caregivers' ideologies—is hostile to good outcomes. For patients and families, as well as their caregivers, the norm is a frequent oscillation between hope for continuing life and acceptance of decline and death. "Acceptance" and "denial" rarely appear in pure form. It is more accurate to think in terms of people's *mixed consciousness*, or what Avery Weisman called "middle knowledge": the simultaneous, even if seemingly incompatible, mental states of denial and preparation for one's impending death.[60] The transition from active treatment (primarily curative or life-prolonging in intent) to palliative treatment (primarily aimed at comfort and support) may happen smoothly and unidirectionally, but more often it is a gradual, confusing, ambivalent process for all concerned. Ideologies and systems of care that require dichotomous thinking and black-and-white choices serve patients and families poorly.

3. High-quality palliative care depends on the personal qualities of caregivers—warmth, technical competence, and stamina—but can be

undermined by systems' constraints. Systemic issues, such as the organization and financing of care, bureaucratic structures, the allocation of resources, and interprofessional rivalries, are significant factors in the effectiveness of individual interventions. The effect of these factors is often amplified by the socioeconomic status, race, ethnicity, and culture of all involved, which can create distance between patients, families, and their professional caregivers.

4. Relationships between patients, families, and caregivers pass through many stages over time. Rapport, empathy, and trust do not spring full-grown at the outset of a caregiver–patient/family relationship. They take time to evolve, and patients and families are frequently selective in identifying a caregiver with whom they feel open enough to share important thoughts.

5. Professional caregivers, as well as patients and families, bring their histories of death and loss into the caring relationship. Sometimes the histories of loss are immediately evident, as with Klara Bergman who was a survivor of the Holocaust. Sometimes they are more hidden, as with the nurse who cared for Jasmine Claude. Having been adopted at the age of two, this nurse experienced intense anxiety whenever she cared for a woman whose death left a grieving child.

6. Rich expressions of spirituality and religious faith abound in our narratives, ranging from the deep-rooted serenity of patients like Jasmine Claude or Martin Roy in Montreal, and Stanley Gray in Lancaster County, to Klara Bergman's fierce arguments with God, a salient feature of her Jewish tradition. Yet patients' expressions of spirituality were frequently met with suspicion or skepticism by members of the palliative care team. It was as if these clinicians had an internalized image of the appropriate emotional and behavioral responses of a person facing death, in which anger, fear, and anxiety were essential elements. To encounter nearly unmixed serenity and calm produced a kind of cognitive dissonance for these clinicians that they found troubling and disconcerting.

7. Growth and change are possible throughout the time of a person's dying, for individuals and for their relationships. Although the dying process can bring out histories of hurt and other fault lines in family relationships the way ultraviolet light exposes letters and words written with invisible ink, it can also mend old wounds and even hatreds. A life of conflict and discouragement can move toward a sense of

integrity and wholeness. It is possible, in the words of Balfour Mount and Michael Kearney, "to die healed."[61]

8. There is considerable variation in how central to their identity an individual makes their self-definition as "dying" over the course of advanced illness. While acknowledging some overlapping across different patients, some of the people in our narratives, such as Richard Johnson, Costas Metrakis, and Miriam Lambert, seemed overwhelmed and at times completely defined by their illness and its fatal course. For others, such as Albert Hoffer, Katie Melnick, Frances Legendre, and Shamira Cook, the sense of themselves as dying—as opposed to getting on with the important projects in their lives—appeared to ebb and flow, sometimes with an abruptness that startled and confused their families, caregivers, and friends. Another group, that included, for example, Leonard Patterson, Jenny Doyle, Sadie Fineman, Martin Roy, Jasmine Claude, and Paula Ferrari, seemed primarily to see themselves as living, or, perhaps, as living while dying—with the emphasis on living—and wanted their lives to remain as normal as possible to the end. "Normal" meant different things to each of them, and their definitions sometimes contrasted greatly with those of their professional caregivers. Yet there was a common thread: a desire to maintain continuity in their sense of who they were as individuals for as long as possible and not be forced to conform to someone else's ideas of what a "dying" person should think, do, or feel. This desire is epitomized in one of the most frequent responses of hospice patients in the National Hospice Demonstration study conducted in 1988, when they were asked how they would like to experience the last three days of their lives: "I want the last three days of my life to be like any other days."[62]

This, then, is some of what our narratives have shown to us. And while this book is by no means a how-to manual for the care of the dying, we think there are also a few useful lessons for caregivers and companions to be gleaned from the narratives by attentive readers, which resonate with our own experience.

1. Bring your full attention.
2. Listen more than you speak.
3. Understand before judging.
4. Prepare to be surprised.

5. Prepare to receive as well as to give.
6. Don't postpone acts of kindness.

Some Personal Words in Conclusion

> I am not seeking an escape from dread but rather proof that dread
> and reverence can exist within us simultaneously.
>
> —Czesław Miłosz[63]

The four of us were profoundly affected by our work and colleagueship in this project. We have different backgrounds and origins (Italo-Canadian, British Canadian, Greek, Jewish American) and different areas of expertise. We mention this not only because we believe these differences have enriched our work, but also to indicate something of the personal standpoints from which we carried it out.

Anna Towers is Associate Professor of Oncology and Family Medicine, McGill University. For the past thirty years she has served as a palliative care physician at the Royal Victoria Hospital, Montreal. She succeeded Dr. Balfour Mount as Director of the McGill Division of Palliative Care (1999–2009). Anna is recognized as a pioneering advocate for the development of supportive care for cancer patients.

Patricia Boston is currently Clinical Professor in the Department of Family Practice at the University of British Columbia. She was Director of the UBC Division of Palliative Care between 2003 and 2012, prior to which she was Associate Director of the McGill Programs in Whole Person Care. Patricia's research and teaching interests include palliative care, grief and bereavement, psychosocial nursing issues, and qualitative research methodologies.

Yanna Lambrinidou is a medical anthropologist and affiliate faculty in the Department of Science, Technology, and Society at Virginia Polytechnic Institute and State University. She is cofounder of the Engineering Ethics and Community Rights Collaborative and of the Campaign for Lead Free Water, a community-led environmental justice initiative. She combines teaching, research, and activism. Yanna's interests include ethnographically grounded pedagogies for engineering ethics education as well as community rights in academic–community collaborations.

David Barnard was University Professor and Chair of the Department of Humanities at the Penn State University College of Medicine during the period of our research. Subsequently, he was Professor at the Center for Bioethics and Health Law at the University of Pittsburgh, where he was also Director of the University of Pittsburgh Institute to Enhance Palliative Care. Now retired, David's teaching and research interests in the medical humanities focused primarily on care at the end of life over a career of nearly forty years. Having moved through life with the advantages, and blind spots, of a White man, he has found this project, with its immersion in the intimate life experiences of a wide range of people, and the collaborative and interactive partnership with his co-authors, to be transformative.

It is not unusual to hear caregivers comment that working in palliative care has improved their own quality of life. This has been true to some extent for us as researchers as well. Through our close contact with the people in these narratives, we learned more about the uncertainty and fragility of life and about getting back to basics—friends, family, and community. There were also personal challenges for us. Once we were invited, we had to go into a dying person's world in some small measure to try to understand it. These moments when we opened ourselves to the reality and inevitability of death were emotionally risky for us, even if the patients were clearly running the greater risks.

The title of this book, *Crossing Over*, is a metaphor for the physical, emotional, and spiritual movements that we witnessed during the three years of our study. All but one of the patients in the following chapters had died when this book first appeared. They had crossed over, leaving this world altogether. Prior to their deaths, these people (and here we include the man who was then still alive) took other kinds of journeys. They reached across old barriers to embrace loved ones, to connect to the past, or to their God. Families crossed over, too. They made efforts to move out of themselves in order truly to understand their dying relatives, to be at their side, and to advocate for them. In bereavement, they had to cross over to a new life without the deceased. Palliative care workers crossed daily from their own bustling, future-oriented lives into the profoundly diminished physical and temporal worlds of their patients, in a way acting as a rejuvenating bridge between the two realms. As co-authors, each of us moved out of the comfort zones of our particular personal and disciplinary standpoints to open ourselves to new ways of relating, thinking, and writing. And we extended ourselves into the lives of patients, families, and caregivers, trying to appreciate their perspectives, their encounters with dread and reverence. We hope this book will help readers make their own crossings.

References

1. Center to Advance Palliative Care. n.d. "About." https://www.capc.org/about/palliat ive-care/. Accessed September 20, 2021.
2. American Academy of Hospice and Palliative Medicine. n.d. "About." (http://aahpm. org/about/about. Accessed September 20, 2021.
3. Cherny N, Fallon M, Kaasa S, Portenoy R, Currow D, eds. *Oxford Textbook of Palliative Medicine*. 6th ed. New York: Oxford University Press; 2021.
4. Ferrell B, Paice J, eds. *Oxford Textbook of Palliative Nursing*. 5th ed. New York: Oxford University Press; 2019.
5. MacDonald S, Herx L, Boyle A, eds. *Palliative Medicine: A Case-Based Manual*. 4th ed. New York: Oxford University Press; 2021.
6. Saunders C. Introduction. In: Saunders C, Sykes N, eds. *The Management of Terminal Malignant Disease*. 3rd ed. London: Edward Arnold; 1993: 1–14.
7. Hutchinson TA, ed. *Whole Person Care: A New Paradigm for the 21st Century*. New York: Springer International; 2011.
8. Hutchinson TA. *Whole Person Care: Transforming Healthcare*. New York: Springer International; 2017.
9. Hooijer G, King D. The racialized pandemic: Wave one of COVID-19 and the reproduction of global north inequalities. Perspect Politics: 1–21. Published online August 11, 2021 by the Cambridge Core. https://doi.org/10.1017/S153759272100195X
10. Center to Advance Palliative Care. 2020. America's Care of Serious Illness: 2019 State-by-State Report Card on Access to Palliative Care in Our Nation's Hospitals. https://reportcard.capc.org/. Accessed November 15, 2021.
11. Center for Medicare and Medicaid Services. 2015. Medicare Choices Model. https://innovation.cms.gov/innovation-models/medicare-care-choices. Accessed November 15, 2021.
12. Brown C. Nothing is real: The slippery art of biography. Times Literary Supplement, September 10, 2021: 4.
13. Elias N. *The Loneliness of the Dying*. Oxford: Blackwell; 1985: 28–29.
14. Jones M, Viswanath O, Peck J, et al. A brief history of the opioid epidemic and strategies for pain medicine. Pain Ther. 2018;7:13–21.
15. Gaertner J, Boehlke C, Simone C, Hui D. Early palliative care and the opioid crisis: Ten pragmatic steps towards a more rational use of opioids. Ann Palliat Med. September 2019;8(4):490–497.
16. National Center for Health Statistics. 2022. Provisional drug overdose death counts, November 7, 2021. https://www.cdc.gov/nchs/nvss/vsrr/drug-overdose-data.htm. Accessed November 17, 2021.
17. Linge-Dahl L, Vranken M, Juenger S, et al. Identification of challenges to the availability and accessibility of opioids in twelve European countries: Conclusions from two ATOME six-country workshops. J Palliat Med. 2015;18:1033–1039.
18. Spooner L, Fernandes K, Martins D, et al. High-dose opioid prescribing and opioid-related hospitalization: A population-based study. PLoS ONE. 2016;11(12):e0167479.
19. Comerci, G, Katzman J, Duhigg, D. Controlling the swing of the opioid pendulum. N Eng J Med. 2018;378(8):691–693.
20. Bruera E, Del Fabbro E. Pain management in the era of the opioid crisis. Am Soc Clin Oncol Educational Book. May 23, 2018;38:807–812.

21. US Department of Labor. National compensation survey: Employee benefits in the United States, March 2020. Bulletin 2793, September 2020. https://www.bls.gov/ncs/ebs/benefits/2020/employee-benefits-in-the-united-states-march-2020.pdf. Accessed July 22, 2022.

22. Government of Canada. September 1, 2019. Compassionate care leave: 808-1-IPG-063. https://www.canada.ca/en/employment-social-development/programs/laws-regulations/labour/interpretations-policies/compassionate-care.html. Accessed November 15, 2021.

23. Yabroff K, Mariotto A, Tangka F, et al. Annual report to the nation on the status of cancer, Part 2: Patient economic burden associated with cancer care. JNCI. 2021:djab192. https://doi.org/10.1093/jnci/djab192.

24. Canadian Virtual Hospice. n.d. https://www.virtualhospice.ca/en_US/Main+Site+Navigation/Home.aspx. Accessed November 15, 2021.

25. National Quality Forum. April, 2012. National Voluntary Consensus Standards for Palliative Care and End-of-Life Care. 2012. https://www.qualityforum.org/Publications/2012/04/Palliative_Care_and_End-of-Life_Care%e2%80%94A_Consensus_Report.aspx. Accessed November 15, 2021.

26. Canadian Hospice Palliative Care Association. The Way Forward National Framework: A Roadmap for an Integrated Palliative Approach to Care. March 2015. http://www.hpcintegration.ca/media/60044/TWF-framework-doc-Eng-2015-final-April1.pdf. Accessed August 10, 2022.

27. Canadian Society of Palliative Care Physicians Human Resources Committee. National palliative medicine survey data report. May 2015. http://www.cspcp.ca/wp-content/uploads/2015/04/PM-Survey-Data-Report-EN.pdf. Accessed November 15, 2021.

28. National Hospice and Palliative Care Organization. August 20, 2020. Facts and figures 2020 edition. https://www.nhpco.org/wp-content/uploads/NHPCO-Facts-Figures-2020-edition.pdf. Accessed November 15, 2021.

29. Medicare Payment Advisory Commission. March 13, 2020. Report to the Congress: Medicare payment policy 2020. Chapter 12: Hospice Services. http://www.medpac.gov/docs/default-source/reports/mar20_medpac_ch12_sec.pdf. Accessed November 15, 2021.

30. Ornstein K, Roth D, Huang J, et al. Evaluation of racial disparities in hospice use and end-of-life treatment intensity in the REGARDS cohort. JAMA Netw Open. 2020;3(8):e2014639.

31. Robert Wood Johnson Foundation. Team customizes, pilots end-of-life curriculum for African-American health care professionals. Program Results Reports, June 18, 2006. https://www.rwjf.org/en/library/research/2006/06/team-customizes--pilots-end-of-life-curriculum-for-african-ameri.html. Accessed November 15, 2021.

32. Payne R, London D, Latson S, eds. *Key Topics on End-of-Life Care for African Americans: An Intellectual Discourse Derived from The Last Miles of the Way Home 2004 National Conference to Improve End-of-Life Care for African Americans*. Durham, NC: Duke Institute on Care at the End of Life; 2006. https://divinity.duke.edu/sites/divinity.duke.edu/files/documents/tmc/KTFULL.pdf. Accessed November 15, 2021.

33. Crawley L, Payne R, Bolden J, et al. Palliative and end-of-life care in the African American community, JAMA. 2000;284(19):2518–2521.

34. Crawley L, Singer MK. Racial, cultural, and ethnic factors affecting the quality of end-of-life care in California. California HealthCare Foundation, 2007. https://www. chcf.org/wp-content/uploads/2017/12/PDF-CulturalFactorsEOL.pdf. Accessed August 10, 2022.

35. Elbaum A. Black lives in a pandemic: Implications of systemic injustice for end-of-life care. Hastings Cent Rep. 2020;50(3):58–60.

36. Schell J, Johnson D. Challenges with providing hospice care for patients undergoing dialysis. CJASN. 2021;16:473–475.

37. Aleccia J. "My time to live": Through novel program, kidney patients get palliative care, dialysis 'til the end. Kaiser Health News, August 30, 2021. https://khn.org/news/ article/chronic-kidney-disease-hospice-patients-palliative-care-dialysis-end-of-life/. Accessed November 15, 2021.

38. Chochinov H, Kristjanson L, Breitbart W, et al. Effect of dignity therapy on distress and end of life in terminally ill patients: A randomized controlled trial. Lancet Oncol. 2011;12(8):753–762.

39. Kredentser MS, Chochinov H. Psychotherapeutic considerations for patients with terminal illness. Am J Psychother. 2020;73(4):137–143.

40. Martínez M, Arantzamendi M, Belar A, et al. "Dignity therapy," a promising intervention in palliative care: A comprehensive systematic literature review. Palliat Med. 2017;6:492–509.

41. Fromme E, Zive D, Schmidt T, et al. Association between physician orders for life-sustaining treatment for scope of treatment and in-hospital death in Oregon. J Am Geriatric Soc. 2014;62(7):1246–1251.

42. Vitaltalk. n.d. https://www.vitaltalk.org/. Accessed November 15, 2021.

43. Advance Care Planning Canada. July 2019. https://www.advancecareplanning. ca/news/advance-care-planning-canada-releases-new-national-poll. Accessed November 15, 2021.

44. Digout C, Lawson B, MacKenzie A. Prevalence of having advance directives and a signed power of attorney in Nova Scotia. J Palliat Care. 2019;34(3):189–196.

45. Yadav K, Gabler N, Cooney E, et al. Approximately one in three US adults completes any type of advance directive for end-of-life care. Health Aff (Millwood). 2017;36(7):1244–1251.

46. Quebec National Assembly, Bill 52: An act respecting end-of-life care, 2014. http:// www.assnat.qc.ca/%20en/travaux-parlementaires/projets-loi/projet-loi-52-40-1.html. Accessed July 22, 2022.

47. Parliament of Canada, Bill C-14: An Act to amend the Criminal Code and to make related amendments to other Acts (medical assistance in dying), June 17, 2016. https://laws-lois.justice.gc.ca/eng/annualstatutes/2016_3/fulltext.html. Accessed July 22,2022.

48. Compassion & Choices. n.d. States where medical aid in dying is authorized. https:// compassionandchoices.org/resource/states-or-territories-where-medical-aid-in-dying-is-authorized/. Accessed November 15, 2021.

49. Government of Quebec. July 8, 2022. Medical aid in dying. https://www.quebec. ca/en/health/health-system-and-services/end-of-life-care/medical-aid-in-dying/. Accessed July 22, 2022.

50. Government of Canada. n.d. Medical assistance in dying. https://www.canada.ca/ en/health-canada/services/medical-assistance-dying.html. Accessed November 15, 2021. Emphasis in original.

51. Parliament of Canada, Bill C-7: An Act to amend the Criminal Code (medical assistance in dying), March 17, 2021. https://parl.ca/DocumentViewer/en/43-2/bill/C-7/royal-assent. Accessed July 22, 2022.

52. Oregon Health Authority. n.d. Death with Dignity Act. (https://www.oregon.gov/oha/PH/PROVIDERPARTNERRESOURCES/EVALUATIONRESEARCH/DEATHWITHDIGNITYACT/Pages/faqs.aspx#exempt. Accessed November 15, 2021.

53. Health Canada. Second Annual Report on Medical Assistance in Dying in Canada, 2020. June 2021. https://www.canada.ca/en/health-canada/services/medical-assistance-dying/annual-report-2020.html. Accessed November 15, 2021.

54. Al Rabadi L, LeBlanc M, Bucy T, et al. Trends in medical aid in dying in Oregon and Washington. JAMA Netw Open. 2019;2(8):e198648.

55. Oregon Health Authority. February 26, 2021. Oregon Death with Dignity Act: 2020 Data Summary. https://www.oregon.gov/oha/PH/PROVIDERPARTNERRESOURCES/EVALUATIONRESEARCH/DEATHWITHDIGNITYACT/Documents/year23.pdf. Accessed November 15, 2021.

56. American Academy of Hospice and Palliative Medicine. Statement on Physician-Assisted Dying, June 24, 2016. http://aahpm.org/positions/pad. Accessed November 15, 2021.

57. Hudson P, Hudson R, Philip J, et al. Legalizing physician-assisted suicide and/or euthanasia: Pragmatic implications. Palliat Supportive Care. 2015;13:1399–1409.

58. Mathews J, Hausner D, Avery J, et al. Impact of medical assistance in dying on palliative care: A qualitative study. Palliat Med 2021;35(2):447–454.

59. Abecassis T. *A Scoping Review of Medical Aid in Dying in Canada and the Potential Implications for Palliative Care Philosophy, Practice, and Teaching.* Unpublished manuscript, McGill University, May 2021.

60. Weisman A. *On Dying and Denying: A Psychiatric Study of Terminality.* New York: Behavioral Publications; 1972.

61. Mount B, Kearney M. Healing and palliative care: Charting our way forward. Palliat Med. 2003;17(8):657–658.

62. Kastenbaum RJ. *Death, Society, and Human Experience.* 11th ed. Oxford: Routledge; 2016.

63. Miłosz C. *To Begin Where I Am: Selected Essays.* New York: Farrar, Straus and Giroux; 2001: 387.

3

Raymond Hynes

When the Storm of a Lifetime Hits in Mid-Dance

Narrated by Anna Towers

Sometimes a family is fortunate enough to have significant resources to face a world that seems to have fallen apart. This was the case for Raymond Hynes and his family when they learned of his incurable cancer. The Hyneses had their way of dealing with this disaster, a way that was different from what the palliative care team wanted to see. The different perspectives may have represented cultural differences between the family and the medical professionals. The members of the Hynes family were practical and stoical; when challenged by life events, they typically sought a common-sense, step-by-step solution, and that is how they preferred to deal with the illness. The team, however, kept expecting more expression of feeling. Silence was a powerful force that informed the family's actions. Nevertheless, the family and the team managed to navigate a course that led to a successful death at home.

Sickness Was Not a Part of His Life

Raymond Hynes loved to dance. In fact, he looked very much like Fred Astaire—tall, slim, and graceful. Even at age 72, he and his wife Margaret went dancing regularly. They were champion ballroom dancers. Mr. Hynes was fun-loving man, always smiling, always welcoming. He was well known for the parties he organized within the Irish community. He was a baseball fanatic who turned televised games into social occasions. He had many good friends through the church, his work, and his golf group. He was a kidder, and he had a twinkle in his eye. He blamed it on his Irish origins.

If Mr. Hynes had worries, he did not share them with others for he didn't want to bother them. He always said that everything was fine. He lived from day to day, was never concerned about his health, and ate and drank what he wanted. He liked to relax and take naps, making it a point to take regular holidays and play golf twice a week.

Margaret thought Raymond was hard on his body. He had smoked heavily for 60 years, and yet he seemed to have no lung problems. He liked his gin and tonic when he got home. He had a great sense of humor and made a lot of people laugh. Sometimes, Margaret would say, his positive attitude about everything went beyond reason, but it was pleasant to live with someone who was as lively as Raymond Hynes.

Mr. and Mrs. Hynes lived in a comfortable detached house in an English-speaking suburb of Montreal and rented a cottage in the country every summer. After retiring as manager of a large furniture company, Mr. Hynes continued to act as a consultant. Mr. Hynes was a very religious man. He went to church every Sunday and served as a lector and warden at the church. He counted the priests among his friends and worked for Catholic charities. He felt that his religion had helped him through a lot of things in life.

Although not one to express affection in words. Mr. Hynes adored his wife. Margaret was a tall, graceful woman who was always impeccably groomed; she was good-looking but unadorned, with short, natural gray hair and tasteful spectacles. Sometimes she wished that her husband could be more expressive, but she realized that he could, in a few words, express a lifetime of love and appreciation. At his 70th birthday party, for example, he had turned to look at her with deep gratitude in his eyes. All he said was, "Oh, Maggie, Maggie"—and that said it all.

The Hyneses had two daughters and one son. They described their family as very close. Mary and Michael lived in Montreal; Jane lived in Florida. Mary was a children's social worker, a lively woman in her mid-forties and tall like her parents. She tended to dress in casual sports clothes and enjoyed exercise and the outdoors. She always seemed to be moving around or saying things to diffuse tension and try to make everyone in the family feel better.

Mary felt very close to her father, describing herself as very much like him. She told me, "I have a lot of Daddy in me. I'm optimistic, but I do talk about it and work things through." In this last respect, Mary differed from her father and felt that her father was in denial about a lot of things. When Mary was a child and was upset about something, her father would be dismissive. He wouldn't sit and talk with her, so Mary didn't go to him if she had problems. She preferred to go to her mother. Now Mary seemed to be the linchpin in the family. When Mr. Hynes became ill, he insisted that Mary be present at every medical and nursing visit, and often she was their spokesperson.

Michael had his own business, which was doing well. He was also close to his father, but in a different way. They played golf together, and although they generally did not say much to each other, their feelings toward each other ran deep. Michael had experienced his share of suffering: he and his wife had raised a handicapped son, who, despite all odds, had just started college. They had received great encouragement from Mr. and Mr. Hynes from the time their son was born. That he had made it to college was a measure of how resourceful this family was. They also knew that good health could not be taken for granted.

Mr. Hynes was very involved in the city's Irish Catholic subculture, and he was proud of his origins, as he was of his family. "Nobody is better than the Hyneses," he would say. Mr. and Mrs. Hynes loved their grandchildren—all ten of them. On vacations the family would meet at their Vermont chalet and rent two houses near each other because it was important for Mr. Hynes to see his family all together. Everyone had come for his 70th birthday party.

The family lived within a culture that limited expressiveness. Although they may have been introspective, they were not open concerning their feelings. They were practical and efficient, they knew how to get a job done, and they had financial resources.

Hearing the Bad News

When the Hyneses began to recount events to me as part of our research project, Mary began, "This isn't a long story, you know." Mr. Hynes was living and dancing full tilt when he began to have epigastric symptoms. In September of 1996, he began to feel ill with abdominal pain; he lost his appetite and started to lose weight. In mid-October he went to see his family physician, Dr. Drummond, a former schoolmate who had been his doctor all his adult life. Mr. Hynes had never been ill before and had never been in a hospital, but four weeks after his symptoms started the doctors told him that he had inoperable cancer of the pancreas. An abdominal scan showed a mass in the pancreas with widespread metastases in the liver and within the abdomen.

When all the tests were in, it was the resident on the medical ward who gave Mr. Hynes the diagnosis. It was late morning, and Mr. Hynes was alone at the time. Mr. Hynes asked a lot of questions. He wanted to know exactly what the tests had shown. The resident told Mr. Hynes that his prognosis was two months to two years. When the resident left, Mr. Hynes tried to hold back his tears. He took some time to consider his situation. What should he tell his family? Was there some way he could spare them the pain? When he was more composed several hours later, he called Margaret and told her the bad news. The family was devastated, and upset that Mr. Hynes had been alone when the physician gave him the news. They would have liked to have been there to support him. Everyone in the family wanted to protect everyone else, to cushion what could perhaps not be cushioned.

Why had this cancer appeared? Mrs. Hynes privately wondered whether her husband's smoking and drinking might have been something to do with it. Mrs. Hynes was not being critical of her husband; his smoking, drinking, and easy-going nature were all of a piece. If anything, she admired his *joie-de-vivre* and felt invigorated by it. But she was looking for a cause. Meanwhile, Mr. Hynes felt guilty at having to impose his illness on the family and thought that he might have been able to prevent it if he had lived differently.

The oncologist offered Mr. Hynes experimental chemotherapy. Mr. Hynes was feeling so shocked and numb that it was hard for him to think. The oncologist told him that the chances that the chemotherapy would prolong his life were not very high, and, in fact, the treatment might not help him at all, but it would give the oncologists information that might help others in the future. Mr. Hynes considered this. He did want to make himself as useful as possible. At the same time, he was finding it hard to think clearly. He told the doctors the next morning that he would go ahead with the treatment, not so much because it might prolong his life, but because the oncologists might learn something. His family supported him and respected his decision.

Unfortunately, Mr. Hynes had a pneumothorax (collapsed lung) as a complication of the liver biopsy he was required to undergo as part of the research protocol, and he needed a temporary chest tube to re-expand his lung. This prolonged his hospitalization by several days. According to his wife, he continued to be cheerful and "a very good patient," and didn't complain about the pneumothorax. Margaret, Mary, and Michael were not as forgiving. They insisted that the staff physician consider very carefully whether tests and procedures were really necessary. They did not want Mr. Hynes to go through any unnecessary tests that would lead to additional suffering—a common dilemma for terminally ill patients who are received highly experimental treatment.

Consulting Palliative Care

The ward physicians told Mr. Hynes that they were going to consult the Palliative Care Service to help him with care at home. Mr. Hynes was eligible to receive this service even though he had opted to receive chemotherapy. It is common in Quebec for cancer patients to get hospice-like home care while they are still receiving palliative or experimental chemotherapy. While on the Home Care Program any patient can also opt to be admitted to a regular acute-care hospital ward and be treated aggressively for any medical or surgical complication if they can find a physician willing to admit them for that.

In cases of patients like Mr. Hynes, the request for a palliative care consultation triggers a visit to the patient and family on the ward. At this stage, the palliative care team acts as a support service. They follow the patient at home, assess his or her symptoms, and provide appropriate symptomatic treatment. They also provide emotional support to the family. As the patient gets sicker, the home care team will mention the resources of the inpatient Palliative Care Unit (PCU). It would be at this point (unless the patient had specifically inquired earlier) that they would talk more about the philosophy of palliative care as it relates to comfort care near the end of life. But the patient and family may choose just to receive the support services and not avail themselves of the PCU—if they opt for aggressive antibiotic intervention for infections, for example. It is only at the point of PCU admission that there is a more formal consent process with discussion of, for example, do-not-resuscitate orders (DNR), the use of transfusions, intravenous antibiotics, or artificial hydration.

When Mr. Hynes met the palliative care consultant, he learned that a nurse from the Palliative Home Care Service would visit him. He was not keen to have a nurse involved. "Why? What is she going to do? Why have someone come to the house?" he asked. He seemed not to want to face the fact that he would get weaker and need help, and he may also have felt that this would be a disruption of their family life. Mrs. Hynes and Mary, however, were very happy that they would be getting help. Dr. Leonard Roget, a resident physician and palliative medicine trainee, was assigned to follow Mr. Hynes.

Leonard was a gentle, soft-spoken man in his early thirties. He had a natural ease in discussing complex issues with patients and families. He came to see Mr. Hynes on the ward and arranged to see him in the oncology clinic as well as to visit him at home as required.

"Maybe Deep Down in His Heart He Was Aware"

After Mr. Hynes went home in early November, Susan, the home care nurse, began to make her visits. She had more than 15 years of experience in palliative care and was cheerful and confident. On her first visit, she noted that Mr. Hynes seemed nervous about palliative care. It scared him; he didn't know what to expect. He seemed stunned by his diagnosis and by the whole medical system. He was very concerned because his symptoms were getting worse. "I can't eat," he would say to Dr. Roget and to Susan. "Why can't you do something about it?" He was trying to force himself to eat and his wife was also pushing him to eat, as she was very anxious about the appetite loss. Although Mr. Hynes was willing to try to eat more, he resisted pressure when it came from Margaret.

It was important to Raymond and Margaret that Mary be present to write down everything that the doctor or nurse said to them. Mary found that she and her mother often had a different understanding of what was said. For example, when Mary heard Susan caution against forcing Mr. Hynes to eat more than he wanted, her mother, who was also listening, said after Susan left, "OK. He can have mashed potatoes and hamburgers."

Mr. Hynes took a ready liking to Susan. Although he was very organized in his thinking and expressed his needs clearly, he was not very talkative. He wrote down all his questions, and when Susan visited him, he would go down his list of questions and jot down the answers. Then he would say, "That's fine. You must be tired. You can go now." Mary also liked Susan for her empathy, but especially because of her practical suggestions. Mary told me, "We needed to know: were we reacting as well as possible or not? We're very practical. We want to know how to fix things. She gave us good advice. She said, 'Go with the ball wherever it leads. If he can't eat, don't force him.'"

Mr. Hynes continued to push himself, to get dressed every day, to come downstairs. He wanted life to carry on as before. Although he was too weak to play golf, he tried to see his friends and play cards or watch baseball on television. But the illness continued, and he had some decisions to make.

He wasn't sure what to do about the chemotherapy. He was begin-ning to doubt his earlier decision to go through with it. He contacted Dr. Drummond, who visited him at home. Dr. Drummond, being up to date on all the test results, said, "It's your decision, Raymond, but you have to think about quality of life. Life isn't going to be easy. Why make it more diffi-cult?" Mr. Hynes considered this opinion, but decided to go ahead with the experimental chemotherapy—not for his own sake, but for the sake of others who might benefit. Mary told me that her dad felt it was his Christian duty to do this.

By the time Mr. Hynes returned to the oncology clinic, however, he had continued to lose weight and was too weak to walk more than a block or so. The oncologist believed that he was now too sick to tolerate chemotherapy. She suggested privately to Mrs. Hynes and to Mary that it was time to call out-of-town family and get them to come. She did not think that Mr. Hynes would make it to Christmas. She did not communicate this opinion to Mr. Hynes, however, preferring to leave this to the family or to the palliative care team. The family decided not to share the oncologist's opinion with Mr. Hynes. No one wanted to say to him, "You have a few weeks at most."

Mrs. Hynes did call her daughter in Florida and asked her to come sooner than she had planned, but she did not discuss the reason with her husband. "I had to make up a story about her coming earlier so her wouldn't worry," Mrs. Hynes told me. Then she continued, "Maybe deep down in his heart he was aware." Mrs. Hynes's concerns about her husband's knowledge and emotions also influenced her feelings about participating in our project. The day I telephoned to arrange my first visit she expressed worry that I might discuss something distressing with her husband. I had to promise to tread gently.

On November 24, I visited them in their comfortable, old stone house on a quiet, tree-lined street. Mrs. Hynes, dressed neatly in a smart skirt and blouse, greeted me at the door. She was cheerful and welcoming, but she looked anx-ious. Mary was also there, energetically rearranging seats in the living room. They had just finished making Mr. Hynes comfortable in his reclining chair. I could see that it had been an effort for him to come downstairs. He was very thin and looked tired. He was a tall man but looked somehow small because of his illness. He, too, was neatly dressed in casual clothes. He jokingly told me how he had taken a lot of trouble to get dressed because I was coming to see him. Even though he was getting very tired, he pushed himself to get dressed every day and to be ready for company. He cheerfully described to me how he was trying to maintain his daily routine: get dressed, come downstairs, read the paper, chat with his wife over breakfast. He smiled. "You know, we have this chat for about 20 minutes every morning, 'How was your night?' You know, things like that. She makes me hot cereal. She takes very good care of me."

I could see how easy it was for Mr. Hynes to maintain his sense of control and be cheerful. It seemed much more difficult for him and his family to communicate about serious concerns. "We joke around a lot," Mary said. "We can't help it. We're Irish." Yet they did have anxieties, especially about Mr. Hynes's diminishing appetite. Their communication with each other became strained over this issue. Susan told me that during one of her visits, Mr. Hynes "blew up at his wife" when, in her frustration and helplessness, Mrs. Hynes coaxed him to eat more. Mr. Hynes acknowledged to me that the stresses and strains were a problem at times. "Sometimes I have a short fuse myself," he said. "That's not like me at all. I want to spare my family. I don't want them to be more stressed than they already are. But I don't know what's happening. I feel lost. I haven't gone through anything like this before."

"How Long Have I Got?"

Mr. Hynes was dying. Everyone in the family knew this, but they did not know how to talk about it. No one wanted to lose control over their feelings, and yet their feelings were sometimes very strong. For example, I had asked Mr. Hynes which persons I could interview for our project, to obtain his consent. He said that his daughter Jane was coming from Florida, but she was very anxious and emotional, so he preferred that I not talk to her. Mr. Hynes was worried that if she talked to me she might get upset and thus upset everyone else. "Mary is okay," he said. "She has feelings, but she can control them." Mrs. Hynes interjected, "We *all* have feelings."

Mr. Hynes simply did not want to express his feelings about his illness within the family. He wanted to live from day to day. Susan continued to advise Mrs. Hynes and Mary: "You have to take the cues from him. He's the boss. However he wants to deal with it, you go with the flow." But Mrs. Hynes would have preferred to talk more.

Instead of talking about Mr. Hynes's illness, they discussed sports. Mr. Hynes continued to watch his baseball games with a passion. They talked about food, and even though Mr. Hynes was no longer eating much they

tried to enjoy their meal times together. In other words, they carried on—
that's how they had always coped with problems.

Mr. Hynes's appetite seemed to be his personal gauge of his condition. As it
continued to dwindle, he became more anxious. He asked everyone he could,
"How long have I got?" No matter whom he asked, the answer was always
the same: "I have no idea. These things can vary." Susan said to him. "You
just have to listen to your body." Dr. Roget told him the same thing; his body
would tell him how he was doing. Mr. Hynes found this advice confusing.
How could he listen to his body? He didn't know how to listen to his body.
This was all very strange and new. He didn't know what was going on, and nobody was giving him a clear answer. He wanted a date! Surely the doctor must
know that much. Was everyone avoiding telling him the truth? He wondered
if the oncologist might have told Mary something more precise. But Mary
said, "They can't tell you, Dad. Everyone has a different body."

Mr. Hynes knew that I was a physician who was familiar with the details
of his illness, and he wanted to discuss prognosis with me also, even though
I was visiting him for our research project and not to provide him with care.
This led to some awkward moments for me. "How will I know how I'm
doing?" he asked me during one conversation. "Susan said you were going
to ask me about pain, but I don't have pain. I don't know what pain is. I feel
something here," he said, pointing to his upper abdomen, "and then I burp,
but I don't have pain. I know I'll get pain—that's what this friend told me."

"It's not inevitable that you will have pain," I answered. "Many people with
this tumor have no pain at all."

"How will I know then?" he asked.

"What do you mean?"

"How do I know when I'm going to die?"

When I paused before answering, he looked angry and impatient.

"You don't know," he said. "Nobody knows."

"Well," I said, "You're weak. But you're eating okay and as long as you're
able to eat you'll be okay."

"How much do I need to eat?"

We talked about calories and eating and the futility of pushing oneself to
eat. Mr. Hynes lit a cigarette. "Sometimes I get full and my wife nags me about
eating," he said. Then he smiled. "But sometimes I can't eat another bite."

I did not want to avoid his direct questions regarding prognosis, but I was
not Mr. Hynes's physician. I found it difficult to be both a researcher and a
physician at this point. I could have gone into a discussion of "weeks rather

than months" in response to his question. But discussions of prognosis are always tricky. We do have patients like him who live on for months, and it does hinge on how good their appetite is. At the same time, force-feeding will not prolong life, as I tried to explain to him. Mr. Hynes had originally been told that his prognosis was two months to two years. One month had now gone by. The practical organizer within him knew that he needed to sort out his affairs and prepare to die, but his feelings had not yet caught up with that.

"We Should Be Saying Things and We're Not"

Mr. Hynes could not bring himself to make the phone calls to get his affairs in order. Mrs. Hynes had not taken over before, but now she felt that she had to do something to prompt him to look after his affairs. But it was hard for them to talk about dying. They would sit in front of the TV and Mrs. Hynes would say, "We should be saying things and we're not."

Mr. Hynes was more open with his family while I was there, as if I acted as a catalyst. Otherwise his wife and daughter did not ask him any questions—they seemed to be waiting for him to initiate the discussion. But he was not a talkative person. Mary told me later,

In the hospital he said to Mom, "You'll go off and marry a rich guy." That's as close as he came to saying anything. We're a pretty upbeat family. It's not that we're in denial, but Dad may have been. The rest of us deal with things. There was a lot of talk, a lot of tears, but not in front of Dad.

And Mrs. Hynes said to me,

He didn't say. "Take care of yourself," to me or anything. He was a man of few words. He would say, "Actions speak louder than words." But we didn't have to talk to each other, because it was *lived*.

But on another occasion she expressed regret that there had been no goodbyes.

Even though Mrs. Hynes often appeared overwhelmed, she did not allow herself to cry in front of her daughter or her husband, and Mary diverted her mother from showing feelings. The family had decided that Susan's role should be to help them with practical rather than psychological or emotional matters. No one in the family was signaling that they wanted to have a private discussion with a member of the team. When Susan spoke with them about how they were coping emotionally, Mary in particular would change the subject.

The Family Gathers

Although Mr. Hynes's strength was also diminishing, he could still walk a few blocks. He was getting thinner, except for his abdomen, which was starting to fill up with fluid. His eyes and complexion were jaundiced. Nevertheless, the Hyneses weren't going around being morbid or sad. Mrs. Hynes was still focusing on getting her husband to eat and drink. What else could she do? Mr. Hynes showed no sign of giving up. He pushed himself to do as much as possible.

Jane had arrived from Florida. She had many questions: What could her father eat? What could be done about the jaundice? How long would this go on? She cried a lot, and the rest of the family seemed uncomfortable with her tears. They were only interested in specific answers to their practical questions. Michael was shy and did not say much. Everyone seemed very scared. Susan wondered: Will they panic as Mr. Hynes gets sicker?

On December 1, Mrs. Hynes phoned Susan to ask her to come to the house: Mr. Hynes was quite jaundiced. When Susan arrived the next afternoon, Mr. Hynes was still in his pajamas—the first time that he had not gotten dressed for her. He was obviously weaker and much quieter than before. He did complain of more discomfort in his abdomen. He seemed very reluctant to consider taking a painkiller, especially when Susan told him that the medication might produce constipation and he would need to take a laxative to go with it. He could not understand why he should take one medication to do one thing and then take another to counteract the effects of the first. When, as usual, he asked Susan how she thought he was doing, she told him that she didn't like seeing him in his pajamas, that it was not a good sign to her. "He seemed to appreciate that," Susan told me later, "because previously I'd always thrown the question back to him. But this time it seemed quite obvious that he had deteriorated."

Mr. Hynes was scheduled for an appointment with his oncologist, who sought to see her patients even when the palliative care team was following them. If the patients were at home, she saw them in the clinic for as long as they were able to come to the hospital. The family wondered if Mr. Hynes would be able to keep the appointment. Although he was too weak to walk, he still wanted to go, and, on December 4, Mary pushed him into the clinic in a wheelchair. He saw the oncologist, who gave him another appointment in two weeks. This oncologist always gave her patients return appointments, though she told me later, "I don't think he'll be able to make it."

After the consultation, I observed that Mrs. Hynes looked anxious as she helped maneuver her husband's wheelchair out of the clinic. She looked like she was trying to avoid her own emotions, putting on a formal front. She spoke in a detached way and was very task-oriented: "Now we have the medications straight. You have to take those pills." The visit had taken almost all of Mr. Hynes's energy and he looked terrible. He looked to me like he was dying. But he had on his baseball cap and he was going home to watch the game on TV.

Mary had taken a leave of absence from work and was now spending most of every day with her parents. Michael continued to work as usual. Jane stayed for one week, but then went back to Florida because her return airline ticket could not be extended. Her mother and sister had advised her to go back home even though she wanted to stay, since no one seemed to know how long this would take.

Preparing to Die at Home

Mr. Hynes was now too weak to go to church, but he had his prayer book on his bedside table. He and Mrs. Hynes discussed calling the priest. They agreed that the priest should come to give Mr. Hynes the Sacrament of the Sick. The priest was one of several who were personal friends of the family. Although Mr. Hynes spent most of his time sleeping, he was awake and alert when the priest came, and he seemed peaceful and accepting after this ritual.

On December 7, Dr. Roget made another home visit. The family asked him to tell Mr. Hynes not to come downstairs anymore, for he was now too weak. The Hyneses had come to trust Leonard, and they were always happy and relieved when he visited them at home. On this day he had to have an important conversation with them: they had to decide now whether they wanted to have Mr. Hynes die at home. Since he did not have any difficult symptoms, both Susan and Leonard felt that it should be possible to keep him at home, which is what Mr. Hynes had already told his wife that he preferred.

Mrs. Hynes tried to be brave, but she was very anxious and found it difficult to make decisions. She wanted so much to respect Mr. Hynes's desire, but doubted whether she could cope. She was afraid of her husband's dying at home. She could not discuss her fears in front of Mary, though. Mary would say, "Mom, listen. Daddy wanted to die at home, and we're going to do all we can. Come on, we've got some things to organize here."

Leonard tried to reassure Mrs. Hynes. "We don't make any hard and fast decisions here. We don't know what's going to happen. We go hour by hour. At one point things could change, and you may say to yourself, this is not working. And then you can call and we can change tack, and sometimes we change tack several times. We might fix the problem in hospital, and he could come home again. So it's a fluid situation, and you should never feel that you're making a hard and fixed decision."

To help Mrs. Hynes cope at night, when she and Mr. Hynes were in the house alone, they hired a night sitter. That first evening, before the sitter arrived, Mrs. Hynes heard a thump while she was in the kitchen. She went upstairs to find that her husband had fallen out of bed. She called her son to come pick him up off the floor, and Michael stayed until 3:00 A.M. The family then decided that they needed 24-hour private nursing to avoid this situation. Mrs. Hynes and Mary organized the nurses for the next day. Since Mr. Hynes had private medical insurance, this was an option for them.

By December 7, the private nurses and sitters were there 24 hours a day. Because they were older nurses and very efficient, Mr. Hynes accepted their presence easily. They looked after Mr. Hynes in shifts, cleaning him, giving him medication, and the like, while Mrs. Hynes returned with relief to activities that gave her comfort, such as baking her husband's favorite muffins. Susan told her that her husband could not eat the muffins; they were too dry, and he might choke on them. She baked them anyway.

When Dr. Roget next visited Mr. Hynes, he saw him in his bedroom. It did not look like a sick room. There were family photographs on the walls, and a large crucifix. There was a large photograph of Mr. and Mrs. Hynes when they were about 50 years old, photographs of the children and grandchildren taken on his 70th birthday, a photograph of him receiving a prize at work, and one of him with the bishop and some of his ordained friends. Mr. Hynes looked frail and small in the large double bed. He was now so weak that he could hardly speak, but he continued to smile. In response to Leonard's questions about his general well-being, he raised two fingers and made the signal for peace. He signaled that his morale was "ten on ten." When Leonard asked him how he thought his wife was doing, he gave the same signal and also managed to indicate that she was a strong woman. Leonard thought at the time that by stating this in front of his wife, Mr. Hynes might have been trying to tell her that she was doing a good job, that he was proud of her. Everyone continued to avoid talking about feelings, though they were a bit more open with each other away from the bedroom.

When Susan visited the next afternoon, the house was full of activity. There were two nurses there, changing shifts. Michael was walking from room to room, conducting business on his cellular phone, while Mary and Margaret dealt with the nurses and the immediate practical affairs. Susan met Mrs. Hynes in the kitchen, and they hugged each other. Mrs. Hynes said, "He is going fast, but he has a strong faith that has helped him through the worst of times, and it is helping him now. I feel comforted by the fact that he seems peaceful and accepting." Mary came into the kitchen and cried in front of Susan for the first time. But she was unable to stay in the room while Susan talked with her mother about what was likely to happen.

Susan explained to Mrs. Hynes how to get in touch with the medical service and what to do if Mr. Hynes should die in the night. Mrs. Hynes called Mary back into the kitchen to hear this information. While Mrs. Hynes listened attentively to Susan's instructions, Mary wrote them all down, trying to control her tears. It was striking to Susan how they really wanted to get things straight. They wanted to know exactly what to do. Reflecting on the scene later, Susan wrote in her journal,

> I felt at that moment how really sad this is, because they were so grateful for that little bit of information. Numbers. That's all I was giving them. Just names and numbers that they will need to know when the time comes. And yet, that was so important to them. It was something that they could hang on to. Something grounding. What they really want is so much more. And I felt humbled by that.

"If It Had to Happen, That Was the Way to Go"

Mr. Hynes was in bed almost all the time now. He still recognized his family and responded to them through signals and facial expressions. He smiled often. Mrs. Hynes kept asking him practical questions: what he wanted to eat or drink, whether he wanted to be in the chair, who had telephoned. It seemed that the only way she had to express her feelings for him was to sit by the bed and hold his hand.

The next evening, December 8, Mary and Michael both decided to stay. They were in the bedroom with their parents. Mr. Hynes said he wanted to get out of bed and sit in his easy chair. He was agitated, and after about five minutes he got back into bed and Mrs. Hynes took hold of his hand. After a few more minutes something seemed to happen with his breathing. Mrs. Hynes asked Michael, "What's happening to your dad?" Mr. Hynes took a last breath and died.

"It was an experience," Mrs. Hynes recalled to me afterward:

He was conscious of everything up to a few minutes before he died. He was happy in his room and in his bed. He knew that we were there and were helping him. I was happy for him because he had his daughter and sons with him. He died peacefully. He didn't appear to be suffering. I'm at peace with the fact that he stayed at home. And I think, for him, absolutely, it was wonderful. He didn't have much pain. He died in his room, with all his pictures.

Mary said to me,

If it had to happen, that was the way to go. He didn't appear to be suffering that much. He even had a smile on his face. There was nothing that could have been done differently. He didn't even bother us by dying in the middle of the night when he would have awakened us. He did it at such an appropriate time. And it was really, really beautiful. My brother felt that it was a really tremendous experience. He wouldn't have changed it for the world.

The First Year: "It's a Case of Trying to Survive"

As was common for the palliative care nurses, Susan attended the funeral that was held three days later. The old church was packed with friends and family, and the service was long because of the many tributes to Mr. Hynes. Mrs. Hynes and Michael came up to Susan and said to her gratefully, "You've been such a good friend." In her journal, Susan reflected,

It seemed that it was more important to say that than to say "You've been a good nurse," or, "You've done a good job." I think the family were grateful that we were there to discuss practical things like what to do if he died at home, who to call. It was an honor for me to be a part of this team.

I visited Mrs. Hynes and Mary two months after the death. Mrs. Hynes saw her husband's relatively quick deterioration as a blessing. On one of their outings together, Mary and her mother had seen an old man struggling along with a walker. Mary said to her mother, "Dad didn't have to go through that." "Yes," Mrs. Hynes had replied, "I'm grateful for that."

Mary showed me a photograph of her dancing with her father. He was tall, in a graceful pose, smiling. This was the way that she wanted to remember him. We then spoke about how the family communicated among themselves while her father was dying. "We let him do it his way," Mary said. "That's who he was. I don't think it should have been different. But it's not as if we had to make up for lost time. He knew. We knew. Daddy didn't say, 'I'm dying—this is what I have to say to you.' He wasn't that type of guy and Mom took her cues from him. I think it would have upset him. He dealt with it himself, in his own way."

Mrs. Hynes, who was crying quietly during much of my visit, still seemed to be concerned with doing things correctly. Only now it was not a question of caring properly for her husband, but of mourning him. She said,

I think about him a lot. I feel it. It's the loneliness, coming back to the house at night. It gives me comfort to continue to sleep in our double bed. I need to keep myself occupied. At the same time, I feel it hasn't hit me so much. Maybe it's because it happened so quickly, I don't know whether I've been grieving or not. Years ago, they would go into mourning for six months. My aunts fell apart when their husbands died. It was the thing to do. I'm inclined to want to keep busy. I want to get out of the house during the day. I go to an exercise program twice a week. If I'm in the house all day long, I can't concentrate, I can't read. I get bored or lonely if I have nothing to do, and when I'm busy I feel guilty because I think somehow I should be grieving. Is this how it should be? Is this the way I should be? Active? I just know that I don't feel good if I don't have something to focus on.

Friends phoned, but no one actually came to the house to see her except her daughter. If she wanted to be with people she had to go out. It was especially hard for her to go back to church. "Raymond and I always used to sit in the front of the church," she said. "Now I prefer to stay at the back of the church because my emotions take over. I don't want people to see me crying. I don't want to talk to the people at church because I feel so emotional. Once I had to leave the church because I could not hold back my tears."

The team originally had some concerns about Michael. He had kept so busy with his work throughout Mr. Hynes's illness, the team wondered how he was going to cope after his father's death. According to his mother, however, "He is emotional. He has a good cry when he needs to." Michael spoke openly of his father's illness and death after the event. He talked about how he missed his dad, especially when he undertook activities, such as golf, that they had previously enjoyed together. Mary said of her brother: "I think that it's made him a gentler guy. I think that it's great that he was there when he died. He couldn't get over how well Daddy died and how he got through his illness." Holiday times were difficult for everyone, especially Christmas and Easter. One of Mrs. Hynes's friends told her, "It's a case of trying to survive."

By summer, Mrs. Hynes was expressing surprise at how strong her feelings were. "There seems to be a bit more reaction with me now than previously," she told me. "I have days when I'm not as up as I used to be. There's just not enough happening now, with it being summer. There's something that's been taken out of my life that I will never recover from. It comes in waves. The least little thing will set it off." About six months after her husband died, Mrs. Hynes began to feel more despondent. She considered getting some help from the bereavement service provided through the hospital Palliative Care Program. For many weeks Mrs. Hynes had kept their number by her telephone. Now Mary suggested that she call, but then things seemed to get better and Mrs. Hynes decided not to.

That summer Mrs. Hynes went back to their country home for the first time since her husband's death. It was a place they had been renting for 35 years, so it brought back a lot of memories. She said, "I find it rough when the memories come. It was hard to see the houses again, the views, the people there, now that I am alone." In spite of her painful feelings, she pushed herself. She saw everyone whom she wanted to see, and people greeted her warmly. She thought it would be so difficult to face everyone now, to speak about her husband, but she managed, one step at a time.

Even one year after the death, Mrs. Hynes had doubts about whether she was doing things right. "Sometimes I think I should sit back and think a little more," she said. "I think of Raymond a lot, believe me, but sometimes

I question whether I shouldn't slow down and give myself time to think about what happened. But I'm a creature of habit. I keep busy." Then, as if to summarize everything she and her family had been through, she said, "We had this illness. There was no way of curing it, and God mercifully took him quickly. So it was a blessing that it happened so quickly. I think that all his good works and kindness paid off in the end. That's the only peaceful thought that I can hold on to."

Authors' Comments

This narrative demonstrates the work of a palliative home care program that is integrated within a hospital-based service. Physicians as well as nurses are involved, and there is seamless transfer to an inpatient unit if there are issues that cannot be dealt with in the home environment. It is our opinion that home care services work best when there is access to an inpatient unit and when a specialized palliative care physician can visit when required and be involved in the home care team. The narrative also features an example of a service where the oncologist continues to be involved even when the patient has been transferred to the palliative care service. In addition, it is useful in an oncology program to have smooth transitions from active treatment to supportive care and, eventually, to terminal care.

One of the themes in this narrative has to do with the issue of cultural influences on emotional reactions to illness and expressions of grief. Some families are comfortable with open communication and expressions of emotion, while others are not. This family was not. Everyone seemed to be trying to protect everyone else. Mrs. Hynes would say, "We should be saying things and we're not." When chemotherapy stopped working, the oncologist communicated the prognosis with the family but not with Mr. Hynes himself. The family then decided not to share this information with Mr. Hynes. This issue of when, how, and with whom prognosis should be discussed is an ethics question that merits careful consideration and is often affected by cultural factors, as we also note the narratives of Sadie Fineman and Costas Metrakis.

There are standard guidelines for how to communicate bad news to patients and families facing life-threatening illness.[1] These guidelines stress that the patient should be asked how they wish important communication communicated and whether they wish a family member present during discussions. Such guidelines were not always followed in this narrative case.

Another topic has to do with the widespread use of experimental clinical trial drugs in the management of advanced cancer and raises a question of research ethics. Mr. Hynes was alone in his hospital room when the medical resident informed him that he had advanced-stage cancer for which there was no cure. Shortly afterward, while Mr. Hynes was still alone and had not yet spoken with his family, the oncologist approached him regarding the possibility of experimental chemotherapy, which might or might not prolong his life. Decisions need to be made quickly, but whose needs were being served here? Was Mr. Hynes in a good state of mind to make an informed decision about undergoing a treatment that was unlikely to benefit him? Could he have felt comfortable to refuse? It could be argued that the suggestion to Mr. Hynes that he participate in a clinical trial, at what was perhaps the most vulnerable moment of his life, had the decided advantage for the investigators that Mr. Hynes would probably say yes.

At one point in the narrative, the nurse Susan says to the family: "You have to take the cues from him. He's the boss. However he wants to deal with it, you go with the flow." Does this kind of attitude, common in palliative care programs, risk leading to a sort of "tyranny of the patient"? Is it patronizing, in the sense that is refuses to ascribe any moral responsibility to the patient for dealing seriously with the needs of those around him or her? Are we putting the person in a kind of moral limbo, excusing them from ordinary social obligations as soon as they are labeled "dying"? We also see this issue playing out when patients insist on remaining home (or on going back home if an inpatient) and the family is ill-equipped to deal with home care or home death, even with palliative care support. A successful death at home requires significant practical and psychological resources on the part of the family. In many jurisdictions, a home death would require financial resources as well to pay for intensive professional home nursing in the last days of life. This family appeared to have adequate resources. Unfortunately, many families do not.

After her husband's death, Mrs. Hynes would have been benefited from a few sessions of bereavement counseling at about six months. The fact that she did not telephone the bereavement service reminds us how difficult it must be for bereaved individuals to ask for the help that they require. In this setting, bereavement counselors only initiated telephone calls for those considered at risk for bereavement complications. All other key persons would receive a letter informing them about the service and an invitation to attend a memorial event at three months and at one year. More research is needed to explore the potential benefits (or harms) of a more proactive approach, either by the palliative care team or by primary care providers.

Reference

1. Baile W, Buckman R, Lenzi R, Glober G, Beale E A, Kudelka A P. SPIKES: A six-step protocol for delivering bad news: Application to the patient with cancer. Oncologist. 2000;5(4):302–311.

4

Albert Hoffer

Bonds Through Thick and Thin

Narrated by Yanna Lambrinidou

Albert Hoffer was 78 years old when he was diagnosed with cancer of the throat. A deeply private man, he found it painful to endure the invasions of his body and the strong feelings he experienced in the last months of his life. He was an opinionated, forthright, and mistrustful person who tested everyone intensely before allowing them to get close. Years of alcohol abuse had cost Mr. Hoffer his career and damaged his relationship with his wife and children. The complex, interwoven medical and family issues in the context of the Hoffer family's limited financial means posed a significant challenge for the hospice team.

"I Never Knew a Man Who Was as Sharp as He Was"

On the eve of my first meeting with Mr. Hoffer, I got a warning from Margaret Gibson, his hospice social worker: if his wife, Julia, disapproved of me, Mr. Hoffer would refuse to participate in our study. Mr. Hoffer's first personal care nurse had been replaced by a second one because she had made Mrs. Hoffer uncomfortable. I found myself wondering what I could do to make a good impression on a woman I had never met. Our first meeting took place on June 26, 1997. When I walked into the Hoffers' home, I found Mrs. Hoffer standing in the kitchen, staring at the floor and stamping her foot. She was struggling to kill a group of ants. Mr. Hoffer finished the job for her and asked her to join us in the living room. He and I sat on the sofa. Mrs. Hoffer sat in an armchair, put her head down, and started flipping through a magazine.

Looking straight ahead, Mr. Hoffer told me that he didn't know why he was still alive. His life had no meaning. He was no longer able to work, he was no longer active, he had no one to talk to about his cancer. His hospice team had given him the phone number of a support line that would connect him with other cancer patients, but he had no energy to place the call. Hospice staff were tactless at times. His nurse cared only about medical symptoms and ignored the complexity of his existence. His chaplain seemed interesting, but Mr. Hoffer was not sure if he was the right person for him. Out of all the people he had met, however, he found him the most likely to rescue him from his depression. And that's what he wanted. "Pain medications are easier to take than Prozac," he said, "because they alleviate your pain right away. Prozac takes time."

Mr. Hoffer, a 78-year-old White American, was a tall, slender man. One could tell from his physique that in his prime he was muscular and strong. His head was covered with thin light hair, and his smile revealed two widely spaced bottom teeth that he half-jokingly called his "fangs." He had a strong presence. He was opinionated, fiercely independent, and hard to read. I thought there was a mystique about him that gave him an air of untouchability. He spoke in riddles. He liked to express himself indirectly with rhetorical questions, sarcasm, and symbolism. The confusion he brought to his listeners was something he seemed to enjoy. It was his way of teasing, but it was also his way of testing who really understood him and who did not.

Mrs. Hoffer was several years younger than her husband and self-effacing. She was stout with short, white hair whose introversion contrasted starkly with her husband's excitability. Mr. and Mrs. Hoffer had been married for 48 years. They had three adult sons, Frank, John, and Peter, all of whom lived in Lancaster County. Mr. Hoffer also had a daughter, Eileen, from his first marriage. He rarely spoke about Eileen. He reported that she had moved to Georgia and was minimally involved in his life.

A retired millwright, Mr. Hoffer had maintained the machinery at a Lancaster County manufacturing company for 33 years. His job had given him pride. Early on, he became the director of his company's service department and the president of his union. His career came to an abrupt end at the age of 51, when it became obvious that he was an alcoholic. He spent the next decade and a half struggling to keep new jobs and overcome his drinking problem.

It took Mr. Hoffer 14 years, many Alcoholics Anonymous meetings, and several detoxification programs to get sober. Before doing so, he hit rock bottom. Finances were tight. The Hoffers moved into a two-bedroom trailer that stood in a small trailer park on the edge of a lush hillside. According to John, his second son, he drank all day, then "inhaled bottles of aspirin" to treat his hangovers, and drank again. John remembered him "ruining" things—holidays, relationships, employment opportunities, and his retirement prospects. He recounted a day when his father "clobbered" him with a cane. "There were times when I hated my dad," he confessed. It was Mrs. Hoffer who took charge of Frank's, John's, and Peter's upbringing, doing the best she could to protect them from their father. The boys experienced her as an endless source of love. Although she kept her feelings to herself, they knew that she disapproved of her husband's drinking and despaired at his inability to keep a job.

In 1983, a close brush with surgery for a bleeding stomach ulcer shook Mr. Hoffer into the realization that his body had suffered from alcohol and that his family had suffered from him. He didn't want to lose either his life or the people he loved. So he stopped drinking. He regained the clarity of mind and the ambition that had pushed him to the top of his manufacturing company years earlier. He started volunteering at a local hospital and enrolled in a university course to become a master gardener. He also felt the need to make up for the time he had lost with his family. Showing utmost respect for his wife, he did everything he could to meet her needs. By the mid-1980s, Frank, John, and Peter had moved out of the trailer and started families of their own. Mr. Hoffer kept himself abreast of their lives, supported them through hard times, and participated with them in activities they enjoyed. A favorite family pastime was fishing. Trips to the water had unified all five of the Hoffers from the time the children were little, giving them unforgettable moments of happiness.

"My father has always lived life to the fullest," the youngest son, Peter, said to me with love evident in his voice, "even to a fault—to the point he loved to eat, he loved to drink, he loved to party, he just loved all those things about life. He is very much a people-person, my father—he always enjoys talking with people as long as he is the one doing all the talking!"

"I never knew a man who was as sharp as he was," said the second son, John. "The alcohol robbed him of a lot of things—it really did. What a meta-morphosis as a dad. I really did get close to him [after he stopped drinking]. He was a lot nicer to be around." But despite his love for people, Mr. Hoffer held his cards close to his chest. He rarely showed vulnerability.

"I Went into the Damnedest Traumatic Shock I Ever Had in My Life"

In June 1996, Mr. Hoffer got a sore throat. After a month of excruciating pain, he lost his ability to swallow and speak. An ear-nose-and-throat specialist diagnosed him with cancer of the nasopharynx. "I went into the damnedest traumatic shock I ever had in my life," he recalled. "Cancer of the throat is the last thing you are afraid of when you are a drinker." He consented to a six-week course of outpatient radiation intended to shrink his tumor and bring his cancer into remission. But, contrary to his expectations, he never regained his ability to eat by mouth again. The radiation stopped his tumor's growth, but it also closed his esophagus. He could not even swallow his own saliva. He had to spit. For nourishment, a feeding tube was inserted directly into his stomach. Through it, he fed himself liquid nutritional formulas. Mr. Hoffer's throat became chronically dry. Prolonged talking and sleeping exac-erbated the problem and caused him pain.

Six months after the radiation, Mrs. Hoffer had a stroke. Suddenly, the pillar of the family was unable to take care of her most basic needs. Her cognitive abilities declined dramatically as well. As much as she tried, she was unable to keep track of day-to-day activities, including her medication schedule, personal hygiene, and nutrition. She began to eat ice-cream—her favorite food—for every meal, which aggravated her diabetes. She became incontinent. It was not unusual for her to soil the furniture or her clothes without even noticing. Mrs. Hoffer spent hours each day sitting quietly in her armchair or sleeping. Her verbal interactions were minimal. But she didn't like to be patronized. The home health aides and nurses from the hos-pital who visited her several times a week sometimes addressed her husband instead of her or walked into her bedroom without her permission. Some questioned the truth of her statements and turned to Mr. Hoffer for confir-mation. Others bathed her with a casualness that humiliated her. Mr. Hoffer became her protector. He took charge of her medications, cooked for her, and cleaned the house as best as he could. Whoever mistreated Mrs. Hoffer was dismissed.

"I Don't Feel Part of Hospice Yet"

In April 1997, a computed tomography scan showed recurring cancer in Mr. Hoffer's supraglottic deep neck structures. Mr. Hoffer was advised to consider hospice. He was told that the benefits of further aggressive treatment would not necessarily outweigh the risks. Surgery would require a permanent tracheostomy and a laryngectomy with a voice box. Moreover, it carried a risk of infection. Chemotherapy often brought side effects that had the potential to compromise the quality of his life. It was up to him to decide what path to pursue.

He chose everything. He agreed to sign up for hospice, but didn't elect the Medicare hospice benefit. This would pay for his medications, but it would also require him to forego aggressive treatments. He wasn't ready for that. Instead, he decided to pay for his palliative care drugs out-of-pocket so that he would be able to explore the possibility of additional interventions.

He reported to his hospice team that he was suffering from pain, weakness, insomnia, and depression. He was losing weight. Just two days earlier he had fallen, knocking out most of his bottom teeth. He stressed his wife's dependence on him. He wanted his caregivers to understand that he was determined to stay put as long as he could. Nursing homes were anathema to him because both his mother and brother had died in one. What he needed was a volunteer to help him keep the trailer clean.

Mr. Hoffer's hospice nurse, Carmen Maloney, collaborated with his attending physician, Julie McCloud, to design a medication regimen that included long-acting morphine suppositories, concentrated liquid morphine for breakthrough pain, the antidepressant fluoxetine, promethazine for nausea, ranitidine to mitigate stomach acid, digoxin for his heart, and atenolol for his blood pressure. She also assigned Mr. Hoffer a volunteer. Margaret, the social worker, took on the responsibility of gathering information about meal services for Mrs. Hoffer and cremation. She also offered Mr. Hoffer chaplain visits, but he declined. "I don't feel part of hospice yet," he said. He expected that he would be open to a spiritual counselor at a later time.

After her first visit to the trailer, Margaret said,

He was testing me—asking me kind of personal questions every once in a while and kind of making little jokes. I think it was to see how I would react to him. I joked back with him a little bit. He was looking for very concrete things—typical man—looking for concrete tasks that I would be doing for him. He had a lot of questions about different things, such as deliverable meals. He was thinking ahead. He just wanted me to gather some information, so he gave me a lot of homework, and I think it was a test. I came back two weeks later, I had all this information, I explained it to him, and he said, "You are someone who gets things done—I like that." He and I have just hit it off ever since.

On the day of his second computed tomography scan, Mr. Hoffer shared with Carmen, his hospice nurse, that his fears about the future tortured him. The hospital's home health agency that was taking care of Mrs. Hoffer had just informed him that they were considering terminating their services because, in their view, Mrs. Hoffer had been satisfactorily stabilized. Who would manage his wife's care if this agency pulled out? Could he afford the aggressive treatments he might want to pursue? He didn't think so.

The scan was negative. Mr. Hoffer's cancer had not metastasized beyond the area of his throat. But before starting him on aggressive treatments, his ear-nose-and-throat doctor requested more tests. He wanted Mr. Hoffer to have a physical examination and a throat biopsy. On May 19, two days prior to his physical examination, Mr. Hoffer asked for chaplain visits. His worries had intensified. He feared that the results of his tests would disqualify him from further treatments. He was experiencing increased drowsiness, weakness, and tenderness in his neck. Plus, the home health agency caring for Mrs. Hoffer had made the decision to terminate their services. In collaboration with Dr. McCloud, Carmen increased the dose of Mr. Hoffer's long-acting morphine suppositories and his breakthrough medication. She also started him on lorazepam for anxiety.

On May 26, Mr. Hoffer requested that his personal care nurse be replaced. I heard three different explanations for Jane's dismissal. One was that she had made the mistake of talking to Mr. Hoffer about Mrs. Hoffer in Mrs. Hoffer's presence. Another was that she had entered Mrs. Hoffer's bedroom without asking her. And the third was that, in a conversation with the Hoffers, she had made the comment that "cancer is a horrible disease." The nurse was replaced with Betty Beasly. Betty saw Mr. Hoffer twice a week and was soon struck by his mercurial moods. "One minute he is very trusting of you," she told me, "the next minute he does not know if he should let you in the door.

He is very opinionated about everything. He is very different. You can never get a straight answer out of him. He can joke with you and the next minute be very mad with you. I cannot read him. He did tell me he is an alcoholic. I don't know what to believe: is it true or not?"

"To Help People to Live Until They Die"

Mr. Hoffer longed for deep and meaningful interactions with someone he could trust. On his first meeting with the chaplain, Carl Flynn, he talked briefly about his love of fishing trips but switched quickly to pressing matters. He asked questions about Carl's agenda as a spiritual counselor. He also talked about his mistrust of organized religion. Carl explained that his work was nondenominational and tailored to the needs and preferences of each patient. Mr. Hoffer was anxious about the decisions that faced him. All he had to do to prevent his bills from pilling up was to stop seeking aggressive treatments. But he was still not ready to give up the possibility of surgery. He asserted that he wanted to do everything he could to stay alive. His wife needed him.

Carl reflected later that he sensed how much Mr. Hoffer was probing him, asking, in effect, "Will this work? Is this a fit?" and, "Can this person support me and walk with me?"

"I might have to see if I can be somebody who can support him," Carl went on. "I said to him, 'So when are you going to go fishing again?'—I kind of threw it out there. I said, 'What hospice is about is to help people to live until they die, and I encourage you to do that.'"

Mr. Hoffer was intrigued by Carl, but he wasn't sure he liked him. He found his question about fishing almost offensive. He couldn't understand how a hospice chaplain could have proposed such a trip when Mr. Hoffer had just explained that he was drowning in outstanding medical bills. But there was something about Carl's idea that he liked. It was almost too crazy to dismiss. In the meantime, he was anxious to hear from his ear-nose-and-throat doctor if and when he was going to schedule him for his throat biopsy.

"Something Is Being Built and I Have Been Called to Have a Hand in That"

Even though the hospital reversed its decision to terminate its home health services to Mrs. Hoffer, Frank, John, and Peter began searching for extended-care facilities that would accommodate both their parents. They knew that the day would come when Mr. and Mrs. Hoffer would be unable to live by themselves, and none of them had the room or resources to take their parents in. Although Mr. Hoffer understood the necessity of such a search, he was devastated by the prospect of moving out of the trailer. Moreover, he had already spent most of his savings on his palliative care medications. In a tender moment with Margaret, the social worker, he confessed that he was used to having "a handle" on every problem that confronted him. This time, though, he felt that his life was beyond his control. He didn't know what to do. He started to cry. Quickly, he turned his face away and asked Margaret to leave. On her way out, Margaret encouraged him to call her if he needed. Warmly, he took hold of her hand and thanked her.

"Even though Albert asked me to leave," said Margaret later, "there was something that happened there, that he trusted me an awful lot, and it was a really neat thing that happened between us. I felt bad for making him cry, but part of me thought he needed to do that, because I think he has really been holding it in. He is a very strong person, and I don't think he cries very easily."

On July 7, Mr. Hoffer asked Carl if he would be willing to help Mrs. Hoffer open up about her feelings. He wanted to know what she was thinking about his illness. Carl answered with a question: Was it possible that his desire to hear his wife's thoughts reflected his own need more than Mrs. Hoffer's? "I laid it out open-endedly," Carl said when he described the incident later, "but I think he saw it." When Mrs. Hoffer entered the living room and sat on the sofa next to her husband, Carl asked her warmly, "What do you think about this guy having cancer? I can only imagine that it would be tough, but I don't know how it is for you."

"I don't like it," responded Mrs. Hoffer flatly. She had nothing more to say.

Carl returned to the topic of fishing. He told Mr. Hoffer that he knew someone who owned a boat and was likely to make it available to him for a weekend. Mr. Hoffer lit up at the idea. He excused himself and a few minutes later returned to the living room with a smile, holding a T-shirt. On it was an old photograph of him and Peter proudly holding a striped bass.

"I am trying to help this man live until he dies," said Carl afterward, "and if going fishing is something I can do to support him, that is what I need to do. Something is being built, and I have been called to have a hand in that."

"If I Don't Get Better Soon, I'll Ask for a Transfer of Heads"

On July 8, Mr. Hoffer had his throat biopsy. July 9 was his birthday. Eileen called from Georgia to tell her father that she loved him. "Okay," he said, and hung up. I called Mr. Hoffer five days later to see if he would be open to a second visit from me. He told me that he couldn't talk. The stitches in his throat caused him extreme pain. "If I don't get better soon, I'll ask for a transfer of heads," he uttered flatly before ending the call.

Mr. Hoffer called Carmen to request a new prescription for liquid morphine. He had run out of his old one. Carmen was surprised. She reminded him that his doctor, Julie McCloud, had ordered liquid morphine only two days earlier and asked if he had picked it up from the pharmacy. He confirmed that he had, but explained that sometimes he spilled it or misplaced it. At other times, he said, the morphine "plain evaporated." It crossed Carmen's mind that Mr. Hoffer might have been abusing his medication. During this conversation, Mr. Hoffer's new personal care nurse, Betty Beasly, happened to be at the trailer and found an unfinished bottle of liquid morphine in the refrigerator. Carmen was relieved by the discovery, but she also asked Mr. Hoffer to keep a record of the morphine he consumed. As his hospice nurse, she explained, she was accountable for the way he used his medications.

On July 17, Mr. Hoffer learned that surgery would require massive tissue removal because of residual cancer in his pharynx. Though the procedure would not cure him, it had the capacity to lengthen his life. But it would probably debilitate him further. Early the next morning, he tripped on a carpet, which resulted in a two-inch laceration over his left eye. In a panic, Mrs. Hoffer knocked on the door of their neighbor, Ben Housler. Ben ran to the trailer, saw Mr. Hoffer bleeding, and called Peter. Peter called hospice. By the time things calmed down, everyone agreed that Mr. Hoffer required round-the-clock care. In fact, he was a good candidate for symptom management at hospice's inpatient unit. But since Mr. Hoffer was not on the hospice benefit, he would have to cover the cost himself. The Hoffers were torn. Was it time to choose palliation over radical surgery? Was Mr. Hoffer really terminal? After a long discussion with his wife and sons, Mr. Hoffer decided to switch to the hospice benefit. His priority was to receive immediate and intensive palliative care. He was admitted to the inpatient unit on the evening of July 18.

"I Am the Captain"

When I visited Mr. Hoffer in the inpatient unit, I had to confirm with a nurse that the person I saw sleeping was indeed Mr. Hoffer. He seemed older and smaller. He had a large blood blister on his right cheekbone. His skin looked flaccid, his hair more white than I remembered. The nurse asked me if I would be interested in meeting Eileen, who had flown in from Georgia. At her father's request, Eileen was now staying at the trailer to look after her stepmother. I told Eileen about our research and asked if she would be willing to participate. She was glad to. We moved to a private room. Tearfully, she said,

> Yesterday, Dad said, "Don't ask me any questions—I don't want to talk about what I don't want to think about," so he did not want any hugging, or anything like that. In April, when the tumor returned, he called my son and said, "Tell Eileen the tumor is back—I cannot talk to her." That is sort of how he had been treating it with me. He would not even let the doctors talk to me on the phone in Georgia. He completely hid any information from me when his first tumor was diagnosed. A year ago, I just showed up. He was surprised to see me and seemed a little angry, but after that he let me take him to his radiation treatments twice a day. But when I left it was, "Bye, Eileen." So I really think that he does not want to get super close.

Later that day, Eileen got the chance to spend time with her father. Following the visit, she wrote me a note. "We had a wonderful visit, Dad and I. He was affectionate and loving, and so was I. I was sad I had to leave." After her return to Georgia, Eileen and I spoke on the phone. She reiterated that her father had been open and affectionate, but added that that was because he thought he was going to die. "Dad asked me when I was coming in again, and I said I don't really know," she said. "I would not come in if his condition got worse. I wanted to be with him when he was alive, so he knew I cared."

During the first few days in the inpatient unit, whenever Mr. Hoffer opened his eyes, he stressed one thing: he wanted to return home. Three days later, I found him in an armchair. "This pain is an encroachment I find," he whispered as he spit in the cup he was holding. "It's forever aggressive. Aggressive." Though it was clear to everyone that he was despondent, he tried to control his emotions as much as he could. A few days later, when Carl asked him why he was holding back his tears, Mr. Hoffer explained that he didn't like to cry. "You might need to cry," Carl suggested, "as there is a lot to cry about." Mr. Hoffer rolled over in his bed and quietly wept.

Mr. Hoffer called his wife every night. According to a nurse, he lit up "like a Christmas tree" at the sound of her voice. Chemotherapy started looking attractive to him again. "I know I will eventually return to the point I am right now," he told a nurse, "but then I'll know I tried it."

Mr. Hoffer was trying to prepare for two scenarios: in one, he would get better; in the other, he would die. During his stay in the inpatient unit he asked Peter, in the presence of one of the nurses, to help him imagine what life would look like with him "in the picture" and with him "out of the picture." Peter responded that if he were to die, he, Frank, and John would place their mother in a nursing home. Mr. Hoffer's eyes filled with tears. He looked angry. He asked the nurse to leave, saying he wanted to talk with his son in private. Later, Peter seemed distraught. "My father is very self-centered," he said to me, "but this is one area where he is not. He is very concerned about what is going to happen to my mom after he is gone, and I can't say I blame him. As a son, that is an awesome responsibility, and I can say, 'Dad, we will do the best we can,' but these are tough decisions we are making right now. These are the toughest decisions I have ever made in my life."

Later, the nurse remarked, "I will not forget that exchange. You hope for your patients everything that they want, and it just seems like at the end of your life, you should have everything that you want. But to have to admit that you cannot take care of someone that you love is just very, very hard. You think that you can do everything, or that you should be able to, and when you can't that feels like a failure."

To another nurse, Mr. Hoffer acknowledged that he wanted to test hospice's limits. "You know, we are not here to restrict you," the nurse responded, "we are here to make you really as free as you can be, but we are really concerned about you." She then touched his shoulder and noticed tears in his eyes. She also recalled when she knelt in front of Mr. Hoffer to adjust his feeding tube, "I am the captain," he said. Right then Mrs. Hoffer walked in. She asked her husband when he would be coming home. He looked first at the nurse and then back at his wife. "Well," he said, "considering I have nurses on their knees in front of me, it might be a few more days."

A Family Meeting

Cassandra Fleming, the inpatient social worker, suggested a family meeting to determine what support Mr. Hoffer would need to return home and who could provide it. Mr. Hoffer agreed to a meeting but, as if he didn't trust his sons, asked for someone from hospice to represent his interests. He chose Carl.

The meeting took place on July 28. It included Frank, John, and Peter, the Hoffers' neighbor Ben Housler, Carl, Carmen, Cassandra, an inpatient unit nurse, a hospital nurse and a social worker involved in Mrs. Hoffer's care, and myself. Mrs. Hoffer was invited, but was unable to attend. Mr. Hoffer announced that he understood that to return home he needed the help of his sons, hospice, and the hospital that looked after his wife. He wanted everyone to know that he had decided to relinquish some control. He was willing to accept the care he required and cooperate with his caregivers. The inpatient unit nurse explained that hospice could make the administration of liquid morphine easier with prefilled syringes that Mr. Hoffer would inject into his feeding tube. Ben volunteered to help. The nurse also suggested that hospice could relieve Mr. Hoffer of the burden of morphine suppositories by replacing them with a transdermal fentanyl patch. Carmen offered to purchase a pill-crusher to ease the way of Mr. Hoffer's pills through the tube. John volunteered to build a handrail to support his father's movement. He would also place bricks under the armchair and sofa to make it easier for his parents to get in and out of them. Mr. Hoffer asked for an elevated toilet seat. And he accepted the suggestion to sign up for meal services for his wife.

Mrs. Hoffer's care providers reported that her blood sugar level had risen dramatically and that she seemed depressed. Perhaps she needed antidepressants. Peter got angry. He did not want his mother to go through another round of humiliating psychological tests just to be drugged further. The tests she was forced to undergo after her stroke were traumatic enough. As far as he was concerned, Mrs. Hoffer had many good reasons to be depressed. More pills were not going to solve the problem. He told me,

> My mother was the one who really raised us, and that is maybe why I feel so passionate about her and the care she gets as she gets older. My mother feels like she is a burden to us, like, "I really hate to bother you boys." Holy cow, mom! When Dad was working and drinking, who was there? *My mother was there,* and this is the least I can do. She had such an active role in our

lives, and after my father stopped drinking, his personality took over and my mother took a back-seat role, and I think she feels kind of bad about this. Is my mother depressed? Probably. That is where I got upset: We will give her some medication so she can be "happy." I don't think that is the appropriate response. I think, as a family, we need to bear her burdens. What better pill can you give your mother than for a son to drop in and say you love her?

After the meeting, Frank, John, and Peter looked exhausted but relieved. On July 30, Peter drove Mr. Hoffer back to the trailer. When Carmen and Ben arrived to go over practical details, Peter was unpacking his father's belongings. Mr. Hoffer was reading the newspaper and ignoring the discussion. Although he hadn't said so, he disapproved of the plan of care that had been put together for him and had decided to take no part in its implementation.

"It Was Almost a Futile Effort"

Two days after Mr. Hoffer's return home, Peter called hospice for help. His father had refused Ben's help in the administration of his medications. Moreover, he complained that he hadn't been consulted about his plan of care. No one had asked him if he wanted Ben's involvement, and Ben was someone he didn't trust. To everyone's surprise, he said that Ben liked to help himself to his morphine. He further insinuated that it was Ben who had encouraged him to call Carmen for extra refills of breakthrough medication earlier that month. Ben, he said, had a chemical dependency. He was the last person he wanted to see in charge of his care. Careful not to incriminate him, Mr. Hoffer withheld further details about his neighbor's actions and even seemed protective of him. He was primarily angry at his sons who had included Ben in his care without consulting him.

Neither Peter nor Frank believed the accusations. They had heard that Ben had a history of drug abuse, but they suspected that the missing morphine was the result of their father's accidental overdosing. Even now Peter doubted that Mr. Hoffer followed his medication schedule as he was supposed to. Defying hospice's request to keep a record of the times and doses of his medications, Mr. Hoffer insisted on doing things his own way. Record keeping made him feel watched over. The last thing he wanted was to be treated as if he wasn't worthy of his caregivers' trust.

"Looking back at the family meeting, it was almost a futile effort," Peter said to me with frustration. "I got so upset with my father, I was ready to just wash my hands of the entire situation and go away. This pattern that Dad showed us at the meeting has been characteristic of a pattern Dad has shown all through his life. He looked at what we did and he said, 'You guys don't really have any clue as to how to do this, do you? Obviously, I need to be in charge of this.'"

In Frank's view, Ben was irreplaceable. Neither he nor his brothers had the time to visit their parents as often as someone who lived next door. And his father was still not prepared to move to an extended-care facility. He seemed determined, in fact, to break ties with anyone who even suggested such a solution. Frank patched things up with Ben by asking him apologetically if he would continue with some household tasks. Ben assured him that he would.

On August 6, Mr. Hoffer severed his relationship with Carmen, his hospice nurse. Alarmed by the possibility of stolen morphine, Carmen had told him that she was obligated to notify Dr. McCloud about Ben. She reemphasized the importance of record keeping and suggested that if Mr. Hoffer continued to fail to keep track of his morphine, he would have to consider moving to a supervised environment.

Mr. Hoffer took offense. He already felt demeaned that the nurses pre-poured his liquid medication in syringes. Now Carmen appeared as a menacing power about to strip him of his autonomy. He told the chaplain, Carl, that he no longer trusted her. Carl agreed that Carmen could have related to him differently, but asserted that the serious problem of the missing medications was not her fault. Mr. Hoffer conceded, but insisted on a new nurse. Hospice complied. Carmen was replaced with Sharon Brown.

Carl took this incident to heart. "My relationship with him is still intact," he said to me, "and yet I am sure there is a possibility that I could do or say something at some point that he would want to blow me off, too." He further reflected,

> I think there are some unresolved personal issues relating to intimacy and trust that might need to express themselves at some point, and they also could be an underlying factor in him not being able to say, "I am afraid to die." It has never felt like to me that he has wanted prayer, and I have not offered that, but I think I need to pursue that a little bit just to see where he may or may not be—of course, not being tied to the results. I don't want to go prematurely. Given some of his life history, there is a lot of distrust there,

and I think some real rapport-building is important. I think we are still running the gauntlet. We are still having to pass his tests in certain ways, and that's okay.

Sharon acknowledged that she was wary about her new assignment, too:

Knowing that his trust in me could also be destroyed quickly, knowing that in this kind of scenario you are always walking on eggshells, you enter the scene with some anxiety. It presents a challenge for us, as staff, to rebuild trust. This is not just staff having trust in an individual, this is an individual having trust in staff as well. It's a two-way street. So I am responsible for rebuilding trust for him, and I think that is why I may say a prayer before I go there. That is my dilemma: how do I build trust in him, yet also remain non-naive?

When Mr. Hoffer met Sharon, he told her that he didn't need prefilled syringes. He preferred to use his medicine droppers. Sharon decided to respect his wishes. She found it more important to gain her patient's trust than to secure the proper doses of his medications. In fact, she suspected that Mr. Hoffer's diminished dexterity would hamper his ability to use his droppers successfully, but that was an issue she didn't want to raise.

"Now It Is Just You and Palliative"

Mr. Hoffer referred to his cancer as "allegedly terminal." He insisted that his goal was to get stronger. His dilemma about aggressive treatment still tortured him. He decided that if he was to live longer, he was going to invest his savings in a dental plate that would give him a full set of bottom teeth. "You don't lose total thoughts about the aesthetics of your face when you look like this," he said. If, on the other hand, he was not eligible for life-prolonging interventions, he wanted to spend his money on a fishing trip with his family. On August 13, Dr. McCloud informed him that the risks of surgery and chemotherapy far outweighed the benefits. In essence, aggressive therapies were no longer an option for him. He dropped his head and wept.

As Sharon was filling Mr. Hoffer's medication box a few days later, she noticed that he was agitated. He was pacing the kitchen floor and casting furtive glances at his wife. Mrs. Hoffer, who was sitting at the table, seemed unaware. Suddenly, Mr. Hoffer looked at her and announced that his disease was terminal. He was going to die. Mrs. Hoffer tensed. Mr. Hoffer's voice cracked. He assured his wife that she would be taken care of no matter what happened to him. After a moment of silence, he turned to Sharon and said, "Now it is just you and palliative."

Leaving no time for anyone to react, he proceeded to his next dilemma: Was it wiser for him to invest in dental work or a fishing trip? "It is certainly up to you," said Mrs. Hoffer nervously. Mr. Hoffer decided to invite his sons, their wives, and their children to join him and Mrs. Hoffer on a weekend trip to the Susquehanna River—all expenses paid.

Sharon left the trailer speechless. "It felt like holy ground," she told me later. "I was not sure why he chose to do it then unless he needed support in the telling. It was an incredible experience. It really did catch me off guard. It even brings tears to my eyes. But it really did seem as though, in some ways, it seemed a relief for him."

"That Will Be the End of My Story"

The next day, I found Mr. Hoffer on the sofa with a pile of old brochures. He was looking for a park by the Susquehanna River that rented cabins. Everyone had agreed to go fishing on the weekend of September 6. "That will be the end of my story," Mr. Hoffer said to me. "Like all stories, a happy ending. What else would there be to talk about?"

At the end of our visit, he asked me to "back off" for a few weeks. He reiterated that he had run out of things to say. I wasn't sure how to interpret his request. With Mr. Hoffer, I was never sure. Had I done something to upset him? Or his wife? He assured me that wasn't the case. He advised me to make sure to continue to interview his sons and attending physician because their stories would complete his. He simply had nothing more to say. Now that his fight was over, his story was over, too. I never interviewed Mr. Hoffer again.

"In a Strange Way, Those Have Been Kind of Tender Moments"

For the second time, Mrs. Hoffer's home health aides announced that they were going to discontinue their services. Their last visit was scheduled for

August 27. Mrs. Hoffer's blood sugar level had been stabilized. It was now up to a public agency for the elderly to decide if they had the capacity to accept Mrs. Hoffer as a patient. Frank was overwhelmed. As the oldest son and the family representative, he had assumed the responsibility of keeping in touch with hospice, the hospital, and all the people involved in his parents' care. He organized meetings, coordinated schedules, and hired services; and he had committed himself to a 40-minute ride each way, two to four times a week, to see his parents and, when needed, mow their lawn. He asked Cassandra if hospice had support groups for family members. Hospice did not. When I saw him, he looked despondent.

"I wind up feeling I am being pulled in three different directions," he said, "and I don't really feel like I am adequately serving my employer, my own family, my mom and dad. I feel like each one of them is only getting a piece of what I would like to give, so that becomes personally stressful." Yet he had also found unexpected satisfactions. He said,

> There have been some very good times as part of all this. It has brought me closer to my brothers in a number of ways, because we have had to work together as a caregiving team. It has brought me closer to both Mom and Dad. I have felt like this has really allowed me to give back to my parents in a way that otherwise I never would have been able to. Strangely enough, it is a kind of intimate thing to be changing somebody's bandages and to be helping someone administer their medications through one of these feeding tubes. Dad has to trust me at a pretty high level, I guess, to allow me to change that bandage. In a strange way, those have been kind of tender moments, which was certainly an unexpected thing. Mom is really pretty child-like, so that, you know, my relationship with her has become loving in a lot of ways that are unexpected. Would it have been better if her stroke had just killed her? For his cancer to have taken him quickly? You would not have that suffering, but you would not have had all of this closeness that has happened in the midst of it all.

"I Still Don't Know What Your Definition of God Is"

Mr. Hoffer told Carl that he knew he was dying and asked him to conduct his funeral service. "I still don't know what your definition of God is," he said to the chaplain. When he returned a few days later, Carl spoke about the struggle of having to "pass the baton" to others. Mr. Hoffer teared up. After a pause, Carl said, "Jesus didn't want to go to Jerusalem either." Mr. Hoffer started to cry. Like Jesus, Carl continued, it was time that Mr. Hoffer allowed his sons to wash his feet. He could use this opportunity to mend fences, grow closer to his loved ones, and not "give up," but "give over" to something that was bigger than himself. At that moment, Mrs. Hoffer walked into the living room. While wiping his tears, Mr. Hoffer followed his wife to the kitchen and offered her a cup of coffee. Somberly, he proceeded to tell her that he wanted Frank, John, and Peter to increase their involvement both in his care and hers.

Carl interrupted. "Can I be 'chaplain' here and help facilitate this conversation a bit?"

"Sure," Mr. Hoffer replied, as if relieved.

Carl addressed Mrs. Hoffer. "Albert knows he is dying, he does not want to die, he is concerned about you, and he knows he is going to miss you, and that is really hard for him. Albert has been the man of the house here and in charge and in control, and he sees he is going to have to pass this baton on, and he does not want to do that, and it is really hard. I bet this guy maybe has not given you as much credit for your ability to care for yourself as you probably can."

"I think I can," Mrs. Hoffer said.

"I think he wants to have closure with you and your sons," Carl went on.

"And she got it," Carl reflected later. "And I did a check with Albert, and I said, 'Is this where you want to go? Is this okay?' and he said, 'Yeah.' But a little bit later he left and sat on the living room sofa. It was just so hard, so hard for him, and I knew he wanted to say it, but because of the depth of his emotion and how large it is as well, he just was not able to do that."

At the end of the visit, Mr. Hoffer took hold of Carl's hand and with teary eyes invited him to the Susquehanna River. If it hadn't been for him, he said, he wouldn't have planned the fishing trip at all. Carl was honored by the invitation, but declined it regretfully. He explained that he saw this trip as an opportunity for him to spend time with his family. Mr. Hoffer understood. The next time Carl visited, Mr. Hoffer offered him a gift: one of his ties and a $20 bill. "It is my way of thanking the Lord that you came by today," he told him.

A few days later Mrs. Hoffer had a blackout. Mr. Hoffer found her on the floor. He, himself, was getting physically and mentally weaker, too. Frank, John, and Peter were losing sleep thinking about their parents' safety. They felt burned out, that something had to change. Frank decided to call another family meeting right after the fishing trip. He was going to be the one to set the agenda.

"It Was a Miraculous, Miraculous Meeting"

The fishing trip did not turn out as planned. The drive to the cabins was long, and the weather was cold and windy. On Saturday morning, Mr. Hoffer woke up with diarrhea that lasted all day. John called hospice and was instructed to discontinue the medication his father was taking for constipation. Everyone, except for Mr. Hoffer, went out to breakfast, but when they returned they found Mr. Hoffer in bed, crying, pleading to be taken home. Frank drove his father back to the trailer park. The rest of the family stayed at the cabins one more night.

On Monday, Mr. Hoffer asked to see Carl. When he arrived, Mr. Hoffer—barely able to whisper because of his sore throat—told him that he had seen his deceased brother. Carl offered to pray with him. Mr. Hoffer declined.

The second family meeting took place three days later. Mr. Hoffer seemed nervous and was tearful from the beginning. Frank and Peter gently expressed their concern for their parents' safety and their worries about themselves. Mr. Hoffer left the room twice, crying quietly. In his absence, the room filled with silence. Carl followed him to the hallway. He told him that neither his family nor his hospice team wanted him to fear that decisions would be made without him. When Mr. Hoffer returned, Frank took the opportunity to introduce the option of an extended-care facility. He had visited one a few days earlier and thought it would meet his parents' needs. To everyone's surprise, Mr. Hoffer agreed to consider the idea. He then stood up, went to the phone, and called the facility himself. He scheduled a family tour for the following day. When he hung up the phone, he asked Carl to accompany him for support.

"It was one of the most incredible turnarounds for the good I think I have seen in this job," Margaret exclaimed to me. "That Albert just finally said, 'Okay, I trust you.' That whole trust issue just had been paramount. He was just fighting the boys tooth and nail, and on that day he finally trusted all of us to do this for him. It was just wonderful." In tears, Frank remarked, "It was a miraculous, miraculous meeting. I personally feel that the Holy Spirit guided that whole process. I have no other explanation for it."

The visit to the extended-care facility went well. On the way back to the car, Carl pulled Frank aside and said, "I think you guys need to understand something here. I don't know what is going to happen, but I have often seen that when the dying person has been struggling with an issue that they need to resolve—whether it is reconciling a broken relationship or making arrangements for a spouse's care once they are gone—that once that issue is resolved, they let go and the end comes fairly quickly."

Three days later, Carl called hospice from the trailer. Mr. Hoffer was nauseous, lethargic, confused, and weak. He couldn't sit up unassisted and had skipped some of his medications. Carl urged that Mr. Hoffer go back to the inpatient unit. Mr. Hoffer agreed. Peter transferred him that day.

"Why Should a Dysfunctional Family Suddenly Function So Well?"

"It is real clear that we are in the final days now," Frank told me soon after Mr. Hoffer's return to the unit. "Last night he was not even strong enough to spit his phlegm into the little dish they have, so he would just stick his tongue out, and I would have a Kleenex and a little rubber-tipped toothbrush thing that I used to swab it out of his mouth. It sounds kind of disgusting, but to be able to do those little things, they take on a significance that I never would have expected."

Mrs. Hoffer insisted that she be brought to the inpatient unit daily. Frank told me how moving it was to watch his parents together.

> You can just see the love between those two people. They just hold hands and look at each other, and she strokes his face. Physical touch is about the only form of communication Dad has left. One time I started to leave without hugging him, and I heard this, "Come back," and I looked around and there he was with his arms out, so I know that's an incredible breakthrough. This whole process has drawn our family closer together in some surprising ways. Given the family history, I do not have any particular answer other than the Holy Spirit. I don't know. Why should a dysfunctional family suddenly function so well?

When I walked into Mr. Hoffer's room on September 24, he was lying in bed, staring quietly at Mrs. Hoffer and Peter who were sitting by his side. Suddenly he extended his hand toward them, and whispered, "Get me out of bed." Peter wrapped his arms around his torso and slowly pulled him up.

"It hurts! It hurts!" cried Mr. Hoffer with every move he made. But the pain did not stop him from sitting up and turning sideways to face his wife. Peter, overwhelmed by his father's fragility, sat next to him to keep him safe. Shaken as he was, he leaned his head against his father's, and they both cried.

"I think Albert is ready, finally," Margaret said to me. "These three boys seem to have all forgiven him, which is incredible, and they have all given so much of their time and effort. So, as many mistakes as Albert must have made, he and Julia must have done something right. I really feel proud about this case. I feel Albert has grown to trust us, and I know that was not easy for him. And it was not easy for Julia, either. And Julia has made tremendous changes. I mean, Julia smiles at me now and talks with me. She never used to do that."

On September 25, Mr. Hoffer stopped speaking. Periodically he opened his eyes and stared at the people sitting by his side—his wife, his sons, and Eileen, who had flown in to pay her final respects. They took turns holding Mr. Hoffer's hand. Eileen told Carl that she worried about her father's salvation. After the difficult life he had led, was he going to Heaven or Hell? Had he accepted God? Had he been forgiven? Carl told her about the gift Mr. Hoffer had given him a month earlier. From that act, Carl said, he had surmised that God was more present in Mr. Hoffer's life than he ever expressed. Eileen seemed reassured.

On September 26, Mr. Hoffer started to moan. He no longer seemed responsive. But when his wife and children arrived to see him, he opened his eyes and puckered his lips. "I love you," he said faintly to each of them as they bent over to receive a kiss. Eileen had never before heard her father speak these words to her. Carl encouraged Mr. Hoffer to lift his fears, doubts, and concerns to God. He blessed his journey and encouraged him to let go when he felt ready. Mr. Hoffer's hands were cool and dusky, his knees mottled. The next day his breathing changed. Nurses noted periods of apnea and gave him morphine to ease his respirations. His wife kissed him goodbye. A few minutes later he died. The family held hands around him and prayed.

"Amazing Grace"

John wasn't sure what he wanted to say at the funeral. His relationship with his father had been complex. The night before the service, he came across an old diary in which Mr. Hoffer confessed his guilt about his alcoholism and abusiveness toward his family. Mr. Hoffer took full responsibility for his actions, including the clobbering of John many years earlier. Now John knew what to say. He spoke about the two people he had known in his father: the one who was an alcoholic and detached, and the other who was sober, caring, and involved in everyone's affairs. He declared that Mr. Hoffer taught him an important lesson: to take responsibility for his own behavior.

Carl officiated at the service, wearing the tie Mr. Hoffer had given him. Frank, John, and Eileen's son sang "Amazing Grace," Mr. Hoffer's favorite hymn. In tears, everyone joined in. People laughed as intensely as they cried. In the background stood Mr. Hoffer's urn, surrounded by photographs and memorabilia. Looming large was an old T-shirt that read: "Pieces of Fatherly Advice: No. Absolutely Not. Never." After the service, Mr. Hoffer's older sister stomped her cane and declared that she was tired of reuniting with her family only when someone died. She invited everyone to join her two weeks later in celebration of her 90th birthday.

When I spoke with Carl a few days later, he recalled,

> I had a little time of closure after the funeral service. I stood underneath a tree and just kind of spoke to Albert from my heart and said goodbye. For Albert to have really given himself over to the process, to have mended fences with his family, and to be reconciled and have healing occur—I counted this as a good death. I think I tend to have more sadness with those who are not open to living until they die. I am planning to go deep-sea fishing in October, and there is no doubt in my mind that Albert Hoffer is going to come to my awareness. I know I will have a few words with him, and maybe it will be praying to St. Albert to help me catch a good fish.

"If You Don't Grow Close to Someone When You're a Child, Their Dying Is a Good Time to Do It"

Before moving to the extended-care facility, Mrs. Hoffer, with the help of her sons, took time to sort through her and her husband's belongings. Frank kept two reference books from his father's gardening classes that were filled with handwritten notes. John selected a pitcher he remembered his mother using for lemonade and iced tea. Peter picked a set of china and a book about the Civil War that he used to browse over and over again as a child. It reminded him, he said, of his father's passion for history. Together they decided that the things Mrs. Hoffer could do without they would auction off to help pay thirteen outstanding bills, including taxes, hospitalizations, and funeral home expenses.

Mrs. Hoffer moved in the beginning of October. At their aunt's 90th birthday party, Frank, John, and Peter were surprised to see her be social and solicitous. The only time she revealed a hint of her feelings about her new life was when Peter referred to the extended-care facility as her "home." "It is not my home," Mrs. Hoffer asserted. "It is just the place where I live."

None of the Hoffers felt the need for follow-up bereavement services from hospice. The times they had needed the most support were when their father was suffering. "Even with all the support that I had through hospice," Frank said, "there were times when it was just very lonely." Six months after Mr. Hoffer's death, Frank and his brothers continued to worry about their mother. Although they saw her often, she didn't remember their visits. Frank brought her photographs of family gatherings to remind her that she wasn't abandoned.

Frank looked back at his father's dying as a time of healing. He was thankful to have reunited with Eileen and vowed to keep in touch with her. Among the objects left behind at the auction was a copy of the New Testament that Mr. Hoffer had been given by his Sunday school teacher in the 1920s. Frank had never seen this book and was thrilled it wasn't sold. He interpreted it as tangible evidence that his father had a relationship with God. "This little Testament," he said, "I am really saving for Eileen. She was so concerned with whether Dad was going to go to Heaven, and I am hoping that it might be comforting for her." He added that he was also grateful for the transformation of his relationship with his father.

Peter felt the same way. Remembering the time in the inpatient unit when he cried alongside Mr. Hoffer, he reflected, "If you don't grow close to someone when you're a child, their dying is a good time to do it."

A year after Mr. Hoffer's death, I was informed that the Hospice of Lancaster County had created a support group for the caregivers of terminally ill patients. The catalyst for this initiative was Frank Hoffer, who had wanted such a group when his father was alive, but had to do without it.

Authors' Comments

A noteworthy aspect of this narrative is the superb work of the hospice chaplain Carl Flynn. Carl was willing to take risks in his persistent search for a language in which to form a supportive bond with Mr. Hoffer. That language turned out to be a fishing trip, as well as a willingness to engage Mr. Hoffer at a serious theological and existential level. As a result, the chaplain was able to cultivate the conditions that, in due time, gave him the role of trusted facilitator during several tense family meetings. The way Carl's relationship with Mr. Hoffer developed illustrates another point. Palliative care trainees are sometimes disappointed when they come to a patient's bedside intending to have a "deep" conversation, only to find that "nothing happens." In fact, patients are often selective in the person or persons with whom they will share personal thoughts and feelings. An intimate, confessional moment often requires a period of relationship-building before it can occur.

The chaplain's role as a trusted facilitator was even more important because Mr. Hoffer was a mistrustful man—something that became very evident when he chose Carl, rather than his own sons, to represent his interests at an important family meeting with hospice. Sharon Brown, one of the hospice nurses, also recognized, and acted upon, the tenuous nature of Mr. Hoffer's trust when she prioritized trust-building over an absolutely by-the-book approach to monitoring her patient's self-administration of pain medication. Given the suspicion of possible opioid abuse in the family or its social circle—a common concern in palliative care, magnified today by the opioid crisis we discussed in the General Introduction—this nurse's choice appears as an act of thoughtful, nuanced professional judgment, despite the risks that it may have involved.

The narrative also reveals two profoundly consequential systemic issues that we will encounter in several later narratives, especially from Lancaster County in the United States. One was the excruciating choice Medicare hospice rules forced Mr. Hoffer to make between insurance coverage for palliative care (including medicine to control his pain) and treatments for his disease. Because he was not ready to give up his efforts to treat his cancer, Mr. Hoffer had no choice but to pay for his pain medications and other palliative care support out of pocket—a serious matter given his relatively limited means and an example of how socioeconomic status plays a large role in the care that people with serious illness can access.[1]

The Hoffers' limited resources also made them dependent on social welfare policies for help for Mrs. Hoffer after her stroke. Had the Hoffers been wealthier, they might have avoided the haphazard, confusing, and seemingly arbitrary coming and going of home health aides that the Hoffers experienced. As it was, in addition to the anxiety and uncertainty of Mr. Hoffer's illness, the couple had to deal with the equally stressful, and even humiliating, inconsistencies of the support available to Mrs. Hoffer in her time of disability. Indeed, the three systems of care at play here—oncology, hospice, and social welfare—are often seen and studied as "separate," when, in real-life situations they can intersect in important ways. The suboptimal care that Mrs. Hoffer got had a clear impact on Mr. Hoffer's ability to come to terms with his dying and reach some state of peace. Mr. Hoffer's decisions and preferences for treatment, and his spiritual journey, were very likely informed by his sense that he, himself, was his wife's best and most consistent caretaker.

Mrs. Hoffer's difficulties reflect the patchwork, siloed nature of supportive services for people dependent on social welfare. It is a feature of the US social welfare system today that both illustrates and perpetuates health inequities. The dichotomous choice Mr. Hoffer faced between palliative care and active anti-cancer treatment, however, has begun to yield to new approaches and would probably not have confronted him today. Thanks to the Medicare Care Choices Model, the demonstration project sponsored by the US Centers for Medicare and Medicaid Services (CMS) that we discussed in the General Introduction, and in which Hospice and Community Care (the new name for Hospice of Lancaster County) is a participant, hospice patients may continue to receive curative or life-prolonging treatment under the Medicare benefit for their underlying terminal condition.

Reflecting on Mr. Hoffer's death, his son Peter said, "If you don't grow close to someone when you're a child, their dying is a good time to do it." Indeed, Mr. Hoffer's death was—in part due to the sensitive, therapeutic presence of Chaplain Carl Flynn and his hospice colleagues—a time of healing for this family. Seeds of hopefulness and reconciliation seemed to have sprouted in the midst of their mourning.

Reference

1. Wachterman MW, Sommers BD. Dying poor in the US-Disparities in end-of-life care. JAMA. 2021;325(5):423–424.

5

Klara Bergman

Burdens from the Past

Narrated by Patricia Boston

When Klara Bergman's doctors told her that she had incurable lung cancer, she did not question the diagnosis. But she felt it was a terrible injustice. She felt that she had been cheated and was being punished for no good reason. Mrs. Bergman, who was 80 years old, had suffered in Nazi concentration camps during World War II and lost most of her loved ones. She had cared for her sick father for many years after they were freed from the camp. Since then she had strived to repair and alleviate the suffering of victims of concentration camps, never thinking of herself or of her own needs. Why had God inflicted such a terrible injustice on her? A good and loving God would not do such a thing. Perhaps there was no God. All her life she had been deeply religious and committed to her Jewish faith. But if God existed, he was not there for her now.

Hurts in the Past

Klara Bergman was a Polish Jew who married and had her first child at age 22, just prior to World War II. After one year of marriage, she was taken along with her husband and child to a German concentration camp. Klara survived. When she returned from the camps, she was 24, having lost her 14-month-old son, her husband, and her mother. Still, she felt lucky because her father had survived. She could now care for him.

A friend in the Polish government helped her find a job, which was to establish an office of the World Jewish Congress in Warsaw. Klara's mission was to bring together Jewish families who had been separated by the war or incarcerated in concentration camps. Hundreds of Jewish families were reunited as a result of her efforts. But then Poland became occupied by the Soviet Union and she and her father had to flee. With the help of people from the World Jewish Congress, she went first to Paris, then to London where Klara met the man who became her second husband. They had a daughter, Ellen, and, when her husband was offered a position in Montreal, the family decided to move to Canada.

All in all, it was a wonderful life in Montreal. Klara was able to find a job right away with a Jewish organization and continued her work of reuniting separated families. She also went to law school, enabling her to help people settle legal problems incurred during the war.

The Bergmans settled into a comfortable suburban neighborhood where they raised Ellen. She was a bright, intelligent girl who excelled at school and later went on to study law at the local university. Klara and Ellen had an especially close relationship, and when Ellen left home to study at the Sorbonne in Paris, Klara found it hard to be without her.

In Ellen's final year at the Sorbonne, her father became ill with cancer and Klara took time away from her law practice to nurse him. After her husband died, it was hard to be without him. But time passed and she gradually took up her law practice again. She enjoyed the company of her friends and traveled to Europe to see Ellen. Life began to have meaning again.

Three years after her husband's death, Klara noticed that she was beginning to have some trouble with breathing. She had smoked cigarettes for 50 years, but now she stopped and saw her family doctor, Dr. Rajesh Gupta. A chest X-ray showed a serious problem and Dr. Gupta referred Mrs. Bergman to an oncologist, Dr. Jacob Lieberman, who told her that her symptoms were due to lung cancer. He was optimistic about her recovery, however, and scheduled her for a right upper lobectomy and biopsy of her lymph nodes. Following the surgery she had four weeks of radiotherapy treatments to decrease the chance of local recurrence.

"Why Now?"

When she heard after the surgery that there was no immediate evidence of metastases, Klara was not only relieved but felt confirmed in her strong belief in God and the Jewish faith. Though she had spent two years in a concentration camp and had lost all of her loved ones except for her father, she had always believed in God's goodness and purpose in all that happened in people's lives. Two months after the radiotherapy, however, she began to have increasing shortness of breath and trouble swallowing liquids. Six months later, Dr. Lieberman told her that a bone scan and X-rays showed that she had multiple bone metastases. He offered external beam radiotherapy to help control her pain.

Mrs. Bergman found it hard to understand why this terrible thing had to happen now, just when she was enjoying the fruits of her labor. For her, dying was the end of everything. When I met her and began talking with her about the onset of her illness, she told me that she couldn't sleep at night for trying, as she put it, "to put together the puzzle." She said,

> Why now, when I could relax and enjoy old age? Because I have really enjoyed old age. Old age was never something I have worried about and been frightened of and all those things people think about getting older. I thought this would be great. I would be old and live to a good age as my father had done. I didn't even look forward to retiring. I didn't feel that my mental powers were in any way diminished, and I liked what I was doing.

When Mrs. Bergman realized that there was no cure for her cancer, it became difficult to continue seeing her clients—not only physically but because of her increasing feelings of resentment. Her clients' problems and grievances became irritating and seemed trivial compared to her own. They were pursuing claims for compensation for losses that resulted from the war; she felt they did not appreciate the life and the wonderful resources they already had. She explained,

> They came to me with measly little complaints. Everybody I saw wanted more money and I couldn't understand it. I knew all of their past histories and that they had more now than ever before. There was no logic to asking for more money. Maybe a friend had told them they had an increase in their pension and that person would want an increase in their pension. People always came to me saying, "Everybody's getting more than me."

Mrs. Bergman could no longer sympathize with these problems. Here she was, "wracked with pain and a dying woman," and "all they wanted was a few dollars!" It was even more frustrating that her clients really did not sympathize with her. They saw themselves as victims of purposely inflicted injustices; to them Mrs. Bergman's situation was different because no one had inflicted her illness upon her. It was no one's fault.

Mrs. Bergman felt that her illness was a punishment, and the injustice of it made her more and more angry and confused. She examined her past life. Was she being punished for something? Had she done some terrible wrong? Certainly, she had been luckier than many; she had come home from the camps. But Mrs. Bergman's memories of the camp were of an intense struggle to keep her strength and health and to survive. Perhaps she had been too lucky. "There were others," she recalled, "many others who were much more damaged by the persecution. People who suffered in three, four different camps—much more difficult camps—who were physically mistreated and who, in spite of that, bore up quite well." She was fortunate by comparison. She had not suffered the same brutality as some.

Yet she had experienced terrible losses. There was a pain in her heart that had remained for the rest of her life. She said:

> You see, my husband and I had a young son when I was taken to the camp. And when we were told we had to go there, there was a chance to leave my son with some friends who were not Jewish and who would have cared for him. I could have left him behind. There was, for that moment, that opportunity. I knew he would be safe. But I was reluctant to part with my child. He was, after all, 14 months old and I thought he needed to be with his mother. So I took him with me to the camp. He didn't survive. He became ill with pneumonia. There was no treatment available for him, and I lost him.

Now, as Klara contemplated her own suffering and death, the memories of her son and the question of whether she should have left him in safe custody plagued her. There were, of course, women who had lost two or three children in the camps and had suffered greatly. To this Klara responded, "I don't think that the loss of two children amounts to more than the loss of one child. Because the pain is always there. And your life is never the same again, especially if you think you could have avoided the loss."

As I listened to her story, I wondered how I, as a mother or as another human being, could ever understand this woman's pain. I had raised two children of my own who were healthy and always full of life and energy. It was hard to relate to her loss. Although my own parents were now dead and I still felt their loss, they had both lived full lives and I had good memories.

Pain: "A Punishment from God"

In the fall of 1995, a few months after Dr. Lieberman told her that she had bone metastases, Klara Bergman began to have gnawing pain in her legs. It was controlled to some extent by acetaminophen, and she could have increased doses if needed. But the thought of increasing her pain medication only increased her anguish. She feared losing control of her mind.

As her pain persisted the whole ordeal felt increasingly like a "punishment from God." It was unfair and could only mean that God was unjust. Perhaps God did not even exist! During the war, she had always held on to her faith. Since being released from the camp, she had tried to lead a good life. Although her faith was tested at times, in the end she had always been able to feel that God was there for her. But now it was impossible to make peace with God when she had been given a terrible punishment for a crime she had not committed. She prayed for God's help. Sometimes she joked that she was preparing a speech "for when I get up there and what I will tell Him." But she doubted whether God was even listening.

Why did she have this terrible cancer? Perhaps it was the result of smoking for so many years. But why wouldn't a loving God protect her after all she had suffered in her life? She could find no answers to these questions. Meanwhile, the pain in her chest increased. The radiological reports showed lesions consistent with metastatic bone disease. Over the next few months, a widespread invasion with pain in her left femur and chest wall developed. She lost weight and didn't feel like eating. Her situation seemed to get more and more hopeless.

I met Mrs. Bergman during this period of her illness, first visiting her home in November 1996. She lived in a cottage-style house in a middle-class neighborhood of Montreal, a comfortable home with many personal mementos scattered throughout the rooms. There were old photographs, some of which might have been taken 60 years before, and souvenirs, most of which came from all the countries she had visited over the years or were the result of Ellen's travels. Mrs. Bergman looked much younger than her 81 years, and it was hard to believe she was as ill as she was. Her face was unwrinkled, with porcelain-like, clearly defined features. Her long, white-blond hair was elegantly rolled into a chignon, giving her a majestic, regal air. She had a pink shawl draped over her shoulders and sat up in bed, propped up by five or six large pillows and floral cushions. Although the bed seemed very large for her tiny, delicate frame, it seemed well suited to the ambiance of grace surrounding her. Two large, soft, stuffed rabbits sat on the bed beside her.

Because of the way she held herself and looked at me through clear blue eyes, she impressed me as a woman of profound dignity, as well as elegance and beauty. She had a way of regarding one intensely with admiration and interest in what one had to say, no matter what it was. She was well-schooled in drawing out information, and I liked talking to her. There were times when I would catch myself enthusiastically chatting about my own life, only to remember that I was the interviewer. I thought she must have been a superbly competent lawyer.

Changing Relationships and Roles

Mrs. Bergman knew she was going to die. Her question was whether she would be able to handle her illness with her accustomed dignity. She wasn't able to talk about it to the people who visited, even though many were old friends. It was not that she was ashamed of her illness, but she didn't "want to make a well person feel embarrassed or anything." "I don't want to make a well person feel that I'm envious or that I feel that he or she should have it and not me," she said.

One December day when I visited, Mrs. Bergman was with an old friend, Sophie, who was also born in Poland. The two women had been close friends for 35 years. Sophie was about to leave for her yearly winter sojourn in Florida. Sophie and Klara knew that this was probably the last time they would see one another. Mrs. Bergman recounted,

> We sort of said good-bye to each other. And she was the one who was crying. And I felt so bad about it. Because I know her. And I know what she thinks and feels. And I felt really bad about having to say good-bye to her because it made her feel she was privileged, you know? I felt that she would feel that I am envious of her position. And I almost said, "so help me God, I'm not." I'm glad that she is in this position. Thank God she has a good life, a good daughter and grandson. She worked hard all her life. She was an immigrant, just like me!

Mrs. Bergman had no biological family to speak of, except for a brother in England, whom she seldom saw. Ellen was all the family she had, and

Ellen had made her life in Israel, where she had an excellent job with the government record office. After leaving for Israel in 1992, Ellen returned to Montreal only to observe religious holidays. For the most part, the friends Klara Bergman had made over the last few years were her family.

Now, her surrogate "family" were coming through for her even though many were even older than she was. It was amazing to her to see how people with crippling arthritis, asthma, or even heart congestion would struggle through the snow and ice in the cold Montreal winter just to come and help her. Mrs. Bergman wasn't sure if she herself could have done it. "Frankly," she said, "If I were going to visit somebody who is sick and as old as I was, or even older, I would probably feel a bit put out. I might think to myself, 'in this weather, why do I, an old woman, have to go out?'" Once her friend Naomi found Mrs. Bergman vomiting on the bedroom floor. It was "demoralizing," throwing up on the floor and then watching her friend, with whom she had only shared philosophical debates and intellectual discussion, mop up the remains of breakfast and lunch. As Mrs. Bergman recalled: "She stood with me, over the sink, holding my head while I was throwing up. She is 83 years old. And I said to myself, I am really fortunate, you know? She was talking to me like one talks to a child, holding my head and stroking my back with the other hand. It's a wonderful feeling."

Palliative Care

Dr. Gupta had cared for Mrs. Bergman for the past 15 years and was more than a family physician to the Bergman family. He and Mrs. Bergman's husband had been friends and colleagues for a number of years before she became his patient. He wanted to continue to care for Klara, but when he saw how ill she was, he felt that the palliative care team should be involved. Dr. Matt Fitzgerald, one of the physicians with the palliative care service, visited Mrs. Bergman at her home to see how he could help and to discern whether she wanted him to take care of her.

It was not a difficult decision for Klara to make. She had heard of Matt from a good friend and knew that he was kind and compassionate. She needed to be able to talk to someone about the thought of dying; it was impossible for her to talk about it to her friends who were well.

Matt visited Klara Bergman regularly. He enjoyed his visits. They would often talk about her life experiences, though she didn't want to talk much about her time in the camps. Dr. Fitzgerald had cared for other patients who had suffered greatly in their past, and sometimes this had a profound impact on the way they reacted to a diagnosis of terminal cancer, but Mrs. Bergman appeared to be a woman who would decide for herself how to respond. Matt recalled,

> She was a firm woman. She was a woman who I felt I could let take the lead on how she was going to handle her situation, maybe more than some other people who had experienced similar events in their lifetime. I thought she was in charge of the things she needed to discuss and would raise quite comfortably whatever needed to be raised. I didn't think it was necessary to push her and to elicit material that either she wasn't ready or had decided not to talk about.

Mrs. Bergman was fully aware that she was going to die within a relatively short period—several weeks or perhaps a few months. She told Matt that she wanted to die in the best way that she could, free from pain, if that was possible. What she asked of him, and what was most important, was that her mind remain clear until the end. She worried that pain medications "would cloud her intellect" and that she would lose control of her mind. Matt prescribed oxycodone, which would help alleviate her pain and yet might have less risk of producing confusion compared with other opioids.

Alone in a Separate World

The oxycodone did not make her drowsy or confused. She was able to read and enjoy her friends. Still, Mrs. Bergman felt alone. The differences in roles and the way people related to her now magnified her sense of isolation. People had busy lives; they had careers and families, they traveled the world. They had lives to look forward to and memories to make. Ellen was young and perhaps would marry. But even if she did, Mrs. Bergman would never know the person.

Whom could she talk to who could really understand? She felt she could not share her grief or her fear of death with even her closest friends. She certainly couldn't talk about these things with Ellen. If she made a remark about dying, Ellen would cut her off, saying, "Oh, stop it." It reminded Klara of when her own father had wanted to talk about his fears and feelings about death, and she had said the same things Ellen was saying to her now: "Oh, don't talk like that!"

Ellen

Ellen took an extended leave from her job in Tel Aviv so she could care for her mother. Klara felt secure and safe when Ellen was around. Although Mrs. Bergman had many helpful friends, good doctors, and the support of home care nurses if needed, Ellen was the person to whom she had delegated most of the responsibility. As her parents' only child, Ellen felt alone with this. She worried continuously, describing herself to me as the "worrying type."

Ellen took up her caretaker role in the midst of another loss: months before Mrs. Bergman was diagnosed with lung cancer, Ellen had hoped to marry a man she had known in Israel for some time, but the relationship fell through. Ellen didn't want to talk much about her broken relationship. She rarely showed extreme emotion. She did say to me once that she would like to marry but now probably would not. She had good friends and an interesting job. "Life could be worse," she said.

Ellen was attractive, soft spoken, slight in build, and looked much younger than 38 years old. Her dark brown, curly hair framed her fine features. I thought she had beautiful eyes that somehow stayed sad when she smiled and even giggled as she told me her story. Mrs. Bergman worried about Ellen not being married. She still felt angry toward the man who had "broken his obligation." "I'd like to see Ellen happy and cheerful," she once said. "She's cheerful enough but I think that it is just a dress-up, for me. I know she is sad and would like to be married with children."

When her father died, Ellen was left with a lot of regrets. He had died while she was studying in Paris, and her mother had cared for him until he died. Ellen felt upset about her own lack of involvement, reasoning that she had not been more involved because she had not been told the full truth about the seriousness of her father's cancer. At the same time, student life at the Sorbonne was full and demanding, and she now wondered if perhaps she hadn't pursued the truth, or even called home, as much as she should have. On her father's birthday, when she had called to speak to him and there was no answer, she had not followed up with further calls. "The next day," she recalled, "I got a message that my father was seriously ill in the hospital. I flew back to Montreal the next day, but three days later he died.

There is a lot of guilt in me, and unfinished business which I can never repair."

Now it was vitally important to her to be in Montreal and to be a "good" caretaker. In the past, Ellen had always felt like a little child in relation to her mother. In spite of her 38 years, her studies at the Sorbonne, her travels to Europe, and the fact that she had an independent life in Israel, she had always felt like the child who was being looked after. Klara Bergman had been strong, always there for her, watching over her. Now the roles were reversed.

Ellen took over the household affairs, paying bills, cleaning, cooking, monitoring medications, and coordinating the doctor's and nurse's visits. She found it very difficult to take any time off from these duties. Once she went for an overnight trip to Ottawa, one of the first full days she was away from the house since her return from Israel several weeks earlier. She worried the entire day she was out and was not able to relax. She knew her mother was anxious and fearful the entire time that she was away. Although her friends had planned a day of sightseeing, she spent the whole day worrying that something could happen if she didn't get back to her mother's bedside. The experience made her feel physically ill.

"If You Cannot Control My Symptoms, You Know What You Can Do"

Klara was receiving oxycodone for chest pain, metoclopramide to prevent nausea, and lactulose, bisacodyl suppositories, and docusate to prevent constipation. But as the days went by, her breathing became more difficult, and she barely managed to eat the kosher food that Ellen prepared. Dr. Fitzgerald began to feel that his patient needed greater access to the palliative care home services. He asked Mary Thompson, another palliative care physician more closely connected with the home care service, to take over Mrs. Bergman's care. Mary began to visit Mrs. Bergman at home regularly.

One day the home care nurse was so worried about Mrs. Bergman's breathing that she called Dr. Thompson and asked her to visit immediately. When Mary arrived, Mrs. Bergman was visibly more short of breath and wheezing. "I am dying," was the first thing she said. Mary's assessment was that Mrs. Bergman had a parenchymal spread of tumor. She ordered oxygen, salbutane, and dexamethasone. She considered that her patient might be anemic, which would also account for her shortness of breath. She thought that if Mrs. Bergman did have anemia a blood transfusion might help. But it would involve a short stay at the hospital.

Mrs. Bergman appeared despondent. "I am dying," she said to Dr. Thompson. "Why do you want to transfuse me?"

Mary recalled that she hesitated for a moment before answering, and Klara said to her, "Don't look at me like that—you know it's true." When Mary explained that her intentions were to make Mrs. Bergman more comfortable, not to prolong her life, Mrs. Bergman agreed to the plan, but added, "I want to go soon. I don't want this to drag on."

Above all, Mrs. Bergman did not want to suffer. She said to Dr. Thompson, "If you cannot control my symptoms, you know what you can do." It was clear to Dr. Thompson, at least at this moment, that her patient was alluding to euthanasia. She responded that she would discuss various treatment options that were available in palliative care, including how to keep her comfortable without prolonging her life. Mrs. Bergman said she would like that, although their conversation did not continue at that time.

Home or the Palliative Care Unit?

A few days following Mary Thompson's home visit, Dr. Gupta called at the house. Mrs. Bergman told him that she now had intense pain over her left hip and could no longer put weight on the left leg. When Mary heard this, she thought it best to admit Mrs. Bergman to the hospital for radiological confirmation of metastases and to assess her overall physical condition. She worried that Mrs. Bergman might have a fracture of her left hip due to her advancing disease. It was also necessary to achieve better control of her pain.

As her mother's pain increased, Ellen felt inadequate and worried that she was not nursing her mother competently enough. When one of the visiting nurses noticed that Klara was beginning to get bedsores, it confirmed Ellen's fears:

> When the nurse mentioned bedsores, I remembered there was some material for bedsores that someone had recommended a week or so back. And I thought I could have got it. I hadn't got round to ordering it. So, I felt really anxious and blamed myself. Because it really was my fault. I should have ordered it right away.

Mrs. Bergman's pain was keeping her awake at night. Ellen worried that if she didn't stay by her mother's bedside all the time, her mother might fall out of bed. She thought of hiring a private nurse "who could be paid to stay up and keep an eye on her." She tried putting a baby monitor in her mother's room so she would hear if Klara called out in the night, but it didn't work properly. The situation was all too much to handle.

The Palliative Care Unit

Klara Bergman was admitted to the Palliative Care Unit in December 1996. Barbara, the nurse who took care of her on the unit, settled her into a sunny, spacious room. Mrs. Bergman liked the colorful, homespun bedcovers on her bed, for they reminded her of the shawls her mother had crocheted many years before. The bed was comfortable, and the bathroom was close by. Being at home in her own bed was nice, but it had meant a difficult walk to the bathroom. Ellen also settled into the room. Though she didn't plan to stay overnight, she spent most of the daytime with her mother and wanted to be fully involved in her care.

Klara impressed the palliative care team with her charm and graciousness. Dr. Lucien Crevier, one of the palliative care doctors who also took care of Mrs. Bergman, recalled,

> In my first meeting with her, I had a hard time believing she was very ill. Her face was almost like that of a young woman. Her eyes were bright and clear. She was alert, poised, and inquisitive about all of us. Her hair was beautifully coiffed. She wore a white crocheted shawl elegantly draped across her shoulders. To me she looked like she should be sitting on a veranda somewhere sipping tea.

"A Special Caregiver Challenge"

Ellen also impressed the team with her industriousness and dedication. She helped give her mother her morning bath, carried the meals, and set up the tray at the bedside. Frequently, Mrs. Bergman went for a stroll, walking slowly up and down the hallway, leaning heavily on Ellen's arm. To me, Ellen still appeared tired and even overwhelmed by her mother's needs, even though she now had direct access to the palliative care team. Mrs. Bergman preferred that Ellen be her caregiver. Once when I was visiting, I noticed Mrs. Bergman seemed a little short of breath. I asked if I might go and ask a nurse to help attach the oxygen mask. "No!" she replied. "It is not necessary, I don't need it just now." But as soon as Ellen came into the room, her mother asked her to fix the mask. Ellen was visibly irritated. "Why didn't you ask someone else?" she said. "Why must it always be me?"

Some of the nurses saw taking care of Mrs. Bergman as "a special caregiver challenge," in part because Ellen also needed a lot of attention. She was so fearful, so anxious to meet her mother's needs. Lena, another nurse, told me,

> Sometimes Ellen will come to us and say, "My mother needs a laxative. I think you should give her a lower dosage than you did last time." Or she'll say, "My mother needs something for pain. But don't give her as much oxycodone this time. You gave her 5 milligrams too much last time." Or Ellen will ask you to try another type of medication that perhaps she heard about from another patient. So you are constantly trying to balance Mrs. Bergman's needs with Ellen's needs and what you are able to do in the nursing role.

Ellen did not want to usurp the nurses. She wanted the team to care for her mother and to provide her with respite from demanding and wearisome tasks. Yet it was important for her to feel that she had explored every option to improve her mother's care. As she explained,

> I will never forgive myself if my mother doesn't get exactly the care she needs. Already I feel I should have been a much better daughter—more competent. My mother has always wanted perfection. And I should be prepared to give her perfection in the way she is cared for.

Managing Pain and Other Symptoms

At times, Mrs. Bergman's pain was excruciating. The pain seemed especially acute in her left hip, though it seemed to be spreading to all her limbs. Radiological studies showed extensive bone metastases. "How much worse will it become?" she asked Dr. Thompson. "I am afraid. I am afraid of pain. I am afraid of this dragging on, of losing my dignity. What will happen to me?"

Mary told Mrs. Bergman that there were a lot of options for controlling her pain. She began by discussing the option of increasing the dose of opioid medication. Mrs. Bergman often chose to live with her pain because she still did not want to be confused or drowsy. As it became absolutely necessary to increase the dosage, Mary tried to increase it so gradually that it would not cause drowsiness or result in Mrs. Bergman feeling out of control. She also arranged for radiotherapy to the painful area, and prescribed lorazepam to calm some of Mrs. Bergman's fears and reduce the anxiety that accompanied the pain.

After a few days, the pain seemed better. Mary urged Mrs. Bergman to let the nurses know when it seemed that the medication was insufficient. But the cancer in her bones was not the only source of Mrs. Bergman's pain. She also had two small bedsores at the base of her spine. Ellen was still worried that they were due to her own previous care of her mother at home. Barbara reassured her that bedsores happen easily with patients who are bedridden for lengthy periods. The nurses cleaned the bedsores with Hibitane and applied regular heat lamp treatments to them. They provided oxygen if Mrs. Bergman needed it to alleviate the distress of feeling short of breath, and she could have the drug dexamethasone to help relieve her breathing difficulties. Klara was impressed. She told me,

> I feel good, now that I am here. Of course, it is not like home. Home is always nicer. But now everything is readily available for me. If I have pain, there is something for it. If I need other things, the nurses are already here.

For a while, Mrs. Bergman experienced some relief from physical discomfort. When it became difficult to breathe, she took salbutamol and oxygen, and these measures helped. She felt in control and chatted with people who stopped by to visit. She always seemed to downplay her own discomforts and concerns when I visited her, focusing instead on other people's worries and misfortunes. One afternoon, after her friend Helga visited, Klara worried that her friend might not go home to a hot meal that evening. Helga's stove had broken and couldn't be fixed until the following day.

Fear of Being Alone

Two months passed. It seemed less and less likely that Mrs. Bergman would go home, even for a short stay. Although her pain was now controlled, she was becoming much weaker. She didn't feel like getting up at all. "I am tired, and my body is weary," she said.

Ellen also seemed weary. She would almost snap at her mother when her mother asked for something. She found more reasons to leave the unit "to do errands." But just as Ellen finally allowed herself to get away, Klara seemed to want her daughter's presence even more. "How long do you think this will go on?" she would ask Mrs. Bergman's various caregivers. No one could say for sure.

The nurses saw how much Ellen needed time away from the unit. They also saw that when Ellen was gone, Mrs. Bergman wanted one of them in the room with her all the time. Often, Barbara would go to Mrs. Bergman's room to turn her onto her side or reposition her pillows. Mrs. Bergman would ask her to linger, then ask for something else, such as changing the water in the flower vases, folding the clothes and towels, or tidying up papers—anything, as long as it involved staying in the room. There was fear in her eyes. But Barbara had four or five other patients in her care who were very ill and dying, and she needed to be there for them as well. This emotional challenge was even more complex than the physical management of Mrs. Bergman's symptoms. Barbara asked one of the volunteers, Linda, if she would sit with Mrs. Bergman. But Mrs. Bergman didn't feel secure with just anyone in the room; she wanted the presence of Ellen, or if not Ellen, then Barbara or Lena.

"I Want to Die with Dignity"

One day, Mrs. Bergman told Dr. Crevier that what she most needed and wanted was "freedom from fear." "How can I get rid of that constant sense of fear inside me?" she asked. To me she said,

> I hate it, I hate it! This sense of being a child again—not in a good sense, for someone like me, but in the sense that I must now depend on others to be sure that I eat without making a mess and that my body functions without making a mess. All the time I think of this and I am afraid of it. For some perhaps, it is not so important, but for me it is impossible to bear.

She continued, "I've always been one for keeping beautiful and elegant. Loss of dignity, there is something ugly about it. I want to keep as beautiful as possible in these circumstances."

Yet now she was losing control of her bladder. On occasion she had to ask Ellen, Barbara, or Lena to change the bed clothes. It was not so bad if Ellen or Barbara were around; they knew her situation. But what if it were one of her friends? One day, when several friends were visiting, her incontinence was especially bothersome. The team thought that she might benefit from a urinary catheter. Mrs. Bergman was pleased with that idea. Anything was better than "wetting the bed and invading my dignity," she said. There was also the advantage that the constant leakage of urine would no longer chafe her skin or irritate the bedsores, which had now begun to heal.

"I Don't Know If There Is a God"

As she lay in her bed, Klara again wondered whether she could trust the religion of her childhood. She struggled with questions such as "Does God exist?" "Who is God?" "What exists after I die?" "Is there a benevolent God?" and "If there is, then why am I suffering?" Sometimes we would be chatting about topics such as a recent visit from a friend or the lunch menu and she would suddenly interrupt with thoughts about her faith. Once she asked me, "Do you believe in God?" I said I did. She replied,

> You see, I don't know if there is a God. So many bad things have happened. What is His logic? It doesn't make sense! How is it He permits so much to happen to people? Why would such a God, if He exists, allow these bad things to happen? I have spent most of my life dedicated to helping others in need. There is no justice in this.

Sometimes she could alleviate her fears by talking to her rabbi or to staff members, such as Kyle, who had impressed her with their own faith. After one of the rabbi's visits, she told me, "His faith in God does not waver. He believes in the goodness of mankind. He told me to focus on the good times I have had, and I have had many." Indeed, she could see the dedication and goodness of so many people on the Palliative Care Unit, she said. Certainly, what the rabbi had said was true for the people she saw working here. She continued:

> I struggle with my fears: fears of losing all of my faith, fears that God does not exist. But my sense of logic—you see, I work on logic—tells me that

there is goodness and compassion in others. These people—the nurses and doctors here—have no reason to be here. They don't have to choose this work, to be with dying people day after day. Such love and such dedication! And it is sincere.

Mrs. Bergman also marveled at the devotion of some family members toward their loved ones on the unit, especially the devotion of adult children toward their parents. She had noticed a young man in his early thirties caring for his mother. He had cared for her unselfishly for four years, she explained to me. Then she said, "I am so impressed by the devotion of the young man. He stays here with his mother all night and then leaves to work and then comes back here. You can't imagine it. He is young with so much life ahead of him, and yet he has made such a great sacrifice." At these times she could relate to her rabbi's argument about the goodness of human beings. Still, she said, if God does exist "it follows that I must be angry with Him for making me afraid and for allowing my and others' suffering."

Looking to the Past

No one on the team knew quite how much pain Klara Bergman had endured in the concentration camp. We all knew that she had suffered and that she had fought to survive. But no one could tell exactly what she had endured. Although she talked freely about the events of her life following her release from the camps, we knew little about her life inside. All she would say was, "My life was difficult in the camp, and I suffered. But everyone suffered and the most fortunate thing for me was that I came home. Many others did not."

She did mention some of her dreams. "Sometimes they are not just ordinary dreams," she said. "They are troubling dreams where I can't seem to control the events." She dreamed she was falling down a steep slope. She couldn't remember the details, but when she awoke, she felt a sense of helplessness. When I asked if she wanted to talk about her dreams to someone on the team who might be able to help, she responded,

I am not interested in speaking with anyone who will try to rationalize my situation. My situation will not improve if I talk about my dreams. I am going to die. I am dying. I hate it, and when I say hate it, I hate it. Of course,

if someone is going to tell me that I am not going to die—well then, it would
be quite another story.

Some members of the team did try to broach the subject of Mrs. Bergman's
past experiences. The music therapist, Sue, asked if she wanted to tell the
story of her past. Mrs. Bergman responded abruptly, "I like to talk, but you
shouldn't talk to me about my Holocaust experiences." She told Sue that she
did not like people who were "Holocaust professionals."

Dr. Thompson thought there was no real evidence of clinical depression
in Mrs. Bergman's case. Mrs. Bergman was eating as well as she could. She
was talkative (if not about past events), she enjoyed the company of many
friends and visitors. When she felt up to it, Mrs. Bergman would read, look at
television, or attend the musical concerts that were available in the palliative
care lounge. She readily acknowledged to Mary that she was sad about what
had been happening to her for the past two years, but she also felt proud of
her many achievements. Besides, even if she were clinically depressed, Klara
Bergman had little interest in seeing a mental health professional. She "didn't
believe much in the benefit of such help," Mary noted. She did take the lorazepam that Mary had prescribed to alleviate anxiety, but her fears seemed to
penetrate the effect of the medication.

"There Will Always Be Someone Here for You"

Most of all, Mrs. Bergman feared dying alone. "There will always be someone
here for you," Barbara told her. "Even if I can't be there on one of the days,
Lena is here." Ellen now began to stay with her mother at night as well as
during the day. She slept in a cot beside her mother's bed, listening for any
sound her mother made. "It is as though my mother knows whether I'm
here or not," she told me. "Even if she's sleeping, as soon as I go out into the
hallway, even for a short walk, she wakes up, I hear her call out my name.
I know that she is really scared."

Sue, the music therapist, tried to work with musical images that would
provide comfort and relief for Mrs. Bergman. To a small extent it worked. As
Sue explained,

I suggested she try putting on some quiet music and really try to imagine
with all her senses that she was back within the beauty of the images she

was experiencing. She thought about the good memories she had had. We created an image of her sitting at home on her favorite chair with her beloved cat on her belly, where the pain was. And I looked at her as she was describing the cat and how much fun she had with this cat and how the cat meowed and how she loved it and the special communication she had with this animal—and for a while, her face looked very relaxed. She enjoyed it and she said she had, at least for those moments, forgotten her pain and her fearfulness.

When Sue returned the next day to try a similar experience, Mrs. Bergman told her, "This form of imagining with music" wasn't for her. After Sue had left the previous day, she had felt "frightened," "isolated," "with a terrible feeling of abandonment." "All my nightmares came flooding back again," she said. Sue offered to make a cassette that Mrs. Bergman could listen to with headphones. Sue made the cassette in which she guided the images, and Mrs. Bergman tried to use it sometimes.

"Maybe I Could Go to Sleep and Simply Stay Asleep?"

One day Klara said to Lucien Crevier, "I don't want this to just drag on and on. I don't want to suffer endlessly. If I am to die, then let it happen soon and quickly." Then she asked, "Maybe I could go to sleep and simply stay asleep?" Her pain was well controlled by hydromorphone, and chloral hydrate, a sedative, also offered some relief. "But I am afraid," she said. "I thought I was above being afraid like this, but I am afraid, all the time, and there it is!"

Even if euthanasia were legal and available, however, which at this time it was not, Ellen made it very clear that *she* was not willing to accept such an option. She was not willing to let her mother go. "I hate it when she talks that way," she said to me. "I told her she needs to try and be strong for my sake, if nothing else." To her mother she said, "We'll manage. I won't leave you alone."

Ellen helped with her mother's morning bath and coaxed her to eat the yolk of an egg and a little juice, no matter how long it took. Every day she brought home her mother's night clothes and special towels to launder and would return within an hour with fresh, clean, scented clothes for her mother to put on. Ellen's eyes looked bloodshot, and they had dark shadows under them. Sometimes I saw her sitting facing the side of her mother's bed with her head resting in her hands. When one of the nurses tried to coax Ellen to sit in the family kitchen and perhaps make herself a cup of coffee, Ellen became irritated. "I am not tired!" she insisted. "I am not in the least bit tired."

Fears of Persecution

In the beginning of February, seven weeks after Klara Bergman was admitted to the Palliative Care Unit, she began to show signs of confusion and suspiciousness. She would hear the sound of footsteps in the corridor and wonder if someone was coming or waiting to give her some order. On one occasion she heard the voices of two of the volunteers chatting as they wheeled the library book cart down the hallway outside her room. "Who is there?" she called out. "Are we under surveillance?" On another occasion she asked me if we should try and get alternative accommodations. "Perhaps," she said, "we won't be able to stay here for too long." If you looked directly at her, she might ask, "What are you looking for?" Even when familiar nurses entered her room to fix her bed or give her a back rub, she would awaken abruptly and ask what they wanted from her. She wanted to know who was waiting outside, what people's names were, why they were there. More often than not, she would refuse to eat the food that was offered.

Dr. Crevier noted,

She is starting to talk about wanting to see the police record of the nurses. She believes that someone wants to come and get her back to the concentration camps. She sees men in her room behind us. Her daughter found her this morning with two coils of oxygen tubing around her neck. She was restless in the bed, moving about and never finding a comfortable spot.

The Last Days

In consultation with the psychiatric consult team, Mary and Lucien worked to ascertain dosages of haloperidol and lorazepam that would alleviate Mrs. Bergman's fearfulness. The drugs worked. Once her mind was clearer, she began again to reiterate that what bothered her most was not knowing what to expect. For her, dying was the end of everything. If her life had to end, then surely it should end quickly. Her list of fears was now enormous.

Despite her previous insistence that she had to remain alert and awake at all times, Mrs. Bergman said she was now ready to sleep. To be able to have a peaceful sleep, free of anxiety, was more important than anything. She was ready to let go. The physicians adjusted the medication so that she slept more and more. Ellen, struggling to come to terms with the reality of her mother's imminent death, stayed constantly beside her mother's bed.

Early on a mid-February morning Mrs. Bergman died. Ellen held her hand during the last hours. It was good, she said, that her mother died with people close beside her. Most of all, she had wanted Ellen to be there with her. Dying on this particular day was, in her own way, "doing a favor to me," Ellen said. According to Jewish custom, the time of Mrs. Bergman's death did make things a little easier for Ellen, for her mother died just before the Sabbath. Had she died on the Sabbath, Ellen would have needed to ask the Palliative Care Service not to allow anyone in the room for 24 hours.

Authors' Comments

Klara Bergman might well have benefitted from psychiatric therapy for the duration of her care, especially given what we know of her history as a Holocaust survivor. She had lost her husband and her baby in the concentration camp. Her anxiety about maintaining her dignity may also have been related to her experiences there. Just over 20 years ago, Dr Harvey Chochinov, a Canadian psychiatrist and palliative care physician, introduced a brief psychotherapy model known as dignity therapy aimed toward the relief of psychological and existential distress at end of life. Since that time, a plethora of research has evolved indicating the benefits of this model, showing that it goes beyond traditional psychiatric variables for treating end-of-life anxiety and depression.[1]

In Klara's last days, we witnessed her extreme fearfulness and delusional state of mind. It is not uncommon for patients to suffer from delusional fears in their last days, which can be greatly helped with haloperidol and lorazepam as was the case with Mrs. Bergman. But perhaps psychiatry could have been involved from the onset of her illness on a continuous basis. In recent years, there has been a move toward including the psychiatrist as a formal member of the multidisciplinary team. Palliative care psychiatry is now being seen as an important subspecialty of psychiatric practice.[2]

Mrs. Bergman also stated openly that she struggled with her faith, saying at one point, "I struggle with my fears: fears of losing all my faith, fears that God does not exist." The content of her spiritual anguish is noteworthy: anger at God and questioning the fairness of what she experienced as God's punishment despite her virtuous life. Arguments with God are part of a long tradition within Judaism,[3,4] while *theodicy*, seeking a justification for suffering at the hands of a benevolent, all-powerful God, is pervasive across many faiths.[5,6] These religious themes appear in several other narratives in this book as well.

Klara did derive some comfort from Kyle, a staff member who, although of a different religion, had a great faith in the existence of God. She also seemed to feel some reassurance through visits from the rabbi. It is possible that she could have benefited from spiritual counseling had it been available on a more continuous basis.

Klara's daughter Ellen worried about taking good care of her mother and questioned her own competency as a caregiver. She often seems overwhelmed by her mother's needs and emotionally exhausted. Although the palliative care team did their best to support Ellen, this chapter highlights the lack of formal structures to support family caregivers. This is still true today. While the Canadian government has committed funds for improved palliative home care, at present there is no consistent implementation plan. There is also emerging literature calling for more attention to the psychological health of family caregivers and a more formal role for mental health professionals.[7-9]

Ellen felt guilty at times that she was not caring for her mother in a way that her mother needed. As she put it, "I should have been a better daughter—more competent. My mother has always wanted perfection. And I should be prepared to give her perfection in the way she is cared for." Here is an example of how people's experiences of dying, and caring for the dying, often reveal and reenact patterns from prior phases of life and relationships.

If Klara Bergman was alluding to a request for euthanasia, it would have been neither legal nor possible twenty years ago. Today, as we have discussed in the General Introduction, requests for euthanasia in Canada can be considered under the legislation for Medical Assistance in Dying (MAID), enacted by the Parliament of Canada in June 2016. We cannot know whether Klara Bergman would have asked directly for MAID if it had been legal, but that option would be available at the present time. For further discussion of this issue, see the Authors' Comments for the narrative of Frances Legendre.

References

1. McClement S, Chochinov HM, Hack T, Hassard T, Kristjanson LJ, Harlos M. Dignity therapy: Family members perspectives. J Palliat Med. 2007;10(5):1076–1982.
2. Fairman N, Scott AI. Palliative care psychiatry: Update on an emerging dimension of psychiatric practice. Curr Psychiatry Rep. 2013;15:Article no. 374. https://doi.org/10.1007/s11920-013-0374-3
3. Weiss D. *Pious Irreverence: Confronting God in Rabbinic Judaism*. Philadelphia: University of Pennsylvania Press; 2016.
4. Laytner AH. *Arguing with God: A Jewish Tradition*. Lanham, MD: Rowman & Littlefield; 2004.
5. Soelle D. *Suffering*. Minneapolis, MN: Fortress Press, 1975.
6. Hauerwas S. *Naming the Silences: God, Medicine, and the Problem of Suffering*. Grand Rapids, MI: Eerdmans; 1990.
7. Kristjanson LJ, Aoun S. Palliative care for families: Remembering the hidden patients. Can J Psychiatry. 2004;49(6):359–365.
8. Hudson P, Trauer T, Kelly B, O'Connor M, Thomas K. Reducing the psychological distress of family caregivers of home-based palliative care patients: Short- term effects from a randomised control trial. Psycho-Oncology. 2013;22:1987–1993.
9. Alam S, Hannon B, Zimmermann C. Palliative care for family caregivers. J Clin Oncol. 2020;38(9):926–936.

6

Frances Legendre

The Price of a Death of One's Own

Narrated by Anna Towers

Frances Legendre was accustomed to being in control. When she came to the Palliative Care Unit suffering from advanced ovarian cancer, she was prepared to die. She exuded acceptance and calm, and she drew her family and the palliative care staff into her plans and images of eternity. But Mrs. Legendre did not die then and, a few weeks later, convinced that it was not yet her time, she launched into a relentless effort to find a cure. She insisted that her oncologists enroll her—against their own judgment—in high-risk experimental treatments, and the palliative care team found itself advocating more aggressive care for their patient. When all the treatments failed, Mrs. Legendre again came back to the Palliative Care Unit to die. This time she and her family wanted the end to come quickly, peacefully, *now*.

Beginnings

Frances Legendre was 51 years old when she learned she had cancer. At that time, she was a businesswoman, married to Jacques Legendre. Like Frances, Jacques was French Canadian, 57 years old, and a wealthy and successful businessman for 30 years. The Legendres had traveled widely. They had four daughters who lived in Montreal, Paris, and the Bahamas. Mrs. and Mrs. Legendre usually spent winters in the Bahamas, the rest of the year enjoying their home a few miles outside Montreal. Mr. Legendre had built the house for their retirement, as a gift to his wife. The tall, majestic, Mediterranean-style villa stood overlooking the fields and hills of the Quebec countryside, flower-filled gardens, and a manmade lake. Mr. Legendre had also built a fountain in the garden, calling it their "wishing well." The home reminded them of Italy, where they had lived for a few years—the best time of her life, Mrs. Legendre recalled.

When she first visited her doctor, complaining of lower abdominal pain, he told her that she had "a little cyst on the ovary." While she was initially reassured, the pains persisted. Her doctor reexamined her and again found nothing of great concern. Eventually her doctor ordered more extensive tests. By the time these tests revealed ovarian cancer, two years had passed since her initial diagnosis of a benign cyst. The news was a terrible shock, but Mrs. Legendre had already known that the pain she was having meant that something must be seriously wrong.

The cancer was already quite advanced, and experimental therapy was all that was available. The couple decided to pursue any treatment that might give her even the slightest chance of remission. It didn't matter how expensive the treatment was or how difficult it might be to find it. "I wanted to fight," Mrs. Legendre said. "I am still a young woman. My life is wonderful. I have a good husband, wonderful children. They all did well and there is so much love in our family. I have a young grandson, everything to live for. I felt cheated. I wanted to keep my good life."

"Something Might Work!"

Although the experimental drug paclitaxel resulted in a slight remission, this lasted only two months, and Mrs. Legendre's tumor progressed. At that point, Mrs. Legendre said, she felt "cheated and mad that my life was being taken from me." She and her husband pressed on with their determined search for a cure, only now they felt that they were alone in their mission for her doctors were offering no more treatments. Mrs. Legendre interpreted this as a loss of interest in her and a withdrawal of support. "We had to take matters into our own hands and think up answers on our own," Mr. Legendre said. They did their own research, pored over New Age type journals, and sent away for literature described in the advertisements. They sought out unpublished information by word of mouth. At times during their quest they felt they were being taken advantage of, Mr. Legendre said, by people who were "probably making a lot of money by giving out 'recipes' to cure cancer." But they were prepared to pay anything, and, besides, Mrs. Legendre asked, "what choice did we have?"

They tried organic foods, nutritional formulas, home remedies, vitamin therapy, herbal remedies. One Chinese herbal remedy, a blend of 170 herbs, proposed, as Mrs. Legendre recalled, that "it could make the tumor melt." It didn't work and it was costly—$300 "under the table." But whenever there was even a chance, the Legendres would find the money. After all, they said, "something might work!"

After several weeks and many thousands of dollars, Mrs. Legendre began to feel sick again, and she was in intense pain. All the treatments, of whatever type and from whatever source, had failed. It appeared that there were no other options. When Dr. Samuel Singer, her oncologist, examined her, he found that the tumor had grown and had spread to her liver. "I'm sorry," he told her, "but your sickness is now at a very advanced stage." "I'm not ready to die," she answered, "what do you have to offer me?" But he had no other suggestions. Moreover, the side effects of the experimental drugs made her feel sicker than she could ever remember. At that point, Mrs. Legendre gave up trying. "I knew I had to stop," she recalled later. "I wanted to live, but I just couldn't take feeling sick."

"That's the Beginning of the End, You Know"

In the fall of 1995, the Legendres returned to their home in the Bahamas. Over the next few weeks Mrs. Legendre's abdominal pain intensified. Dr. Singer had prepared her for the symptoms that were to come. As Mrs. Legendre understood what he said, "You are now in the terminal phase, first the bowel, then your stomach gets hard like a rock, you have nausea and your stomach is not able to process food anymore." Dr. Singer prescribed morphine for her pain, but Mrs. Legendre was reluctant to take it. She was like many patients with advanced cancer who resist taking pain medication as a way to stave off the reality that their disease has progressed. To take the medication was to admit that the pain was getting worse. To admit that the pain was getting worse was to admit that the cancer was getting worse. And to admit that the cancer was getting worse was to begin to look into the face of death. Mr. Legendre, relieved that at least something could be done for his wife's pain, argued with her. "Why suffer?" he would ask. "It's there for you."

Mrs. Legendre took the morphine but thought to herself, "Well, that's the beginning of the end, you know."

The morphine Dr. Singer had prescribed was not enough to control her pain. He suggested to the Legendres that they return to Canada where services to manage her pain and other distressing symptoms would be more readily available. At the end of December, Mrs. Legendre flew back to Montreal, accompanied by her daughter Lily. She arrived at the hospital's emergency department late on a Saturday afternoon, certain that the end was near.

When Dr. Michael Raymond, a physician from the Palliative Care Service, met Mrs. Legendre for the first time, she was lying on a stretcher in the emergency department, with Lily sitting beside her. Michael could see immediately that Mrs. Legendre was in pain and that she had a look of panic in her eyes. He had already spoken with Dr. Singer and the resident in the emergency department, who had told him that Mrs. Legendre had a small bowel obstruction. The cancer in her abdomen was too far advanced for her to have surgery to relieve the obstruction. Michael knew that there was a 50% chance that the obstruction might resolve on its own or with the help of steroid medication, only to recur again within a couple of months. In the worst-case scenario, if things did not improve now, she would not be able to nourish herself and she would probably die within a few weeks.

Though he was a young man, Michael Raymond was an experienced palliative care physician. He had seen many patients die under these circumstances, and it was hard for him, even though he knew he could control his patients' pain. He thought it was probably easier caring for soldiers at the front in wartime than caring for a patient who was alert and aware, knowing she was starving to death, because at least he would not have come to know the soldiers as intimately as he knew his patients on the Palliative Care Unit (PCU). No matter how much experience you had with dying persons, Michael had once said, and no matter how much could be done to relieve their distress, "when people are dying, for those last days and hours and minutes, you must be close to them in a human and very compassionate way. And sometimes there can be three or four deaths in the space of one or two days. You get to be with the families, you are closely involved in the lives of those families, and there is a relationship that is highly significant for them and for you."

Now, however, Dr. Raymond's responsibility was to reassure Mrs. Legendre. What could he offer her? Seeing how panicked she was, Michael guessed that Mrs. Legendre expected to die within a few days. In fact, the actual time of her death was not easy to predict, "You know," he said to her, "I don't work for any psychic alliance, but in my experience I've learned one thing: I cannot make predictions. I've also learned that for people who are quite sure when they will die, very often life will do something else." At the moment, he continued, there was much he could do to make her more comfortable. Dr. Raymond arranged immediately for Mrs. Legendre to be admitted to the PCU and ordered adequate morphine for her pain and intravenous dexamethasone and metoclopramide to try to get her intestines working again.

"I Am Going to a Beautiful Place"

People seemed kind and friendly on the PCU. Her nurse, Ena, settled Mrs. Legendre into a bright, sunny room. The 16 rooms on the unit are especially designed to be cheerful and bright with pastel-colored furnishings, homespun-style bedcovers and blankets, and brightly colored curtains. Mrs. Legendre's room was situated at one end of a carpeted hallway. At the other end was a small kitchen and dining area where families and friends could cook and visit if they liked. Near the kitchen was a spacious carpeted lounge with colorful easy chairs, floral-covered sofas, coffee tables, and a large grand piano that occupied a central space. The lounge looked out onto a large woodland area and provided an impressive aerial view of the city. Mrs. Legendre felt good here. It wasn't like the hospital wards she had experienced before. In fact, "it wasn't really like a hospital at all," she said. "People had time."

It was at this point, in early January 1996 and just a few days after her admission, that I met Mrs. Legendre. Dr. Raymond had explained our project to her, and she was very open to participating in it. The Legendres told me about their earlier experiences with Mrs. Legendre's illness and the events that had led to her present admission to the PCU.

When I first saw her, she was sitting up in bed, propped up by colorful pillows and dressed in a floral pink nightgown. I thought there was a radiance about her. Her pain was now under control. She seemed vivacious and happy. She looked like a strong, well-built woman, and her tanned and ruddy complexion made her appear younger and much healthier than she actually was. She laughed often, and, even when she was serious, her eyes twinkled as though she were ready to break out into laughter.

Mr. Legendre was sitting on the bed holding Mrs. Legendre's hand. He was a rather short, strong-looking man. His sunburnt, weather-beaten complexion led one to think that he worked outdoors a lot. He was a quiet man who didn't smile or laugh as much as his wife. Whereas Mrs. Legendre chatted animatedly and easily, Mr. Legendre looked at the floor when he spoke or just simply stared ahead. He often seemed thoughtful, sometimes hesitating before answering a question. His slightly drawn face often showed sadness and concern when the conversation revolved around his wife's illness. When Mrs. Legendre seemed to be in pain, he would rub her back or massage the back of her neck and shoulders. They often sat together just holding hands.

That day the atmosphere in the room felt warm and serene. Mrs. Legendre's family had brought in pillows, bedcovers, pictures, and mementos from home, as all families on the PCU were encouraged to do. The Legendres, however, had gone further than most families; they filled the walls with family photographs, scenic posters, religious pictures, and Catholic icons. A crucifix hung over the bed, and a large photograph of the Legendres' grandson, André, stood on the night table.

André was the eight-year-old son of the Legendres' daughter Josée, who spent much of her time in Europe. Despite the long distance between them, André occupied a very special place in his grandmother's life. This may have been because the Legendres had lost a son in infancy, and when André was born it was as if their loss had been made good. Mrs. Legendre saw herself as one of André's teachers, a source of special wisdom and experience for him.

Pinned onto the back of Mrs. Legendre's door was a large, poster-sized map of the Milky Way with several red stickers on it in the shape of stars. Periodically a new red sticker would appear on the map, and, after a while, I saw that the map was quite full of stickers, each with someone's name written on it. For her the map "had a very special purpose," which was clearly connected to her death. The map showed the constellations of the stars, and the red stickers represented all the people who were surrounding her. "Those people will always be close, we will always be running in the same constellation . . . so we cannot say death is the end, but the beginning of something," she explained. After my third visit, Mrs. Legendre asked me to take a red sticker from her night table, put my name on it, and place it on the map.

Mrs. Legendre told me that she was ready to die. Why did she look so bright and happy? "Because I am going to a beautiful place," she explained. "There is a place I am close to in Italy called Monte Stelle—'Monte' for the mountain and 'Stelle' for the star—and between the two peaks of the mountain, there is a bright, bright star." She believed that her soul "would go and get installed on that bright star" and that every time people thought of her she would be glistening there. That is how she would remain close to her loved ones.

The religious beliefs Mrs. Legendre expressed were an eclectic mix of traditional Catholicism and personal and idiosyncratic ideas, such as when she spoke about becoming a shining star in the galaxy. She spoke with assurance, firmly believing that what she had worked out in her mind was true for both herself and all people. For the Legendre family her beliefs also rang true. The family had asked their mother "to give a code or something" so they could be in touch when she had gone. "That's where my mother came out with this most extraordinary plan," Lily said, referring to the map of the galaxy and to all the named stickers surrounding her star. "My mother is going to come back and watch over us, so you see she will always be with us. I feel very comfortable with the idea of my mother visiting all of us after she dies, and I don't doubt it."

During a time when André was in Montreal, he told the PCU psychologist that he would be able to keep a spiritual contact with his grandmother by means of a star (as well as through a pendant she had given to him, which he would keep forever as a symbol of their close bond). Lily added, "It would give continuity. You know that saying—'in the world, something is created, nothing is destroyed . . . matter can be transformed but never destroyed.'"

Acceptance or Denial?

Mrs. Legendre's doctors, nurses, and other caregivers did not know how to interpret her beliefs and her way of preparing for death. They were grappling with a challenge in caring for Mrs. Legendre that was, as in the care of many palliative care patients, more confusing and complicated than the management of her physical symptoms. How should they respond to Mrs. Legendre's serene and calm acceptance of imminent death? Her attitude was particularly puzzling to some of the staff because it abruptly followed the Legendres' ferocious pursuit of a cure. Were the staff witnessing a profound transformation in Mrs. Legendre's attitudes and outlook, or was her serenity a façade? Should they attempt to probe beneath the surface in case Mrs. Legendre was denying her true situation?

Whatever their private suspicions, outwardly the team fully supported Mrs. Legendre's needs and wishes. More and more stickers appeared on her galaxy map, most being placed there by caregivers. A nurse or volunteer might give Mrs. Legendre a special bit of help on a particular day, and, as that person was leaving, Mrs. Legendre would ask, "Have you put your star there yet?" To my knowledge, no person declined. Some caregivers went even further, adding their own creative contributions to Mrs. Legendre's beliefs—one of the volunteers found a poem about the constellation of the stars; the music therapist found a song called "There Is a Star for You."

While Dr. Raymond also wanted to support Mrs. Legendre, his past experience as a palliative care physician made him cautious. Her dying was almost too easy. Everything was planned out, and he saw no sign of any sadness or regret that her illness was now truly terminal. Why the sudden change to full acceptance of dying? He thought it was important to "really listen attentively to what was happening" and asked the psychologist to have a talk with Mrs. Legendre. The psychologist described the patient as "healthy with a good outlook" on her coming death. Her notes from this visit read,

> She has a very special spiritual way of seeing her death. We rarely hear and witness this particular kind of rapport with death. There is a mixture of strength, peace, joy, poetry, realistic, and idealistic views. This kind of view is difficult to share as some people automatically expect to experience suffering in the process of saying good-bye.

Nonetheless, Dr. Raymond was concerned, for there was something that didn't quite fit for him. It was hard to accept Mrs. Legendre's sudden readiness to die, when, only a few day ago, with her pain under control, it had seemed so important to her to enjoy life.

To the Legendre family, the relief of Mrs. Legendre's pain and the security of being on the PCU had given Mrs. Legendre a special opportunity to organize her death. Indeed, Mrs. Legendre said that she felt "secure and safe now." She envisioned the afterlife as another dimension to the life she was leading now, but first she had to prepare for her death properly. "I'm the one who has to control and organize my death before going to the other dimensions of my life," she explained. The pastoral counselor who visited with Mrs. Legendre heard her express these thoughts, and he, too, wondered if Mrs. Legendre was not "*too* organized." He would have expected more uncertainty, more grappling with the unknown, or at least some signs of sadness at the prospect of saying final good-byes. On the other hand, he said, "She was a manager in her own life and she was managing death as though she were managing her own business."

Going Home Again

A month passed, and Mrs. Legendre did not die. It was now the first week of February 1996. She had begun to drink and then eat more, and her intestinal obstruction slowly resolved. Although she sometimes complained of pain, this was usually alleviated by morphine in varying dosages. She was comfortable enough to receive many visits from friends and family, and when she was alone she was usually chatting, often laughing, on the telephone. During a one-hour visit I made, the phone rang at least five times. While everyone seemed to like her company and it was easy to be with her, we felt as though we were all waiting with her for death to happen.

Occasionally Mrs. Legendre would cry, and she told the psychologist that she sometimes felt depressed. The psychologist's notes continue:

> We explored the fact that one can face death with trust, or healthy curiosity, and at the same time be in touch with sadness and fear. She is now in a slow process of negotiating contradictions within herself in facing the final phase. She is afraid to go back home, which in her mind represents going back to life, and again, in her mind, being here means preparation for dying, as if she would practice the act of dying ahead of time.

Ordinarily, however, Mrs. Legendre almost never talked about dying. She seemed relatively well in comparison to other patients on the unit. Mr. Legendre said, "She wants it to happen now, just now, but maybe it's up to God." Her daughters Yvonne and Lily began to feel the strain of waiting for their mother's death while also enjoying the time they still had with her. "It's hard," Lily told me at this time. "We are waiting in one way, but we don't want her to leave. We want to know she's happy and we're happy for her." She paused. "But we're feeling it, you know?"

One day, toward the middle of the month, Dr. Raymond went to see his patient to tell her he would be going away from the unit for a week. "I won't be here when you get back," Mrs. Legendre responded. Michael tried to convince her that, in truth, she was not dying that fast. "Loss of control is terrible," he reflected later. "You need to be able to make plans even if it is to die. It's very difficult to abandon that."

When I talked with Mrs. Legendre during the week that Michael was away, she didn't seem quite as radiant and spontaneous as before. She still smiled, but it seemed to be an effort. Mrs. Legendre missed Michael's presence on the unit, even it if was only for a week. She remembered his talk with her before he left and she seemed to be thinking about it. "Dr. Raymond understands me," she said. Moreover, she trusted him. He was "human and kind" with a "good philosophy;" he was "a very extraordinary man."

A naturally open and sociable woman, she had started to get to know some of the other patients and their families. "I feel sorry for them," she said, "to see them suffer, and you feel bad for the families." The unit was busier than usual; there had been 21 deaths on the unit in the past 17 days. Gentle crying, sometimes sobbing, could be heard in the hallway not too far from Mrs. Legendre's room.

When Dr. Raymond returned, Mrs. Legendre informed him that she had thought her situation over. "It is not time to die yet," she said. She wanted to go home. On February 20, Mrs. Legendre returned to her home in the Bahamas. I spoke to her on the telephone from time to time over the next several weeks, and she sounded active and happy, "busy driving my car and enjoying the ocean." Michael kept in close touch with the Legendres and observed, "She doesn't see herself as sick anymore. The last time I talked to her she was giggling, laughing, busy in her house, doing her household chores."

Mrs. Legendre began to talk again about treatment to arrest her cancer. The PCU was far from her thoughts now, though she still relied heavily on Dr. Raymond's support. In her mind she had moved into a new and different place, and it was as if I, and our project, had become part of an old memory. Her talks with me were still enthusiastic but they were now totally centered on pursuing the means to live "by any way possible." She laughed a lot during our conversations. "My tummy is full of tumor," she said. "I look nine months pregnant and my feet are swollen." But she felt good. "The morphine is working!"

"Dying a Third Time"

In May, Mrs. Legendre came back to her home in Quebec and immediately contacted Dr. Singer to get information about an experimental "vaccine" she had learned about from a television program. He offered to find out what he could. At the same time, he contacted Michael Raymond, who was still managing Mrs. Legendre's symptoms. Mrs. Legendre was experiencing more abdominal pain and swelling in her legs. Michael suggested a readmission to the PCU. Mrs. Legendre agreed to go back to the unit to try to relieve her symptoms, but she still wanted to pursue information regarding the new treatment. At least she might get one more winter in the Bahamas and she could spend most of it with André.

Mrs. Legendre returned to the unit on May 18, and Dr. Singer and Dr. Raymond began to work as a team. Dr. Singer was experimenting with a new cytotoxic chemotherapy agent, and he arranged for Mrs. Legendre to receive the drug. Dr. Raymond continued to try to manage her symptoms, using large doses of diuretics to try to relieve her massive leg and abdominal swelling. Although the swelling was reduced, her pain got worse. It was unclear whether this was a side effect of the chemotherapy or whether it was from growth of her tumor. Whatever the reason, her symptoms became very difficult to manage at this point. She vomited and suffered intense abdominal pain that her nurse Ena described as "horrible to watch." Ena would go into her room to find her screaming, crying, holding onto her stomach. All Ena could do was to sit with her, rub her abdomen or back, or apply a heating pad. She felt helpless, but Mrs. Legendre would look up at her appreciatively through her pain. Later she would smile and even laugh in spite of her pain, saying, "I don't care what it takes. Something is still being done."

Jean, a volunteer who had worked with Mrs. Legendre, also noticed an air of defiance, even joy, despite Mrs. Legendre's symptoms. For example, when Jean saw that the room was no longer elaborately decorated with the posters and the map of the galaxy and asked Mrs. Legendre where the decorations were, Mrs. Legendre replied, "Well, I'm not going to die, so I know I'll go back home and so I don't need to decorate."

Dr. Raymond not only cooperated with Dr. Singer in managing Mrs. Legendre's symptoms, he also often took Mrs. Legendre's side in urging Dr. Singer to continue an aggressive treatment plan, sensing how much it meant to her to feel she was actively fighting her disease. While this approach permitted Mrs. Legendre to benefit from palliative and active treatment simultaneously, everyone paid a price for it. Mrs. Legendre paid in the form of her intense suffering, though at this point it was a price she was willing to pay. Dr. Raymond and the others on the palliative care team had to witness Mrs. Legendre's suffering, which they believed would prove futile in the long run.

And they had to remain on the tense boundary between the goals and effects of active treatment and palliative care, experiencing the intense ambivalence inherent in Mrs. Legendre' situation.

Mrs. Legendre saw what was happening to those around her. "I know Ena doesn't want me to suffer and I know my family doesn't want to see it and I know it hurts my husband," she told me, "but I want to take this drug as long as they will give it. I want to take up all possibilities [of experimentation] and the doctors do have them."

Ena felt a special closeness to her patient. She felt she understood her and wanted to protect her. Yet it often took a special effort for Ena not to react personally to Mrs. Legendre's anger, especially when, in the last few weeks of her life, Mrs. Legendre became very demanding and short-tempered. One day, as Mrs. Legendre asked Ena to help her into the bathroom, Mrs. Legendre looked up at her and asked, "Are all your patients like me?" "What do you mean?" Ena replied. "Oh," Mrs. Legendre said, "demanding." Ena answered, "You're not demanding. You're going through a rough time. And everyone is different." As far as Ena was concerned, her own reactions were beside the point. "I never let her feel that I felt that," Ena recalled. "Because I don't know how I would feel to be dying a third time."

Sometimes Mrs. Legendre expressed anger and frustration toward her doctors, feeling that they had been too hesitant to prescribe or search out more experimental therapies. When further treatments were not immediately forthcoming, she sometimes expressed a feeling of injustice. She "felt abandoned," she claimed, and "not listened to." One day she complained bitterly to me, "I feel like they [the doctors] don't give a damn for me. I'm here to die and that's it and so let's pass to the next one."

One day Mrs. Legendre asked Dr. Singer why he had not responded to her request for treatment earlier. "Why do you turn your back on me?" she said. When he tried to explain how risky any further treatments were in light of her very advanced disease, she replied, "I know I'm a bad risk . . . but I'm just 54 years old. . . . You see, I have the energy inside. I have to stop those tumors." Then she told Dr. Singer, "You know what? My ashes will come back to haunt you if I die and the day after they discover something good for tumors!"

Mr. Legendre also paid a price for his wife's determination to fight. One day early in June I saw him crying openly in the hallway as he walked toward the elevators. He stopped for a moment to say, "You shouldn't go into her room right now. My wife is very bad, to watch her suffer like that, to look in her face, it is too difficult." Watching his wife scream out in pain was unbearable; he couldn't stay in the room. He would come back later.

Later that same day, Mr. Legendre reflected more on his wife's condition. Her choice to put herself through the anguish and pain puzzled him. "I don't know why she has to go on suffering, she's been through so much already," he said. "You just go on watching her suffer, but she doesn't want to give up." He went on, "She's a strong woman, and always very determined. But I don't know why she wants to go through all this . . . too much suffering. . . it's not humane."

Meanwhile, Dr. Raymond was observing his patient closely and trying to manage her pain the best he could. He felt that her pain was more than physical, that she had "total anguish" as she now truly faced the reality of dying. In addition, Mrs. Legendre had always been a woman to whom physical appearance was important. It was very difficult for her to accept the swelling and the other physical changes that were occurring. Mrs. Legendre had been able to share some of her feeling with Dr. Raymond: "She was feeling more and more disfigured," Michael recalled, "all that was very difficult for her." At the same time, she continued to have hopes of remission. But the treatments did not work.

Trying to Control the End

On June 14, Mrs. Legendre went home for a short period, but she had to come back to the PCU two weeks later because of her steadily worsening abdominal pain and the swelling in her legs. When I went to see her on the unit this time, a sign on her door confronted me: "No Visitors Please. Please Ask the Primary Nurse." I requested to see Mrs. Legendre when I saw Linda, her nurse for that day. Linda knew Mrs. Legendre was not doing well. Her breathing was more difficult now, and she needed oxygen most of the time.

"She seems to have given up this time around," Linda said. "She's different—not so feisty, and it's like she feels there's no hope anymore. She's not fighting." Mr. Legendre was finding it hard also, Linda said. "He feels there is very little hope, and that waiting there, just waiting, is long and painful." Linda mentioned that Mr. Legendre was now talking about selling their house in the Bahamas and tidying up their affairs.

I knocked gently on Mrs. Legendre's door and entered the room. The walls were nearly bare, so different from the richly adorned walls I had seen seven months ago. There were no decorations from home: no pictures or photographs, no map or stars—nothing except some pictures the unit provided. The room was large, bright, and spacious, but at that moment it seemed clinical and lifeless. There was something forlorn and lonely about the woman who lay flat on the bed with her eyes closed, breathing quietly with oxygen prongs in her nose. After a few moments, Mrs. Legendre opened her eyes and looked at me. "It's no good," she said. "I'm not going to make it this time. This is it. They couldn't do it. They couldn't get me the drugs. There's nothing left for me . . . no hope." She pointed to her stomach. "I can feel the tumor here. I can feel it pressing. It's pressing on my chest and I'm having trouble breathing. I just don't think I can go on like this anymore."

Mrs. Legendre was very weak now and almost completely bedbound. Though her physicians were able to control her pain, she began to have periods when she would lose complete control of her bowel functions. "An absolute affront to her dignity," her husband said. She began to talk openly about wanting her doctors to help her die. On July 8, she asked Dr. Marie Clermont, a fellow in training on the PCU, to give her something to end her life. Marie explained that she was unable to do that. Euthanasia was illegal, he said, and beyond that, Mrs. Legendre was so weak at this point that it was not possible to have an extended conversation with her to explore the meanings and ramifications of her request. What Maurice could offer, however, was to help her sleep comfortably, so she would not suffer.

This was not good enough for Mrs. Legendre. She had made another decision. She told Linda, "I'm as good as dead. I want them to give me something so I can go now." Just as she had decided to fight for her life despite all the odds, and before that, to take her leave and settle among the stars, now she had decided the fight was over and it was time to die—now.

Sedation or Euthanasia?

For the next 10 days, Mr. Legendre fluctuated between demands for immediate action to help his wife die and equally fervent hopes that chemotherapy would extend her life. In the last week of July, Dr. Raymond had to be absent from the unit, and Mary Thompson, another palliative care physician, took over Mrs. Legendre's care. Mary was an experienced palliative care physician who had cared for people with terminal illnesses for many years. Patients and families liked her and expressed confidence in her. She was easy for the

Legendres to talk to—"caring, a good listener, kind. You felt secure with her," Mr. Legendre later recalled.

Dr. Thompson got to know the Legendres over a period of a few days. During this time Mrs. Legendre's breathing had become worse. Mary believed that this was probably due to pulmonary emboli and that Mrs. Legendre would probably not live more than another week or two. Mary also felt that when Mrs. Legendre said, "This is it, I can't take it anymore," she was expressing her frustration, the affront to her dignity caused by the loss of control of her bowels, and the anxiety of her increasing shortness of breath. Mrs. Legendre had not asked Dr. Thompson directly for help to die, though she had readily agreed to Mary's suggestion that she be made to sleep so she would not experience respiratory distress or anxiety. Mary's offer was to provide Mrs. Legendre with "palliative sedation," which was not the same as complying with her earlier request to Dr. Clermont to just "end it." Dr. Thompson could give Mrs. Legendre the drug midazolam and maintain her in a state of sleep from which she could be aroused, if necessary, to permit further interaction with her family, though only if she could tolerate being awake without an increase in suffering from her symptoms.

Mary discussed her plan with Mr. Legendre and the Legendres' daughters, Lily and Yvonne, on August 2. She said that she herself had not received a specific request from Mrs. Legendre to do anything beyond helping her sleep. She related to the family that Dr. Clermont had received such a request and explained why Marie believed he could not agree to it. Dr. Thompson also observed that, while there certainly appeared to have been some days when Mrs. Legendre was so frustrated by her struggle that she just wanted to give up and have it all come to an end, there were other times when she still hoped to gain a little more time to live.

Mr. Legendre said he found it very hard to witness his wife's discomfort. There were some very difficult times, he believed, when euthanasia was the best possible course of action. He remembered, in relation to other family members, when it would have been best for them if they hadn't been forced to stay alive. (In Mr. Legendre's mind, refusing to grant his wife's request for euthanasia seemed to be the same as "forcing her to stay alive.") Both he and Mrs. Legendre had watched her mother and father being kept alive by artificial tubes even though there was no hope for recovery. "That was totally unnecessary suffering," he said, "it was not humane."

Dr. Thompson explained that the medicines they would give Mrs. Legendre would keep her comfortably sedated so that she would not suffer from either respiratory distress or general anguish. Yet the sedatives would allow for her to wake up at any time so she would be able to communicate with her loved ones. She wouldn't be unconscious or so heavily sedated that she could not awaken. It might still be possible in a good, comfortable moment to have a brief conversation, perhaps to speak some last thoughts. And it allowed for any of her family to say things they needed to say to her.

Mr. Legendre and his daughters agreed to the sedation, though they were adamant that Mrs. Legendre not suffer. Mr. Legendre was especially concerned about the possibility of his wife's choking when her last hours came. Even if it were only for two seconds, he said, that was really her worst worry. Dr. Raymond had assured Mr. Legendre that they could almost certainly prevent that from happening, and Dr. Thompson repeated this reassurance now. She said she would go ahead and give Mrs. Legendre the midazolam.

The Last Hours of Life

Mrs. Legendre's physical condition rapidly deteriorated over the next two days. She became more short of breath, so Dr. Thompson increased the midazolam dose. Her daughters, Yvonne, Lily, and Marie, traveled from their respective homes to be at their mother's bedside. Mr. Legendre was there all the time. They sat together in Mrs. Legendre's room for hours. They brought food and warmed it in the kitchen. They tried to relax in the lounge, where they met other people going through a similar experience. As Marie recalled to me later, it sometimes just helped to talk to someone who was "going through the same kind of sorrow." Mr. Legendre telephoned their fourth daughter, Josée, at her home in Paris and told her of the gravity of her mother's condition. Josée arranged to travel to Montreal as soon as she could.

On August 4, Dr. Thompson came to Mrs. Legendre's bedside and found her sleeping peacefully. Her breathing had been made easier with the drug scopolamine, which helped to reduce the secretions in her upper respiratory tract. Lily was at the foot of the bed and seemed relaxed. Mrs. Legendre's brother came to say goodbye. Now all the family were there except for Josée, who was delayed on the last part of her journey from Paris. Josée had telephoned and said she would make it to the hospital within the next two hours. Mrs. Legendre had asked for Josée several times in the last days. Mr. Legendre moved closer to his wife and said, "Try and wait. Hang in. Stick with it. Josée is on her way. She just called me." But his wife shook her head. "I can't wait," she said, and died a few minutes later.

The family stayed in the room with Mrs. Legendre's body for about three hours after she died. Josée arrived during this time. "It was not painful to see her dead," Mr. Legendre recalled. "She had a smile on her face. She always had that same smile on her face, even after she had gone."

Looking Back

I spoke with members of Mrs. Legendre's family several times in the months following her death. Despite their uncertainties about Mrs. Legendre's wishes for euthanasia, and the periods of great suffering she endured during her last fight against her disease, the family expressed genuine satisfaction and gratitude for the way Mrs. Legendre had died. To Mr. Legendre, his wife had died in a way that was ideal. "She died the way I'd like to go," he said to me: dying in the company of all one's loved ones and surrounded by kind and caring people. He felt that at the end his wife had not suffered as her father had, which had been one of their greatest fears. "The way they were doing things [on the Palliative Care Unit], that was good for her and good, 100%, for us. You know people are going to die anyway when they are there. They are ready for it. I knew my wife was going to die . . . even about eight days before. But to take such good care, right up to the last moment of death like that, it was marvelous."

In another conversation months later, when Josée was also present, Mr. Legendre returned to the same theme. Having the palliative care support "was a big thing for us," he said. There was a difference, he thought, between dying in a hospital and dying on the unit. "Because on the Palliative Care Unit," he explained, "you know what happens and the moment, almost the moment, that it happens. You don't panic because you know what will happen ahead of time from the people who are specially trained to do the job. It is an enormous help. Maybe as a family, yes, you are suffering [because you are losing somebody], but with that support, you are sure everything will go well."

Mr. Legendre also reminded me of Mrs. Legendre's wishes and plans for life after death. She had made her last plans calmly and without fear, he said. Mrs. Legendre had wanted to be cremated. She wanted to have her ashes placed in Italy, close to Monte Stelle, the mountain she had often spoken about when she first came to the Palliative Care Unit. "That's what I did," Mr.

Legendre said. "I took her ashes to Italy and I put them there. Everything was orchestrated to be like that."

She knew exactly what would happen, he continued, and it was clear that at the very end she had no fear. "She gave that big smile, a beautiful smile, and that's how it stayed," he concluded. "She died the way I'd like to go when I die. Because I'll die with all my people around me, the way she did. And I'll be looking at them and saying goodbye."

Authors' Comments

In the past 25 years, palliative oncologic treatments have become almost universal. Patients often receive treatments to try to control tumor growth until the last weeks of life. Therefore, palliative care has become more and more integrated within oncology practice, with the patient benefitting from the expertise of both services. This requires good communication among the professionals involved, as exemplified by Dr. Raymond and Dr. Singer in this narrative.

We do not have details of the many discussions that must have ensued between them following Mrs. Legendre's change of mind regarding her care. Nevertheless, it is clear that each physician worked through and beyond his personal and professional philosophy and approach to care. However it was done, both physicians managed to eliminate any potential communication problems such as control issues, competition, or power plays in favor of joint problem-solving, mutual understanding, and open communication in the pursuit of common goals.

As her terminal illness progressed, Mrs. Legendre asked for euthanasia. At the time, euthanasia, now known as medical aid in dying (MAID) in Canada, was still criminalized. Even if euthanasia had been legal, the person must be competent when making the demand. Mrs. Legendre would probably not have been eligible for MAID even today unless she had made the request earlier, when she was more alert and aware. *Would* she have made the request earlier? We cannot know. In fact, Mrs. Legendre received palliative sedation with a benzodiazepine, midazolam. In the terms currently used in Quebec, besides MAID there are "intermittent sedation" and "continuous palliative sedation." In the latter case, where the person is sedated until they die, regulatory bodies now ask for prior written consent from the patient or their proxy. Although exceptions could be defended, continuous sedation is only meant to be administered when prognosis is in the order of a couple of weeks or less.

Some have argued that there is little or no difference, clinically or morally, between continuous palliative sedation and active euthanasia, even referring to the former as "slow euthanasia."[1] Family members, especially, may ask why, once the decision has been taken to maintain the patient in a continuous state of sedation, and thus unable to eat or drink as well, they and the patient must endure a prolonged period of waiting for the inevitable end. Would it not be more "humane," as Mr. Legendre expressed it, to bring the dying process to an immediate conclusion? These questions become more acute in an environment of legal MAID.

A full analysis of this complicated ethical issue is beyond the scope of this commentary. I can, however, offer these thoughts. First, I think I speak for my colleagues when I say that continuous palliative sedation does not feel like aiding suicide, or euthanasia, to those of us who provide it. The matter of *intent*—to maintain comfort, as opposed to ending life—seems to be the crucial factor for those who maintain the distinction. Second, intermittent sedation, but not active euthanasia, seems more commensurate with the frequently encountered ambivalence and uncertainty in both patients and families when they deliberate about MAID. Even Mr. Legendre, who at points was pleading with the palliative care team to bring his wife's suffering to an end *now,* pleaded equally fervently with her to "Try and wait. Hang in. Stick with it," when their daughter was en route to the hospital in the very last hours of Mrs. Legendre's life. Following Mrs. Legendre's death, her husband seemed satisfied that the sedation had prevented her from suffering the way his own father had suffered at the end of his life, without the benefit of palliative care.

Reference

1. Billings JA, Block SD. Slow euthanasia. J Palliat Care. 1996;12(4):21–30.

7

Shamira Cook

"I Want People to Know Who I Am"

Narrated by Yanna Lambrinidou

Shamira Cook, a poor, Black, single mother with a history of heroin addiction, was 34 years old when diagnosed with cancer. She saw her illness as an urgent call to share her story with the world and set the record
straight on who she really was. She was also determined to do everything
possible to extend her life. For some members of her hospice team, her
unwillingness to surrender to the institutionally preferred plan of care
was a challenge. It raised questions about whether she understood the
gravity of her condition, and it created disagreements about whether she
was "hospice-appropriate" or a "drain" on the system. Underneath the
tensions that arose lay conflicting ideologies about hospice's obligation to
patients who do not fit the dominant patient profile. Is it to "nudge" them
into an end-of-life path that complies with institutional ideals or to accompany them on a journey that might be less familiar to hospice staff but
that grants them more control? This case offers a glimpse of end-of-life
care when institutions take positions that contradict the patient's wishes.
It also raises questions about institutional racism and classism as well as
discrimination against people with substance abuse pasts.

"I Got Clean to Die"

Shamira Cook had been a heroin addict from the time she was 13. By the
age of 33, her dilapidated group home in western Pennsylvania had turned
into a crack house. She had been incarcerated several times. Her 12-year-old

daughter, Rowena, would hide every time she heard the police. Ms. Cook decided she had had enough. She moved to Lancaster County, placed Rowena in foster care, and entered a drug rehabilitation center. In February 1996, she walked out clean. She got a job at a convenience store, rented a small apartment in a subsidized housing complex, and regained custody of Rowena.

Ms. Cook relished every moment of her new life. Lancaster County came to symbolize her rebirth. She saw her transformation as a divine gift and her second chance to show herself, Rowena, and the rest of the world that she was worthy of a good life. More importantly, she saw it as her second chance to be a good mother. But the day before Christmas 1996, severe respiratory distress brought her to the emergency room. She was diagnosed with non-small-cell lung cancer with metastases in her lymph nodes, kidney, and abdomen.

Ms. Cook arranged with her next-door neighbor to look after Rowena so that she could begin inpatient chemotherapy and radiation. The radiation impeded her ability to swallow, requiring her to get a percutaneous endoscopic gastrostomy (PEG) tube for her nutrition. The chemotherapy gave her nausea and made her lose her hair. She returned home bald, weak, pale, and exhausted. Rowena was so frightened to see her that she extended her stay with the neighbor for a week.

Visits from fellow members of Ms. Cook's Narcotics Anonymous group, co-workers from the convenience store, nurses from a home care agency, and the hospital's chaplain-in-training, Yolanda Dixon, gave her comfort. Ms. Dixon, a friendly and energetic woman in her forties, met Ms. Cook at the hospital and bonded with her instantly. It did not take her long to notice that Ms. Cook rarely slept—she either cried through the night or held her eyes open for fear of dying in her sleep. Ms. Dixon promised to stand by Ms. Cook's side no matter how her illness evolved. "I worry about Shamira every day, every minute," she reflected. "When she started relaying her life to me, I realized I cannot let this woman die alone. I don't want this woman to go out of this world and people not to know the goodness of her, regardless of the badness that was there." From her second day in the hospital, Ms. Cook adopted Ms. Dixon as her advocate. She refused to make decisions without her and requested her presence every time she felt depressed.

Looking back at her life, Ms. Cook decided that it was filled with lessons, which needed passing on. She had advice for drug abusers, thoughts for cancer patients, and motherly stories for Rowena. She bought a small cassette player and a box of blank tapes, and, when she had the physical strength, she spoke memories into the recorder.

For better control of her symptoms, hospital staff offered to refer her to the Hospice of Lancaster County. On February 5, 1997, Ms. Cook, Ms. Dixon, and a hospice admission nurse met in Ms. Cook's apartment. "I got clean to die," said Ms. Cook solemnly. She proceeded to talk about her family. Her mother had passed away seven years earlier, her brother was killed two weeks after her mother's funeral, her father was absent from her life—she did not know if he was alive or dead—and her 18 half-siblings were scattered in different parts of the country. One of her sisters, Keisha, lived in neighboring Dauphin County. Because she was a hard worker and a good disciplinarian, Ms. Cook had called her to discuss transferring to her Rowena's guardianship.

Ms. Cook left a lasting impression on the hospice admission nurse. "I was overwhelmed with Shamira's courage and bravery and her awareness of what was happening to her," she told me. "At some point she took me back to her bedroom. She wanted to show me her PEG tube; then she broke down. She started to cry and apologized then for crying. I just remember saying to her that I thought she was so brave and so open. I just think she is a courageous person."

At the recommendation of Ms. Cook's attending physician, hospice nurse Elly White supplied Ms. Cook with medications for pain, anxiety, depression, nausea, and diarrhea, as well as injections of filgrastim to increase her white blood cell count. At the request of Ms. Cook, Elly locked all medications—except for the morphine she needed for breakthrough pain—in a lockbox. This way, Ms. Cook was assured that her substance-dependent friends would stay away from her prescription drugs. The hospice social worker, Barry Prout, connected Ms. Cook to a hospice volunteer. He also asked her if she wanted to participate in our project. Ms. Cook was enthusiastic about the opportunity to tell her story. The idea of helping others through her experiences gave her both pride and purpose. If her life's journey could be shared with a wider readership, she thought, she had a better chance of making a difference in the world.

I met Ms. Cook on a joint visit with Barry a week after her admission to the hospice home care program. She greeted us warmly at the top of a long flight of stairs. She was a tall, thin woman with prominent cheekbones and big, expressive eyes. A blue bandanna was tied around her head. Without wasting time, she led us to the living room, sat down on the couch, and started talking. She wanted to spend the time she had left away from drugs, so that she would be able to smell the flowers, feel the sun on her skin, and nourish a new relationship with her daughter.

"Rowena and I don't know each other," she said. "I've always been high." Rowena was acting out, skipping school, and asking her mother for large amounts of money. Ms. Cook knew no other way to show her daughter that she loved her except to give her everything she wanted. Her preference, however, was to spend "quality time" with her. It was time, she explained, to put her own pain aside and work on creating better relationships. She wanted to show the people who had hurt her, blamed her, rejected her, and lacked faith in her that she loved them. "I want people to know who I am," she asserted.

As I was listening to Ms. Cook, I found myself both moved and perplexed by her openness. She was speaking to Barry and me as if we were old friends. She was sharing with us painful, personal information without any sign of discomfort. Did her behavior mean that she trusted us? Did it signify that she was bonding with us? Or did it lack a relational quality? In her cassette tapes, she spoke about her desire to show the world that she was a good person.

In retrospect, I think that Barry, myself, and everyone else who walked into her life near its end presented her with another opportunity to start with a clean slate—to shed the parts of her past she didn't like and build herself anew as the person she wanted to be. With her permission, I quote here a composite of excerpts from her personal tape recordings:

Hi. My name is Shamira Cook. I came to Lancaster County because I wanted to get my life together. I am not using today, and I am very proud of myself. Since I have learned that I have cancer, I have not given up the fight. It is very hard. The hospitals and all of the needles and all of the tests— just so much for me to handle in such a short time. I have a lot of wonderful, caring people in my life today, such as Yolanda Dixon, who is just one of my dearest, dearest friends. Then there is the hospice team that works with me. I just feel like I am so loved and that is something that I always wanted, but I did not think that I would get it this way—being sick. But love is love, and I guess it does not matter when you get it.

I am just thinking back when I was a child how I always just wanted someone to love me. I just got beat every day, and I got beat so much that I thought it was normal. I thought it was love. I thought, "Well, if my mom is beating me, she must love me." My life was centered on drugs, sex, alcohol, lying, cheating, deceiving and whatever other slimy thing that I could do because I was an addict. And that is thanks to my father. My parents were both addicted to alcohol and drugs. I loved my father very much. I wanted to be with him all the time. That turned out to be a bad idea, because [when I was] seven he molested me and turned me onto drugs, and that went on for seven years.

They say when you are an addict you only have three things to look forward to, and that is jail, institutions, and death. For the last few days, I have not been able to pray, and I have not been able to thank God for the days of living and the days that I have not used. I don't want to go astray again. And that is so easy for me, being a recovering addict. When things get tough, I usually run, and I'm not going to do that. I want to live each day to the fullest without the use of drugs.

I don't want no enemies. I don't want to die knowing that no one likes me. With or without hair, I am still a beautiful person. I did not give up on using when I was out there, I am not going to give up on living now that I am sick. So I, myself, I choose life over death, although I know, when my Heavenly Father calls me home, I am going.

Rowena

Although she did show love for Ms. Cook, Rowena didn't seem overly attached to her. For the biggest part of her life, her mother had brought her more trouble than good. I saw Rowena only a few times. She was a tall and radiant young woman with high cheekbones and a very sweet smile. I heard that she was a troublemaker, that she got into fights with her classmates, and that she was expelled from school on a regular basis. But every time I ran into her, she either disappeared into her bedroom or sat quietly in the living room with her mother and me. What I remember of Rowena is her warmth. She was quick to smile with every affectionate comment and quick to laugh at every joke. Ms. Cook seemed to fill with joy when she saw her daughter's face light up. I lost count of the times she told me about the day when she brought Rowena to her knees with laughter by taking off her bandanna, putting a shiny earring on one ear, and proceeding to clean her entire apartment while singing the song of "Mr. Clean."

In the middle of February, Ms. Cook decided that she owed it to Rowena to host a belated Christmas dinner. Never before had she been able to do that.

"My addiction was so bad," she recalled, "at one time, I used to sell my baby's Christmas toys." Now, Shamira was going to buy a Christmas tree, Christmas ornaments, and Christmas presents, and she was going to make ham, sweet potatoes, and beans. Her guests would be Rowena, Ms. Dixon, and a few other friends. She scheduled the gathering for February 21, three days before her next chemotherapy.

"I Wish I Could Fly"

I never heard the details about the Christmas dinner. Ms. Cook became so nauseated that she wasn't able to enjoy it. Three days later, she was taken to the hospital with excruciating pain. Her oncologist, Dr. Mark Jenks, cancelled her chemotherapy and scheduled her for a computed tomography scan that revealed metastases in her retroperitoneum. The tumors in her lungs and mediastinum, however, had shrunk.

When I visited Ms. Cook at the hospital on February 25, she was lying in bed half-conscious. Her morphine had been doubled, her eyes were three-quarters of the way closed, and she was mumbling. "I am taking 21 pills a day, and that is way too much," she said. "I am tired of this. I am really tired of this. I wish I could fly." I couldn't tell if she was talking to me, or if she cared for a response. But her demeanor changed instantly when Rowena entered the room. At the sound of Rowena's voice, Ms. Cook opened her eyes and broke into a big smile. Rowena sat at the foot of the bed. Mother and daughter teased each other and laughed. "C'mon, man!" exclaimed Rowena in response to one of Ms. Cook's jokes. "How come you're calling me 'man'?" asked Ms. Cook strictly. "Do I have a beard on my face?" Rowena laughed. "Do I have a moustache?" Rowena laughed again. Still, when it was time to leave, she hopped off the bed and walked toward the door without saying goodbye. "Where do you think you're going?" asked Ms. Cook with affection. "Come over here and give me a kiss!" Playfully, Rowena approached her, kissed her on the cheek, and left.

On March 10, Dr. Jenks told Ms. Cook that most of the areas to which her cancer had metastasized were inoperable. During our interview two days later she reflected that, "Two years ago, if I would have found I had cancer, I would have been dead. I would have overdosed myself. I would have went and got me a bag of dope, shot it up—all the liquor and beer I could get. See, that is the first thing we do as addicts when we cannot handle something or something is not going right in our life: we go get high." The phone rang and interrupted us. Ms. Cook answered to the screams of an angry mother on the other end of the line who informed her that Rowena had just hit her child with a bag of ice. The caller threatened to beat up not only Rowena but also Ms. Cook. Shamira put down the phone in dismay. In her tape that day, she said,

> I need to say that I have been having a hard time with my child and her acting out in different ways, because she does not understand, really, what I'm going through. That reminds me of when I was a child, when my mom was busy drinking and drugging and not having time for me. I feel as though, since I have been sick, it is like I have been paying myself a lot more attention than I have her, even though I'm not using. It seems like we don't really have a relationship going on, and that is something that I really want, because like I said, only God knows how much time I have left here. I just feel helpless and one thing I have learned by doing the First Step before is that I am really powerless right now, and I need to keep my health together, if not for me, for Rowena.

Several hospice nurses wondered why Ms. Cook insisted on chemotherapy when it compromised the quality of her life. A few suspected that she was in denial. Others expressed a more nuanced view. "She knows that she has a terminal disease," said one nurse, "but I don't know if she has a real hard-and-fast awareness that she is going to die. There is probably some denial there, and I have to say that maybe the system is almost feeding into it somewhat. I asked the attending physician when I first met Shamira what his thoughts were as far as prognosis, and he said, 'Probably about three months, but I would not tell the patient that.'"

Chloe Maxwell, Ms. Cook's personal care nurse, spent hours watching television with her, discussing topics that concerned her, and lifting up her spirits with humor. She recalled,

> The first time I met Shamira she said, "You can come in, but I don't want you to talk to me about dying because every time the other nurses [from a previous home care agency] came here they never, ever gave me hope. It was always, 'You are dying, you are dying, you are dying.' If I want to talk about it, fine. You can be open with me. But I don't always want to hear I am dying because I still need hope."

The nurses were particularly concerned about how Ms. Cook would cope when her needs increased. Ms. Dixon said that she would take her into her own home. Although she hadn't secured her family's permission to do that, she was confident that her proposal was feasible. Barry was impressed by Ms. Dixon's commitment, but he also worried that her offer might have been an indication of an unhealthy "enmeshment" with Shamira. Did Yolanda realize what she getting herself into?

"She Had to Be a Survivor to Get Where She Was"

On March 21, mother and daughter had a fight. In the heat of the argument, Rowena left. Panicked, Ms. Cook decided that she didn't have the strength to raise Rowena and that it was time to let her go. She called Keisha to ask if she could take Rowena in. That evening, she vomited uncontrollably. She reported severe abdominal pain and dysuria. In the morning, when Rowena returned home, she found her mother in unbearable pain. Yolanda was out of town, so a family friend gave her a ride to the emergency room. A doctor assessed that she had either a urinary tract infection or further metastasis. He performed a urine test and gave her medications for pain. Ms. Cook's Baptist pastor, Rev. Anthony Johnson, took her back home. An African American community leader in his fifties, Rev. Johnson had never spent time with Ms. Cook before. But he knew about her and had held prayer for her at church.

On March 23, Keisha brought Rowena to her home in Dauphin County, about 40 miles away. The next day, Ms. Cook was rehospitalized at the recommendation of her oncologist, Dr. Jenks. A scan showed that her retroperitoneal metastases had increased greatly. It was clear to Dr. Jenks that the chemotherapy had not worked. Upon hearing the news, Ms. Cook appeared accepting. But she announced that she wanted to continue with her treatment. More than ever, she was interested in any interventions that had the potential to prolong her life. Surprised by her calmness and concerned that she was in denial, a medical resident asked the hospital psychologist to see her for an evaluation. The hospital social worker had a different view. "[Shamira] had to be a survivor to get where she was," she said, "so she did not lay in bed and ask for pity. She knew she was sick and would recognize it, but then not focus on it. I don't know how you can be in denial when people keep telling you what is wrong. I mean, she was alert enough to hear it—how she chose to interpret it, I think, would be more of a coping way, not a denial way."

With encouragement from Barry, the hospice social worker, and Elly, the hospice nurse, Ms. Cook contemplated leaving her apartment. If indeed she was in need of round-the-clock care, where would she prefer to go? Ms. Dixon had already told Barry that she wasn't going to be able to take Ms. Cook in after all, because her husband had recently lost a young relative and wasn't ready to relive another death. Barry and Elly encouraged Ms. Cook to consider a nursing home. The inpatient unit of hospice was not an option for her because she continued to desire chemotherapy and cardiopulmonary resuscitation. Ms. Cook told me that the idea of moving to an extended-care facility at the age of 34 shocked her. But if she were to rely solely on hospice, she would need to give up aggressive treatments and would die. She felt torn. Hesitantly, she asked Barry to help her fill out an application for the nearest nursing home.

"Do I Look Like I Need 24-Hour Care to You?"

"Shamira feels as if decisions are being made behind her back," Ms. Dixon said to me when she returned to Lancaster. "She does not want to die in an institution. She has made that very clear. I hate nursing homes. I would personally like to see her stay in [her] apartment if that is where she wants to be. If we have to set a 24-hour vigil with all the people that I know, we will do that."

On the eve of her hospital discharge, Ms. Cook asked Elly if, once she were to enter a nursing home, she would be allowed back home. Like all members of Ms. Cook's hospice team, Elly saw Shamira's potential transfer as permanent. She realized, however, that her patient wasn't ready for this perspective, so she recommended that she take one day at a time. Ms. Cook exploded in anger. "You never say what I want to hear!" she cried. Later, Elly said,

> I truly empathize with her. She says she wants to deal with reality, but she does not really want to. It is sort of like a no-win situation, and I know that anger is part of the grieving process. I mean, she has to go through this anger before she can reach acceptance. I try not to be negative, but I also would not play into what she wanted to hear, and that just made her furious. I don't think that we could any longer follow her if she stays in her apartment, because it would be an unsafe situation. I am not sure her physician

would follow her. We try to follow what a patient wants, but in this case, because of the circumstances of her life, it may not be possible.

On April 1, Ms. Cook was discharged from the hospital, but because the nursing home had still not reached a financial agreement with her medical assistance program, she returned home. She was delighted to be back in her apartment. She assured Barry that she understood the severity of her condition, but she emphasized that she wanted to live positively. Again and again, she declared that she wasn't ready to move to a nursing home. Sandy Glass, her hospice volunteer, took this statement to mean that she didn't realize she was dying. "I let her have her fantasy," she said. "I figure that she is entitled to that. She is 34 years old, and this is a hard enough thing to be dealing with. One day I did say that death is something we must all face, and then I dropped it. I did not want to depress her."

The following day, Ms. Cook's pain was under control. She felt so well that she decided to go shopping. But first she called Elly to apologize for her outburst. When I visited her, she was in a hurry to visit Rowena in Dauphin County. Excitedly, she led me to her bedroom and showed me her new outfit—green athletic pants with a matching jacket and a pair of white sneakers. Without notifying her friends, her neighbor, Ms. Dixon, or hospice, she arranged for a taxi to take her to the bus station. I was struck by the quickness with which she erased her caretakers from her mind. Although she appreciated their help, it was as if she wished that they, like her cancer, were part of a bad dream she could leave behind. When I asked her about her pain crisis, she started to cry. "I thought I was going to die," she said. And she continued,

> That is the scariest feeling, because when you have a disease, like I have that cannot be cured and it is spreading, it is very scary. They kept throwing hospice at me, like that is where they wanted me to go, but see, when you go to hospice you have to be getting ready to die, and when you go there, they stop all your treatment, and all they do is pain management until you die. One of the nurses from hospice kept pushing the nursing home on me, because she felt like I needed more care—24-hour care. Do I look like I need 24-hour care to you? I don't think so! This nurse has gotten overprotective of me. Every time I am feeling good and I tell her how wonderful I feel, she is like, "Well, you know that you can get sicker. . . ." I know that! I have a

serious disease of cancer. I know it is serious! That is why I'm doing everything in my power right now to keep my health up!

Ms. Cook's outlook elicited strong reactions from hospice staff. Some nurses stated that if she was indeed averse to the idea of receiving only palliative care, hospice had no role in her life. If all that Ms. Cook wanted was someone to fill her pill box, another nurse agreed, then a home health agency would serve her better. Other staff believed that Ms. Cook was both hospice-appropriate and realistic; she had a right to die in the way that she saw fit, even if that involved avoidable hospitalizations and preventable pain crises. They felt that some of her caregivers were trying to push Ms. Cook to decisions more in keeping with an institutional ideology of "the good death" than with her own values. One nurse said,

> I just think not all cases go smoothly. I mean, I know there is probably going to be a crisis again, but that is Shamira's choice, and I think we just have to deal with that. She wants to be able to focus on what living she has left. She knows she is going to die. She does not need someone coming into her room and telling her, "You are going to a nursing home, and you are not going to come out." I certainly do not feel that we should pull out [of her care]. She is terminally ill. I think we need to realize that when we walk into families there are problems that have been there a long, long time, and we are not going to be able to fix that. Not all cases are going to be your white, middle-class, *Leave It to Beaver* or *Ozzie and Harriet* family. So part of me is really frustrated when they say she is not hospice-appropriate just because she does not do exactly what we tell her to do.

I asked Dr. Jenks for his opinion. He said that in cancer care the distinction between "palliative" and "curative" is not always meaningful. In Ms. Cook's case, for example, her cancer was incurable. It was not going to go away with treatments. But this didn't mean that it was untreatable. He told me that her chance for complete remission was less than 5% and for partial remission, between 25% and 30%. Therefore, the prolongation of her life was a possibility, albeit slim. I never learned if Mark had shared these numbers with Ms. Cook, but I could see why she seemed to like him. In his words, I heard hope.

When Ms. Cook told Felicia Johnson, Rev. Johnson's wife, that Elly squelched her optimism, Ms. Johnson called hospice. Shamira knew she was dying, Ms. Johnson said, but she was not yet ready to stop fighting for her life.

Ms. Johnson told me, "We know Shamira is terminal; Shamira knows she is terminal; but Shamira is not *being* terminal; she is not dying right at this moment. I think when hospice goes into a home [they should] assess it: assess the needs, assess where the people are, assess where the families are, and don't come in with their preconceived ideas of how it ought to be."

"Don't Ever, *Ever* Come to Me with Negative Shit No More"

Upon her return from Dauphin County, Ms. Cook was informed that Chloe, her personal care nurse, had been removed from her case. Since she was able to meet her basic needs, hospice deemed personal care services unnecessary. She was assured, however, that if this were to change, Chloe would come back. Shamira liked Chloe and would miss her. "So I have to act like I'm dying to get you back?" she asked Chloe in frustration.

When I visited her a few days later, Ms. Cook rummaged through her drawers to find an enlarged photograph of her and Rowena. It had been taken two years earlier at the drug rehabilitation center. Shamira had a full head of hair and wore a colorful outfit. For her, this picture symbolized victory: her triumph over her addiction and her reunification with her child. Now, Ms. Cook said, the mere thought of hospice brought a "black cloud" over her head.

> I know God is not going to take me away yet, because I do not think I was put here to live the life that I lived. I think He had better plans for me. That is another reason why I hate to be around the negative hospice nurses. I had agreed to go into the nursing home until Elly said I might not come out. I don't need that negative crap, even if I won't be put in remission! Let me live the rest of my life, whatever it might be, in peace!
>
> Elly thinks that I think I'm going to get better and better. I know better than that! I know that cancer is a very serious disease! Especially since I have it in my lungs, I got it in my kidney, now something is going on in my stomach and my back. What makes her think that I am that naïve or that damn stupid that I am not thinking about the death part either? How does she know how I feel when I am here by myself at night? How many nights I have cried myself to sleep? How many times I have asked God to have mercy on me because I am not ready to die? I told her, "Don't ever, *ever* come to me with negative shit no more." So, *shoot!* They better leave me alone!

A Tense Team Meeting at Hospice

The following week, Ms. Cook's fatigue increased. She reported severe pain in her back. Every day she appeared more lethargic. She ate little and lost weight. Her apartment was in disarray. Dirty dishes were piled up in the kitchen sink, and her medications were scattered across the living room. Elly felt that her death was imminent. In the weekly meeting of hospice providers, a nurse supervisor announced that Ms. Cook's health plan did not cover hospice inpatient stays, nor would it pay for additional inpatient chemotherapy. The nurse supervisor expressed frustration, stating once again that she did not understand why Ms. Cook was in hospice. She viewed her as someone who was so eager to fight her disease that she sought treatments uncritically. "Any time she has a crisis, it becomes our problem," she said to the team.

Elly argued that Dr. Jenks kept giving Ms. Cook false hope and leaving it to hospice to deliver bad news. Barry, the social worker, who had listened to some of Shamira's tapes, asserted that Ms. Cook was fully aware of her condition. He did not think she was in denial. When someone mentioned Ms. Dixon's promise to keep Ms. Cook out of a nursing home, tension flared around the table. One nurse asserted, "If Yolanda made this promise, then *Yolanda* has to deal with Shamira." Another staff member exclaimed, "This is not our problem anymore!" And a third declared, "We are not responsible for the promises Yolanda is making."

The meeting closed uneasily. Barry seemed perplexed. He told me that his own impression of Ms. Cook differed significantly from the way she was presented by other hospice staff. He did not see Shamira as unrealistic. He just thought that her way of dying was different. And he wanted to find a way to respect it. He had even come to admire Ms. Dixon for her support. "At first, I thought, 'Yolanda, you are so enmeshed,'" he said. "So what? This is what the world needs sometimes—for people to reach out and do a little more. So I scolded myself."

"They Don't Bother Me and I Don't Bother Them"

When I visited Ms. Cook on April 22, I asked her how things were with hospice. "They don't bother me and I don't bother them," she answered. Three days later, she arrived at the office of Mark Jenks, her oncologist. She was weak and pale. During her examination, she coughed up blood. She was immediately admitted to the hospital. She felt increasing back pain, dyspnea, weakness, unsteadiness, and a tender abdomen. Her chest X-ray revealed radiation pneumonitis—an inflammation of her lungs that was caused by her treatment three months earlier.

In the hospital, Ms. Cook's pain peaked. She rolled in bed, screaming. Everyone thought that she was going to die. Her attending physician placed her on intravenous morphine. Dr. Jenks informed her that her white blood count had dropped dramatically. Under these circumstances, he could not possibly keep her on chemotherapy. There was nothing more he could do for her. Mark then told Elly that it was time to transfer Ms. Cook to the hospice inpatient unit. He didn't think she had much time left. In fact, he wasn't certain if she was going to be able to leave the hospital alive. Still in pain, Ms. Cook agreed to the transfer.

"We thought we were on a roll with it," Ms. Dixon recalled. When she walked into Ms. Cook's hospital room the next day, she found her surrounded by her family from Dauphin County. Ms. Cook looked jovial at first, but when her eyes caught Yolanda her mood changed. She appeared indignant. "I am leaving for Dauphin County," she announced. "I am going with my family. I want to be out of here today! Get it moving!" Ms. Dixon walked out into the hall and cried.

When she learned that Ms. Cook had not been officially discharged from the hospital and would not be able to leave as quickly as she wanted, Ms. Dixon returned hesitantly to her room to give her the news. She found her lying in bed, alone. Keisha and her family had left. Before she had the chance to speak, Ms. Cook apologized for her behavior. She explained that her relatives had brought the "street" out in her. She confessed that she depended on Yolanda's friendship. She did not want to lose her. She was scared. Gently, she took hold of Yolanda's hand, and they both cried. With tears rolling down her cheeks, she closed her eyes and fell asleep.

I saw Ms. Cook two days later. She was lying in her hospital bed, looking frazzled. With her address book in her hand, she was making arrangements for her departure. She was excited to move in with Keisha, but was also upset. "I imagine that it is going to be kind of strange," she said. "You know, being in a house and your sister is telling your daughter what to do. But I have been there. I am not going to take over. I had my chance for that, you know. I had my chance to be a mom twice. The first time, Rowena got put in the foster home, the second time, I am sick. Yolanda and me been crying all morning. She don't want me to leave here."

I realized there was a possibility that I would never see Shamira again. Even if she were to outlive Dr. Jenks's prognosis, I wasn't sure if my schedule and the goals of our project would permit me to make the trip to Dauphin County. Still, I asked her if she would be interested in having me visit her in her new home. She said that she would: "Because I want to give," she explained. "I want to give all that I can after everything that has been given to me."

I was struck by her answer, as I felt that, in the turmoil of her life, her generosity was often overlooked. In the few months I had known her, she was seen more as a drain on the system than an asset of any sort. We agreed that I would try my best to proceed with our work, even if that entailed only periodic phone interviews. Not knowing if this was a feasible plan, however, I asked her if there was anything she wanted me to make sure to include in the story I would write about her.

She paused for a while, and said: "That I was not the bad person that even my family tried to make me out to be. That I was really a loving and caring person—it was just that I was always directing my love in the wrong way to the wrong people. And that if you do have kids, make them your number one priority."

To Dauphin County

On May 1, Ms. Cook's care was officially transferred to a hospice in Dauphin County. When I arrived for my last visit to her apartment, I found her in the living room watching a horror film on TV. She looked drowsy, but insisted that I watch the most gruesome scene. Her eyes narrowed and her eyeballs rolled back. One moment she was looking at me and participating in our conversation, and the next, she was gone. She observed that her new medication regimen gave her the same high that she experienced when she abused drugs. I didn't stay long that day. We already knew that I would, after all, be able to visit her in Dauphin County, so we agreed to see each other in her new home.

Keisha arrived in the early afternoon. She found Elly, Barry, and Yolanda ready to carry her sister's suitcases to her car. Elly and Barry said their goodbyes. Ms. Cook promised to write to them. The last one to leave was Yolanda. The hospital chaplain assured Shamira that she would visit her soon. The two embraced, and Yolanda left. That evening Ms. Cook crossed the border of

Lancaster County for the last time. Yolanda told herself that no matter how attached she felt to Shamira, Shamira still saw her as a stranger. "I think Shamira will die in a hospital in Dauphin County," she remarked. "I feel maybe a little bit jealous, because I wish I would be able to be there with her. I would like to be with her when she dies, I would like to be sitting with her. I think that when she gets closer to her death, she is going to be a lot more scared. It would not surprise me if she calls and asks me to come. I hope she does."

"Patient Denies the Cancer"

Ms. Cook turned down personal care visits from her new hospice, insisting that she could manage her hygiene without assistance. She did, however, accept a bedside commode, a walker, and a shower bench. She reported weakness, unsteadiness in her gate, a distended abdomen, and increased shortness of breath on exertion. An oxygen cannula became a permanent part of her attire. To gain strength, she began eating wholesome foods and supplementing her diet with vitamins. Marilyn Beck, her new hospice social worker, found this worrisome. She did not want Ms. Cook to develop false hopes of a recovery. She told her that her weakness resulted from the progression of her disease and was not likely to dissipate with improved nutrition. Ms. Cook was outraged. Keisha's adult daughter called hospice to say that visiting staff did not have permission to talk to her aunt about the seriousness of her condition. "Patient denies the cancer. Does not want to talk about the 'D-word,'" a hospice nurse wrote in Ms. Cook's chart.

Dr. Robert Bridges, her new attending physician, was left with the same impression. "She is in big denial with her terminal illness," he told me. Ms. Cook requested aggressive treatments, which surprised him. She also complained of pain in her back and neck, reporting that a lymph node in her clavicle had grown so large that it bothered her. Aware that she was receiving an unusually high dose of morphine, Robert consulted a pain specialist. Never before had he worked with a patient who had such a high tolerance for narcotics. The pain specialist, Dr. Michael Neff, switched Ms. Cook from long-acting morphine to 50 mg of liquid hydromorphone every 4–6 hours. But, feeling that her pain was still not managed adequately, Ms. Cook requested a visit with an oncologist to explore the possibility of surgery. She wanted her lymph node removed.

Life in Keisha's home struck the new hospice team as chaotic. Keisha's small row house accommodated Keisha, Keisha's three adult children, four grandchildren, Rowena, and Ms. Cook. "They have Rowena babysitting all of the little kids," said Marilyn Beck, "and every time any of our staff goes in, they are all in there running around naked and screaming, and it has been pretty wild. There are casts of thousands in there most of the time." Ms. Dixon, who visited Ms. Cook soon after her move to Dauphin County, wasn't pleased with the new arrangements either. Ms. Cook's hospital bed stood in the dining room, next to a television set. Ms. Cook was smoking in bed while feeling so drowsy that she could barely keep her eyes open. Ms. Dixon found Keisha's home entirely inappropriate for a terminally ill patient. The only advantage she saw to the new setup was that it rejoined Ms. Cook with her family. "I think she [felt] close to that Black family," she remarked. "I think the blackness of that environment [felt] good to her. They understood her, whereas we were just caregivers to her."

When I saw Ms. Cook on June 3, I found her alone. She was lying in her bed, watching television. The enlarged photograph of herself and Rowena was the only decoration on the living room walls. I noticed that she had lost weight. Her eyes seemed more prominent than I remembered. And she was scared. "It's rough," she said as she cried. "I don't know if people realize how serious my cancer is." Later, speaking into her tape-recorder, she noted, "If it wasn't for my sister Keisha, I would probably be dead right now, because I was not going to go to no [nursing] home, no way. I was not going to go in a [nursing] home because if I went to a [nursing] home that is where I was going to die at—and I probably would have killed myself anyway." The following day, she told me, she was scheduled to see her new oncologist.

Dr. Allison Hopkins explained that there was nothing she could do to contain Shamira's cancer, but, to control her neuropathic pain, she doubled her dose of gabapentin from 300 to 600 mg three times daily. "I don't want to die!" exclaimed Ms. Cook in agony when she saw her nurse Faye the next day. "I'm so scared!"

"We Don't Have Time No More to Be Playing—I Am Dying!"

When Ms. Cook saw Dr. Neff, the pain specialist, the next day, she could barely walk, appearing lethargic and confused. She asserted that her disease was God's way of telling her to "clean up" her life. She wondered why Dr. Neff had referred her to Dr. Hopkins when Dr. Hopkins could do nothing to control her cancer. Gently, Dr. Neff reminded her that her disease was untreatable. Like Dr. Hopkins, he didn't know of any treatments that would help her. Ms. Cook looked shocked. She burst into tears, stood up, and walked out of Dr. Neff's office as fast as she could. "I don't think I was the first one to tell her," reflected Dr. Neff later, "but it was the first time it really stuck. That was hard on me."

When I phoned Ms. Cook on June 26, she sounded alarmed. She had forgotten that I was going to be away for three weeks. "We don't have time no more to be playing—I am dying!" she exclaimed. And she continued,

> There is nothing else they can do for me. They can't stop my cancer no more. My sister already knew. Everybody else already knew but me. I told them it was best not to tell me yet, because I was not ready. What they should know is that you never get ready to hear that you're going to die. It is at the point now, we were discussing the dress that I am going to be buried in. Since I have been told, it seems like I just became sick. It could be mind over matter, you know. I was feeling so healthy again, until [Dr. Neff] told me, "Well you know, you are dying, there is nothing else we can do for you, period, besides keep you comfortable." I don't know how to feel, Yanna! I just don't know what to think, what to do. I feel like a piece of glass. I feel like if I move the wrong way that I am going to go to pieces.

There was a pause, and I heard a rustling. She then resumed,

> Excuse me, I am sweating and I'm trying to wipe the phone off. I don't feel like I'm ready to go nowhere yet, so death better go ahead on and find somebody else, because I ain't ready. Because I don't think God brought me this far to drop me on my head. Because I think there is something He wants me to do before I leave here. I just don't know what the plan is, and I ain't going to worry about it, because when it comes to God, you ain't got to worry about nothing.

I found the agony in Ms. Cook's voice jarring. Until then, I had been fooled. Her feistiness, good humor, and youth had convinced me, to a certain degree, that she was going to make it—that somehow she was stronger than her disease. Now I felt sad and close to her. I knew that

I would miss her. I told her that I wanted to see her soon. We agreed to meet on July 3.

When I arrived that day, I was struck by the change in her appearance. Her face was swollen from steroids, her eyes were bulging, and a thin layer of facial hair covered her cheeks. The wig she had chosen to wear in her coffin was on display at the foot of her bed. It was a set of long, straight black hair with bangs. She looked tired and upset. She was struggling, especially with the fact that Rowena continued to avoid her. "I can't get no sleep," she said. "I try to be everybody's everything, and I can't do it. I am only one person, and I don't even know who I am. For real, I don't even know who Shamira is. I know my name is Shamira, I know I am not a dumb woman, I know I have a beautiful child, I know I am dying, I know I have taken care of all the responsibilities as a mother for when I die. I want to go back to Lancaster County, because I don't think my daughter wants me here. It's like I spoiled something for her when I came."

A few days later, Ms. Cook reported pressure from her distended abdomen, back pain, swelling of her left foot, increased weakness, tightness in her chest, confusion, and forgetfulness. Dr. Hopkins doubled the dose of her breakthrough morphine from 100 mg to 200 mg every two hours as needed. Keisha worried. She told hospice that her sister had started to hallucinate. Three times she had seen her deceased mother. Ms. Cook recalled those moments vividly. Her mother had appeared so suddenly that it had scared her. With her was a small child who was playing peek-a-boo behind the living room chair. Shamira's mother looked proud. "She was looking at me," Ms. Cook recalled, "like she was saying, 'Well, you look like you doing pretty good, like you are handling it,' and, 'Just keep on doing what you're doing.' That is how I took it, and that is how I feel—I am doing the best I can."

On July 9, Keisha called hospice in a panic. Ms. Cook had heard threatening voices and, suspecting that people were trying to attack her, she placed a knife under her pillow for protection. Keisha feared for the safety of both her grandchildren and Rowena. Dr. Hopkins suggested hospitalization for a psychiatric evaluation. Wanting the scary voices to quiet down, Ms. Cook agreed to go. A few days later, she returned with a diagnosis of "psychotic depression." Her revised prescription included an increased dosage of antidepressant medication, an antipsychotic, and a new antibiotic. Keisha wasn't happy about her sister's presence at home. Her deterioration scared her. She worried every time she left for work.

On July 21, Ms. Cook agreed to go back to the hospital for a reevalua-tion. Dr. Hopkins instructed her attending physician to decrease her pain medications until he felt confident that he had struck a balance between pain control and mental clarity. Four days after her admission, Shamira seemed stable. Though depressed, she was alert, oriented, and reported no pain. She was scheduled to be discharged on July 26. On the eve of her departure, she spoke with Yolanda and told her that she loved her. The two women laughed about some photographs they had taken together and agreed to meet at Keisha's home the next day.

In the morning, a hospice nurse found Ms. Cook "wildly anxious." She was refusing to be discharged, crying that she was afraid to die. When Keisha arrived to pick her up, she found her rolling restlessly in her bed. She had lost control of her urine and defecated involuntarily. Frightened and agitated, Ms. Cook asked Keisha to hold her hand. She looked like she was struggling to breathe. "Can't you make this stop?" she asked Keisha in panic. Keisha tried to calm her. Gently, she encouraged her to close her eyes and rest. As she started to rub her leg for comfort, Shamira stopped moving. A few minutes later, Keisha realized that she was dead.

"They Brought Her Out of the Morgue, Put Her in a Box, and That Was It"

When Yolanda arrived at Keisha's house, she was shocked to hear the news. Dr. Hopkins had called Keisha to apologize for her poor judgment in autho-rizing her sister's discharge. She explained that she hadn't expected Shamira to die so quickly and wasn't even certain about the immediate cause of her death. Yolanda sensed that Keisha was frazzled. When she asked her what the matter was, she was shocked anew. Keisha told her that she wasn't Shamira's sister. She was a friend Shamira had met and grown to admire while still in her addiction. Ms. Cook's only blood relative was Rowena. Now someone needed to take responsibility for organizing the funeral, but Keisha could not afford it. Yet the hospital was pressuring her to take Ms. Cook's body from the morgue. Yolanda offered to make the arrangements herself.

The next day, Ms. Dixon raised $800 at her church. This would cover the cost of a gravesite. Other funeral expenses amounted to $1,500, which Ms. Dixon paid from her savings and additional donations she received in the mail. When Keisha called the funeral home to ask who would dress Ms. Cook in her new outfit, she was told that no one was available. Since Ms. Cook was not going to be embalmed, the funeral home refused to touch her. "So what they did," Yolanda told me, "is they brought her out of the morgue, put her in a box, and that was it. They really didn't do anything."

Ms. Cook's funeral took place in Dauphin County, seven months after her admission to hospice. It was July 30. Rowena, Keisha, Keisha's children and grandchildren, and a few friends from Lancaster County gathered under a small, maroon tent. The two rows of chairs set up by the funeral home faced Ms. Cook's light blue casket, which was decorated with a bouquet of white flowers. Against the casket leaned the photograph of Ms. Cook and Rowena. Rowena sat in front of her mother's casket, crying on Keisha's shoulder. At the service, Yolanda recounted her first meeting with Ms. Cook. Rev. Johnson spoke about the time when he and his wife encouraged Ms. Cook to fight for her life until the end. He admired Shamira for having done just that. The Reverend then announced that he and Yolanda were going to hold a memorial service in Lancaster County and that everyone was welcome.

Two weeks later, around one hundred people attended the service: Ms. Cook's extended family, former co-workers, friends from the drug rehabilitation center and her Narcotics Anonymous group, and members of her church and Yolanda's religious community. Looking around me, I couldn't help but notice the diversity of people Ms. Cook had touched, directly or indirectly. Young and old, rich and poor, Black and White had all gathered under one roof to honor a person they had grown to love as a relative, or recovering drug addict, or conscientious employee, or cancer patient. Toward the end of the service, one of Ms. Cook's co-workers stepped forward with a large envelope. He announced that Ms. Cook had asked for his help to write a letter. She had then dictated a message for Rowena. Her words were in the envelope, which he handed to Rowena and sat back down. I never learned what the letter said.

Rowena and Yolanda

Following her mother's death, Rowena visited Lancaster County often. She saw her friends during the day and spent the nights with Ms. Dixon. She told Yolanda that life with her mother had been difficult, and, in many ways, she didn't miss it. Yolanda was convinced that Rowena needed counseling, but doubted if Keisha would offer it to her. She contemplated raising Rowena herself, but questioned the cultural appropriateness of such an arrangement. She invited Rowena to spend holidays with her family and volunteered to buy her clothes. On one of her visits, Rowena gave her a copy of the hope-filled photograph with her mother and herself at the drug rehabilitation center. Yolanda displayed it prominently in her office.

As time passed, Ms. Dixon saw less and less of Rowena. But she spoke about her with an intensity that did not waver. She reminisced about Ms. Cook as well. She told me that she thought about her every day. No matter how much she tried, she could not accept her death as a good one. If only the doctors had explained to her that her disease was incurable, Yolanda reflected, she would have been able to enjoy the last few months of her life, not suffer through them.

The Reverend and Ms. Johnson

"Our attitude affects our physical condition," Rev. Johnson commented when I spoke with him after Ms. Cook's death. As a pastor, he had seen patients outlive their prognosis—and even defeat their disease—because they fought to live. The Reverend made a distinction between accepting one's diagnosis and resigning to it. He believed that Ms. Cook had accepted the seriousness of her condition without giving in to the inevitability of her death. Ms. Johnson concurred. She asserted that the last few months of her life gave Ms. Cook the opportunity to grow spiritually. In the end, she left this world with an improved relationship with God, a renewed relationship with Rowena, and a newfound relationship with her loved ones in Dauphin County. Reflecting on people's tendency to assume Shamira was in denial, Ms. Johnson said, "I was intimidated by Shamira [at first] because I had to change my whole mindset. I had to change my whole thinking about this girl. I had to just shut up, and look at her, and try to go where she was. I think about her because she was such an influence to me, because now when I look at death and dying, I think of it differently. And I will tell people, 'It is not over until it's over.'" She then recalled a time when Shamira had mustered the strength to attend a Sunday service. The Reverend saw her sitting in the balcony and asked her to rise and greet the congregation. Slowly, she stood up and smiled. Everyone turned toward her and applauded.

Authors' Comments

At the time of our research, African Americans made up fewer than 10% of patients served by hospice in the United States. As we noted in the General Introduction, this is still true today.[1,2] The preamble to a resolution on health equity adopted by the Council of Representatives of the American Psychological Association in October 2021 puts the matter succinctly: "[T]rauma exposure, discrimination, and racism have resulted in people of color experiencing barriers of distrust toward health care and its professionals."[3] Some Black patients may mistrust the hospice approach in particular because its requirement to forego life-prolonging treatments as a condition of enrolment contradicts their preferred plan of action, limits options they might want available to them, or appears simply to replicate patterns of control, neglect, and harm that African Americans have experienced at the hands of health professionals for centuries.[4,5] Although these restrictive regulations provoke mistrust and resistance far beyond the African American community, to be sure—and as we note in the General Introduction, Medicare is experimenting with rules that permit combining palliative and life-prolonging treatment—for African Americans, the experience of systemic racism in healthcare amplifies their chilling effect.[6,7]

The overwhelmingly White, middle-class population of hospice beneficiaries not only reflects the dominant culture in the United States; it also matches the demographic profile of the hospice and palliative care workforce. It is not surprising, then, that the comfort zone for hospice providers—the lens through which they see their patients and respond to their needs—is heavily inflected by race and class. At a time of intensified awareness of America's racial divides, we want to emphasize the powerful effects—whether intended or not—of the prevailing image of the hospice patient as a White, middle-class individual who conforms to the dominant culture's social norms, aspirations, and nuclear family structure and who embraces an ideology and ethos of "accepting" their incurable condition, while exhibiting gratitude for the help hospice provides to, as the 18th-century physician Thomas Percival put it, "smooth the bed of death."[8]

Shamira Cook challenged every dimension of this paradigm: a poor, Black, single mother with a long history of substance abuse, she resisted her disease with all her power to the end and pushed against all of the boundaries—bureaucratic and ideological—that hospice tried to impose on her as conditions of providing care. Many, though not all, members of the hospice team assumed that her insistence on life-prolonging treatment showed that she was "in denial" and vehemently questioned her appropriateness as a hospice patient. The team's interpretation actually reveals the inadequacy of dichotomous notions of "denial" and "acceptance." As Shamira often said, it was precisely her awareness that she was likely to die soon that fueled her urgent struggle for enough time to find out—and tell the world—who she really was.

The constant questioning of Ms. Cook's "appropriateness" as a hospice patient and rigid application of rules and regulations, even in gray areas where there was room for flexibility and judgment, had the effect—even if not by conscious intention—of curtailing Ms. Cook's autonomy in choosing how to live her life while trying to combat her disease. Even her efforts to eat healthy foods were dismissed as troubling evidence of "denial." Would Ms. Cook have experienced these attitudes had she fit the hospice paradigm more closely? The contrast between her journey with hospice and the journeys of the Hoffers, the Courts, and Stanley Gray in other narratives in this book is striking. For both Mr. Hoffer and Mr. Gray, the hospice team seemed to bend over backward to accommodate their idiosyncrasies and special needs—and in Mr. Gray's case stretched the definition of hospice "appropriateness" to the limit in order to continue to serve a man whose symptom burden (apart from his underlying shortness of breath) was far lighter than Ms. Cook's. In the case of the Courts, we can note the extraordinary, and truly impressive, support hospice offered to Joey's younger brother Mike—even overlooking the institution's own age requirement for a child's participation in a support group—while seeming to ignore completely the obvious needs for attention and support of Ms. Cook's daughter Rowena as she struggled with the stress and confusion of her mother's illness.

A further example reinforces the interpretation that these shortcomings and contradictions in hospice's work with Shamira Cook demonstrated failures of empathy, attentiveness, and care that stemmed at least in part from race-based, class-based, and ideological prejudices—the often unconscious but nevertheless systemic biases and assumptions about the way the world is or should be that significantly determine how we all "see" and respond to what is in front of us. After Ms. Cook moved to the Dauphin County home of her friend Keisha, reports from her new hospice team about life in Keisha's home started reaching her new hospice social worker, Marilyn Beck. Marilyn was told that the place was small and chaotic, housing not only Keisha and Shamira, but also Keisha's three adult children, four grandchildren, and

Rowena, who often served as the babysitter. Marilyn could have seen in this environment—as the Lancaster County hospital's chaplain-in-training Yolanda Dixon saw—a challenging and complex situation that called for more thorough assessment and remediation of the sort that social workers carry out as a matter of course. What Ms. Beck "saw," however, was that "they have Rowena babysitting all of the little kids, and every time any of our staff goes in, they are all in there running around naked and screaming, and it has been pretty wild. There are casts of thousands in there most of the time." We have no evidence that the hospice took any steps either in further investigation or amelioration of Shamira's living condition. It was as if, having pathologized it in such demeaning and caricaturing language, the social worker had written the situation off as a self-evidently intractable problem that was beyond the reach, or even unworthy, of her attention.

Other challenges in Ms. Cook's care resulted from the inherent complexity of her medical needs. The clearest example was the management of her pain. Ms. Cook received very large doses of opioid drugs for pain related to her retroperitoneal tumors and, possibly, her chest tumors. Cancer at these sites usually produces pain of a mixed type, including neuropathic pain, that requires multiple therapeutic approaches, including one or more co-analgesics and, often, anesthetic interventions. Had Ms. Cook received these treatments, she might not have required such large doses of opioids, with their accompanying effects on her cognitive functioning. Anesthetic procedures like epidural analgesia can be safe and effective in cases such as these. Although the patient is usually hospitalized, it is possible to manage epidural catheters and medication in the home. That Ms. Cook did not receive such treatments might well reflect the relative lack of specialized physician involvement in the care of Hospice of Lancaster County patients at that time. As we have noted in the General Introduction, such expertise is very well provided for today.

It is also worth noting that, at points in the narrative, it appeared that Ms. Cook was using the opioids to get "high" as well as to control her pain. If this was the case—and not accidental overdosing that could have occurred due to confusion or while she was experiencing unbearable pain—the dosages she used could have been significantly higher than what was prescribed. Although there are different tactics to address this challenge—such as, for example, the use of methadone, which is now recognized to be more effective for neuropathic pain; the minimization of long-acting opioids with reliance, instead, on regular four-hourly opioid doses; and psychological, music, or art therapy—the reality is that terminally ill patients with a present or past history of drug abuse tend to experience difficulty having their pain adequately controlled.

References

1. National Hospice and Palliative Care Organization. Facts and Figures 2020 Edition. 2020. https://www.nhpco.org/wp-content/uploads/NHPCO-Facts-Figures-2020-edit ion.pdf. Accessed November 15, 2021.
2. Ornstein KA, Roth DL, Huang J, Levitan EB, Rhodes JD, Fabius CD, Safford MM, Sheehan OC. Evaluation of racial disparities in hospice use and end-of-life treatment intensity in the REGARDS cohort. JAMA Netw Open. 2020;3(8):e2014639.
3. Advancing Health Equity in Psychology: Resolution adopted by the APA Council of Representatives on October 29, 2021. American Psychological Association. https://www.apa.org/about/policy/advancing-health-equity-psychology.   Accessed November 11, 2021.
4. Elbaum A. Black lives in a pandemic: Implications of systemic injustice for end-of-life care. Hastings Cent Rep. 2020;50(3):58–60.
5. Crawley L, Payne R, Bolden J, Payne T, Washington P, Williams S; Initiative to Improve Palliative and End-of-Life Care in the African American Community. Palliative and end-of-life care in the African American community. JAMA. 2000;284(19):2518–2521.
6. Benkert R, Peters RM, Clark R, Keves-Foster K. Effects of perceived racism, cultural mistrust and trust in providers on satisfaction with care. J Natl Med Assoc. 2006;98(9):1532–1540.
7. Clark MA, Person SD, Gosline A, Gawande AA, Block SD. Racial and ethnic differences in advance care planning: Results of a statewide population-based survey. J Palliat Med. 2018;8:1078–1085.
8. Percival T. *Medical Ethics: Or a Code of Institutes and Precept Adapted to the Professional Conduct of Physicians and Surgeons.* Manchester, England: J Johnson; 1803.

8

Rose Picard

"I'm Allowed to Be Happy Even Though I'm Dying"

Narrated by Anna Towers

Rose Picard had led a full and happy life. When, at the age of 72, the gynecologist told her that she had ovarian cancer, she adapted quickly to the news. When chemotherapy failed and she transferred to the Palliative Care Unit, she did so with equanimity. Her husband and children had more difficulty. Mrs. Picard had an unshakable faith and *joie de vivre* that impressed her healthcare givers. She prepared for her death; when she was ready, however, death did not come quickly.

A Life of Joy and Gratitude

Rose Picard was a tiny woman with straight, naturally gray hair, a prominent beaked nose, and lively, large brown eyes. She seemed always to be smiling, joking, and inquiring after the welfare of those around her. She and her husband Philip had been married for 52 years, since they were both 21. They had two daughters, Mary and Linda; a son, Mark; and six grandchildren. The family got together almost every Sunday. In between, the men played golf together and the women went out for lunch or shopping for clothes.

Mr. Picard had been manager of a plastics factory. He was a well-built man with a gray moustache and was soft-spoken. Although talking about feelings did not come easily to him, he was an affectionate man, and I often witnessed him holding his wife's hand and doing little favors for her comfort. He was a sentimental man who valued family and religious rituals and special occasions. Anniversaries were important to him.

"What I lived with my children and my husband is exceptional, exceptional," Mrs. Picard told me one day, after she became ill and had agreed to participate in our project. "It's beautiful! I will never forget this. I hope they, too, will remember after I'm gone." The love that she had experienced in this life she also linked with the afterlife. She was Roman Catholic, and her faith was "very, very important" to her. Philip and the children were also practicing Catholics. "God helps us a lot," she would say. "We might leave this life but we go to another one. I will go to another life. I don't know when. He above knows, and I accept it."

"I always tried to be a good spouse," Mrs. Picard said, "but it doesn't mean that I always was. We have ups and downs in life. There are good days and bad days." In fact, Mrs. Picard would have said that her daughter Mary was her best friend and confidante. Mary told me that her parents supported each other in practical ways, but they never really talked. Mr. Picard was not one to talk through problems or share feelings easily. So Mrs. Picard would confide in Mary instead.

Mrs. Picard came from an Irish-French family of 14 children. She was the youngest daughter and looked after her four younger brothers. She started working at age 12. Though her family went through a difficult time during the Depression, Mrs. Picard was never bitter and learned to be grateful. She had a deep respect for the individuality of others. She would say that each of her children was very different, and she had allowed them to be who they were. This came back to her later, in that the children respected her in the same way. For example, Mrs. Picard explained, "When my children were growing up, I never pushed them to eat. It's normal for children to be hungry one day and not hungry the next. That's how I brought them up. So they don't push me to eat when I don't feel like it. They just say, 'Mom is ill and not hungry right now.'"

Mrs. Picard was a natural mother. Throughout her life she was open to others and attentive to their needs. She was an affectionate person, with a great sense of humor. She enjoyed gatherings, parties, and traveling on business with her husband. Whenever people got together, she wanted to speak with everyone there, showing genuine interest and enthusiasm. At any gathering, Mrs. Picard could be heard above the crowd when she laughed, which she did often. Her husband said to me, "I don't know what it is about her, but everyone wants to be around her. Even in our apartment block, when she went to the laundry room, it was time for a big party."

Illness Comes

Mrs. Picard had been well all her life. Then, at age 72, she began to have abdominal discomfort and, in February 1995, was found to have cancer of the ovary. The tumor was advanced at the time of diagnosis. The gynecologist told her after surgery that 50% of the tumor was still there. He said to Mr. Picard, "We'll try to prolong her life. I don't know how long she has—two months, four months, six months, a year—I don't know." Mr. Picard said of the gynecologist, "He was frank. And I respect that, when the doctor is honest enough to tell us the truth. He couldn't do more. He did what was possible."

The oncologist did not encourage Mrs. Picard to have systemic chemotherapy, and she and the family accepted this. They understood that the aim was to keep her as comfortable as possible in the time that remained. However, the oncologist did give her intraperitoneal mitoxantrone, a local anti-cancer agent. By September, she was requiring paracentesis every two weeks to remove fluid from her abdominal cavity. She was also referred to the Palliative Care Service at this time for pain control. As she lived in a rural area where palliative home care was not available, Dr. Denise Morin, the palliative care physician, followed her via telephone, along with the family physician who visited her at home. Her abdominal pain was soon controlled.

By December, however, the ascites had become a very significant problem. Mrs. Picard's abdomen was heavy and uncomfortable. She still needed peritoneal taps every two weeks, but she decided that she did not want the intraperitoneal chemotherapy anymore, since it didn't seem to be working. She did agree to try oral cyclophosphamide, another chemotherapy agent. In mid-January 1996, Mrs. Picard was admitted to the gynecology ward with vomiting due to a small bowel obstruction. She was treated conservatively with a nasogastric tube and IV rehydration. She very quickly became the "darling" of the ward. She was considerate of the nurses and would make them laugh.

Within a few days, Mrs. Picard's symptoms settled, but she was not well enough to go home. The gynecology staff and Denise Morin, the palliative care physician, discussed with Mrs. Picard and her family the possibility of a transfer to the Palliative Care Unit (PCU) where the palliative care staff would try to control her symptoms. Denise explained to the family that bowel obstruction was a serious complication but occasionally the symptoms resolved and the person could go home again. Mr. and Mrs. Picard and their daughter Mary were visibly upset, but then seemed to accept the situation. Linda, on the other hand, was constantly in tears when she came to see her mother. She would stay for a few minutes but then had to leave because she was so upset.

Mary and Linda

Mary, who was 50 years old, was Mrs. Picard's oldest daughter. She was a remarkably good-looking woman, with long blond hair kept tidily coifed. She was warm and open about her feelings and also concerned about the welfare of others. She seemed to me to be a "natural carer," like her mother. I often saw Mary and Mrs. Picard chatting quietly, holding hands on the hospital ward. They had spoken openly about the cancer from the time of diagnosis. Mary felt prepared. She said to me, "We have known for a year now that she is dying, and I went through it with her. You know, the asking 'Why me?' and feeling angry. And then she would feel like crying and I would say, 'It's okay to cry'. So we would cry together. And then she would feel better."

Linda, who was a year younger, was more withdrawn and had great difficulty accepting the diagnosis. She would not talk about it and would not come with her mother to the oncology clinic for treatments. Later, when her mother was sicker, I would see her rushing into the hospital to see her mother. She walked very fast, looking very anxious and upset, and never stayed very long. Linda was somewhat overweight, had long black hair, and always seemed a bit disheveled compared to her sister. She never looked me straight in the eye and could never chat easily, as Mary could. Linda had always been closer to her father, and she found it difficult now to speak with her mother.

Mr. Picard and Mark did not say much either, though they supported Mrs. Picard in a practical way. It was clear that Mrs. Picard was able to share her feelings with Mary in a way that she could with no one else. Mary had an explanation for this. "I've been through suffering in my life," she told me, "so it's easier for me to accept this than it is for my sister or my father perhaps. When I was 33, I developed a colon infection that led to perforation of the bowel. I almost died. I was in intensive care for a couple of weeks. I went part way into the other world. It took me months to recover. I had two young children at that time. So I came face to face with death then. It made me unafraid. I'm no longer afraid of the dying process."

"It changed my life," Mary continued. "I learned to live 24 hours at a time, and to appreciate what is beautiful in the world. When I love someone, I tell them. I'm a grandmother now, and when I'm with my granddaughter, we talk about the lovely flowers and how nice they smell, and the sounds of the birds. We have a great time together, just appreciating what's around us. So my mother and I spoke about that. My mother said, 'I'm afraid of dying.' 'So?' I said. 'That's normal.' Then she said, 'What was it like when you were sick?' And I explained to her that it felt very peaceful and was a beautiful experience. So she had a dream and she said that she dreamt that she was dying and she saw stars. And it was so beautiful, she said. She said, 'I'm not afraid anymore.' "

"I'd Like to Call You Rose"

On January 20, Mrs. Picard was transferred to the PCU, in a separate wing of the same hospital, and settled into a private room overlooking a wooded park. Within a few days her windowsill was full of cards, and her grandchildren's drawings adorned the walls. The nurses from the gynecology service came to visit Mrs. Picard often. They had become fond of her and would come during their lunch break or after their shift.

Most patients find a nasogastric tube uncomfortable, and as soon as Mrs. Picard arrived on the PCU, Dr. Morin ordered it removed. Denise tried to relieve the symptoms of bowel obstruction with medication, including antiemetics, somatostatin or anticholinergics, and steroids. These medications prevent nausea and minimize gastrointestinal secretions, thus reducing vomiting.

Mrs. Picard never demanded anything and tended not to complain so the nurses quickly learned that they had to ask her if she had pain. She tried to be as active as possible, walking in the hallways aided by her husband or one of her children. She enjoyed sitting in the solarium or in the family kitchen, chatting with other patients, family members, and staff.

At one point, Mrs. Picard became disoriented, and she was afraid; she woke up and thought she was dead. Mostly, however, she was serene in her outlook, exhibiting great openness in discussing her terminal illness. She spoke calmly to the priest of her decision to refuse treatment. "Life is a pilgrimage," she said to him. "When the time comes to finish, it comes." But she wanted to enjoy a good quality of life for as long as possible. For her, this meant being able to enjoy her family and feeling supported by them.

Mrs. Picard developed a very warm and friendly relationship with Father Francis, the pastoral worker who was assigned to the ward. Despite a 30-year age difference between them, Father Francis, who was normally quite formal, was moved to ask her, "May I call you by your first name—Rose? It's a beautiful name. I'd like to call you Rose." She said, "Of course," and started to call him by his first name also. Father Francis came to see her regularly. She appreciated his visits and received Communion almost every day. She commented that Father Francis had been to Haiti and that "he has seen a lot of suffering." She was obviously fond of him.

As January drew to an end, Mrs. Picard began vomiting again, evidence that she might be developing bowel obstruction once more. Mrs. Picard asked the oncologist directly what her prognosis was and was told that it was approximately four weeks. She took the news with equanimity, continuing to say that she was not afraid of death.

Preparations

Mrs. Picard grew weaker over the next few days. Although the symptoms of her bowel obstruction were controlled with metoclopramide (which prevents nausea and aids gastric emptying) and prochlorperazine (a second antiemetic), she was unable to eat much. She asked to go home to spend a final day there. "I want to see my things," she said.

Her family organized themselves to bring her home by car. Mark had to carry her up the front stairs. She immediately went to lie down on the cot in her conservatory, in the sun, among her favorite plants. She lay there happily and fell asleep. A few hours later, her family brought her back to hospital. They would have liked to have kept her at home, but she still had intermittent vomiting and was so weak that she needed total care. Mr. Picard felt more secure with her being in hospital. Although Mary was willing to take time off, she did not feel that she would have enough support in looking after her mother. Linda was too upset and anxious to give practical help. Nonetheless, Mr. Picard wanted to try to bring his wife home on day passes as often as possible. Mrs. Picard accepted that her family did not have the resources to care for her at home and did not put any pressure on them to keep her there.

Formal Catholic rituals were important to the Picards, and, on February 8, Father Francis asked Mrs. Picard if she wanted to receive the Sacrament of the Sick. She agreed. She wanted all her children to be there, but Mark said that he could not take time off work, and Linda didn't come because she was too anxious. Mr. Picard and Mary were present, along with two volunteers from pastoral services. Father Francis later told me that it was one of the most beautiful ceremonies that he had ever experienced. Mrs. Picard participated fully in spite of her suffering and weakness, and she embraced and kissed everyone at the end.

The music therapist visited, and Mrs. Picard requested that she play Schubert's "Ave Maria." Mrs. Picard was very moved by this and said that she wanted this played at her funeral. She was clearly preparing herself for her death.

Mrs. Picard also expressed an interest in having a video made of herself speaking to her family. The staff found a video filmmaker who volunteered to do this for her. Mrs. Picard had a brief prepared text in which she thanked her caregivers and addressed her family. "The time has arrived for me to leave you," she read into the camera, "without regret, but with a lot of serenity. For you, Philip, good-bye and I hope to see you soon. And similarly, for Mary, my daughter and confidante, and Linda, who has learned to adapt to the situation even though you are going through a lot of grief. We have all had a lot of grief. And Mark, you were a joy in my life." Mrs. Picard quickly came to the end of her prepared text and then wasn't quite sure what to say. The music therapist asked her, "What makes it possible for you to be so accepting of what is happening? I find it remarkable." Mrs. Picard smiled and replied,

I am not afraid of dying. I am facing it with serenity. I want it to be beautiful. I want it to be me. Then, in the church, I don't want any fanfare. All I want is for the ones I love to be there. I have accepted this, but it hasn't been easy. I don't want to flinch too much, but it hurts. Like, for my children—Linda in particular—she can't be there when I talk about dying. And my son, too. It's hard for them to be with me.

Mrs. Picard was pleased to have made the video and wanted all her family to look at it with her right away. She would ask caregivers who came into the room, "Have you seen my video?"

By this time, she needed multiple medications to prevent vomiting, as she had total bowel obstruction. She received a cocktail of subcutaneous medication consisting of 20 mg famotidine, 40 mg metoclopramide, 20 mg morphine, 300 micrograms somatostatin, 100 mg dimenhydrinate, and 2 mg haloperidol via a syringe driver. Another syringe driver contained 16 mg dexamethasone. In addition, she took laxatives by mouth. With the aid of this medication, she was relatively comfortable. She was still able to walk slowly, with help, wearing the two syringe drivers in small, fitted pouches strapped to her shoulder. Despite all this, she still managed to look cheerful. One day, as she was returning from the whirlpool bath, I saw her wearing a big smile.

Decreasing the Life-Prolonging Medication

By mid-February, Mrs. Picard was too weak to walk. At this point she said to Dr. Morin, "I'm tired and fed up. I have done everything I need to do, and I want it to be over." Denise considered the situation, realizing that her patient was now dying. The bowel obstruction had not resolved, and Mrs. Picard had a lot of tumor in her abdomen. Denise explained to Mrs. Picard the medication she was on, and what the dexamethasone was doing. Perhaps it was prolonging her life by keeping her bowels open. Mrs. Picard told Denise that she wanted the dexamethasone decreased, thinking that this might bring death sooner. Denise began to taper it in accordance with her wishes; she would increase the medication for pain control and nausea if required.

On February 22, Mary visited her mother in the afternoon as usual. The two of them were alone, which made it easier for Mary to speak with her mother about dying. Mrs. Picard felt very comfortable having this discussion. "Don't think about us," Mary said to her. "We will be all right."

Mark started talking to me about his mother's death. He said that he hoped to take a trip with his dad after this was all over. Linda still seemed more fragile. She was often tearful and would say to me, "This is so difficult."

When I saw Mrs. Picard around this time, she was amazingly cheerful. She said, "I have some Irish blood in me so I'm allowed to be happy even though I'm dying. It's like *pfft!*" She made a sound like a fire going out, then laughed out loud.

A couple of days later it was quiet on the ward. Mrs. Picard looked the most tired that I had seen her. She was having some periods of confusion and some frightening dreams. She had some visual hallucinations, seeing mice and ducks in her room, but she seemed not to be too bothered. (Dr. Morin believed that this could be from the morphine, so she adjusted the medication.) Mrs. Picard said to me, "It's like I wish it were all over. Because I'm so tired. It's long, always waiting, waiting, waiting. And I'm always afraid that

I might choke. I've never choked, but I'm afraid! I'm afraid because I had a friend, and she choked to death. As soon as she drank water, she would choke."

Mr. Picard was anxious to help in whatever way he could. He said to his wife, "I gave you a bit of ice just now, and you were able to suck on it. That helped, didn't it?" He turned to me. "And I helped her clean her teeth and her mouth, and that helped."

"Uh-huh," she agreed. Then her thoughts drifted to her home, which she might never see again. "It's so quiet," she said. "Many patients have left for the weekend, eh? But it's not easy for the families, it's hard for them to get organized. But maybe I can spend a little time at home tomorrow."

"If you're strong enough," Mr. Picard said. "We did it last week because you were a little bit stronger than this week."

Mrs. Picard seemed to drift off a few times during our conversation. Then she would perk up for a few minutes. She spoke about her video. She had viewed it once and wanted to see it again. Several other patients and families on the ward had seen it, and she was very happy about that. Each of the children had their own copy.

We sat silently for a few moments. Mr. Picard was holding his wife's hand and looking at her. Then he turned to me and said slowly and deliberately:

> When you've been married almost 53 years, and you see that your wife is in the hospital, it does something to you. To see her suffer, it does something. I can't help her, but she says my being here helps, so every day I come to see her. We spoke this week, and she told me that she's tired of living, because of all the physical symptoms. So she made me promise not to hold on to her. Then she said that when she's up there, she's going to speak with me every day. So that's what helps me. And the children support me, too. I hope that God comes to take her as fast as possible, because she tells me she's tired of suffering.

Mrs. Picard, who had been listening to this, added, "It looks that way."

It impressed me how this couple, who had been together for so long, could speak so openly about letting go of their earthly relationship. I could sense their deep faith in a relationship that could continue in the afterlife. Mr. Picard continued, "We said everything that we had to say to each other. And our children were there, too. So, this week she received the Last Rites, and we were here. So she's ready to go in peace. That's what we wish with all our hearts. And as far as we're concerned, it's understood that we'll talk to her every day and she'll monitor us, eh, Ma?" Mr. Picard said, turning to address his wife.

Mrs. Picard replied, with no hesitation, "There'll be nothing to monitor."

"You'll keep an eye on us, anyway."

Mrs. Picard said, with a twinkle, "You're old enough to do your own monitoring." This made Mr. Picard laugh.

"Don't Worry, I'm Here Beside You"

Father Francis commented to me that Mrs. Picard seemed to bear her physical decline with an unwavering faith. "It's surprising to me," he said, "because the more she declines physically, the stronger her faith. But it is a balanced faith, not an exuberant faith. It isn't, 'I believe in God no matter what, everything rests with Him, and you'll see—He will save me.' It isn't the kind of faith that's like a lifesaver."

Mrs. Picard was not expecting a miracle. When she saw her children and her husband now, she made them promise that they would let her go, that they would not try to hold on. Linda continued to have difficulty with this and was very tearful whenever she saw her mother. Mary, on the other hand, was able to be more realistic and cool about the situation. The next day, February 25, Mary asked whether the dexamethasone might be decreased further. She felt that the dexamethasone might be prolonging suffering now, rather than prolonging useful life. "She wants to die and is exhausted," Mary said. "It's so hard to see her this way."

Dr. Morin continued to taper the dexamethasone. There seemed to be no conflict in her mind: her patient was dying and her goal was to keep her comfortable, not to try to get her to eat or drink again.

Mrs. Picard found it difficult to be alone at night now. She had had nightmares the day before that were possibly related to her medication. Mr. Picard was afraid that she would have them again, so he said that he would stay with her and keep an eye on her. He could help Dr. Morin by observing his wife and reporting back what happened during the night.

The nurses prepared a cot so he could sleep beside his wife, but he did not sleep much that night, having never slept in a hospital before. He would get up every hour or so to check on his wife. "Don't worry, I'm here beside you," he would say if he saw that she, too, was awake.

Periodically, Mr. Picard would listen to her breathing. "And when I couldn't hear her breathe," he explained to me, "I would get up to have a look. Then suddenly, she would start breathing again. So, I would say to myself, 'She's still alive.'" Mr. Picard found it impossible to rest. Mrs. Picard woke up many times, too. Mr. Picard would say, "Don't worry, I'm next to you. I'm sleeping." Finally, at 7 A.M., having hardy slept, he went home. He slept for a few hours and then came back because he knew that his wife needed him to be there.

Linda was too anxious to spend nights with her mother, and Mary had been admitted to the hospital with pain from kidney stones. The family decided not to tell Mrs. Picard about this. Mr. Picard did not dare ask his son to stay the night because Mark had his work and his own family, and he had not offered to stay. The ward staff tried to ensure that there was a volunteer to sit with Mrs. Picard late into the evening.

"She's so tired," Mr. Picard said to me around this time. "I don't know what keeps her going. She wanted to see Peter, one of our grandchildren, and she was so happy to see him. She was holding on for that. And then, it's her birthday in five days. I think she's waiting for her birthday to come. Is she waiting for her birthday, to die on her birthday? I don't know. Only God knows. But I hope that she goes soon, because to see her suffer—she hasn't eaten, she feels sick to her stomach. If only I could be the one to suffer, to spare her, but she's the one that has to suffer."

He sobbed. Then he continued,

I can't say that the nurses and doctors aren't doing their job. It's extraordinary what they do. But it's difficult anyway, to see her day after day and to see that she's still alive but that her color's changed and she's lost so much weight. She weighed 126 when she came in hospital and now she can't weigh more than 100 pounds. In the summer, she weighed 170 pounds. Yesterday we stopped by the Oratory and we prayed God to take her because it's difficult for us to see her suffer. The doctors can't do more than what they're doing. No, I can't ask more of them. They're doing their best, but she's the one who's suffering.

Mr. Picard had trouble containing his tears. The family looked exhausted. They had many questions about what would happen now. How was she going to die? Mrs. Picard had been weaker and confused for a few days but occasionally she seemed to perk up and be able to sit up in bed. Mary said, "She is such a lively person, always smiling. Even now, we were in the solarium and she wanted to talk with everyone, to touch everyone. She enjoys touching people. So do I. There was a Spanish-speaking woman there and she tried to talk to her in Spanish! She was so lively."

Whenever the music therapist came now, Mrs. Picard only wanted to hear the "Ave Maria." She looked sadder now, though she smiled occasionally. Death did not come.

Tired of Waiting

It was early March and Mrs. Picard again expressed frustration—she was tired of the whole situation. She started to feel anxious that the dying process was taking so long, and she was afraid that she might have more pain. When she asked Dr. Morin to give her a sedative so that she could sleep more during the day, Denise decided to increase the midazolam. Mrs. Picard now needed small amounts of medication (15 mg each of morphine and midazolam subcutaneously over 24 hours) to keep her asleep; the dexamethasone had been stopped.

By March 4, Mrs. Picard was obviously dying. She mostly slept, and she ate very little. She complained of thirst at one point, but this was alleviated by increasing her mouth care. I tried to talk with her but could not get a response. Mr. Picard, Linda, and Linda's husband were at the bedside. Linda was visibly upset and was not able to talk to me. She either paced in the hallway, her eyes red from crying, or she sat by her mother's bedside, holding her hand. She was trying her best to control her strong feelings and spend more time at her mother's bedside, especially since Mary was still in another hospital with her kidney stone problem. Mrs. Picard was so somnolent and confused that she seemed not to notice that Mary was absent. Still, Mr. Picard wanted his wife to receive even more sedation. "Mary and I spoke with Dr. Morin about it," he told me. "To give her an injection to relieve her—not euthanasia, but to relieve her. My wife also spoke to Dr. Morin about it. She is thinking about me, saying, 'You'd be better off at home.' I am staying with her all the time and she didn't want to bother anyone. She always thinks of others before thinking of herself."

In one of her rare wakeful moments, Mrs. Picard said again, "I'm tired. I'm fed up, let me go." By this time, she was not eating anything. Linda and her father wanted the nurse to give Mrs. Picard more tranquilizer, as their tolerance for any sign that she might be in discomfort or confused was low. They wanted her completely asleep. Although the nurse was very busy she understood their anxiety and gave Mrs. Picard another injection, even though to the nurse the degree of agitation was minor. Mrs. Picard was now receiving 5 mg midazolam every 4 hours, as required, to keep her asleep.

Mr. Picard was now the most anxious that I had seen him. He said that Mrs. Picard seemed uncomfortable in the bed, and he kept ringing the bell for the nurse to come. He got impatient when the nurse was not immediately available to help reposition his wife, whose legs were rubbing against the bed rails. He was trying to be polite, but his anxiety came through. He paced in the room. If he got upset, he would pace in the hallway. He said to me: "It is her 75th birthday today. She will have lived through it, but not experienced it. I have brought her flowers, but she is not aware of this. I am praying the Lord to take her today. I have been speaking with Linda over the weekend. I've told her, 'You have to accept that your mother is dying. You have to let her go.'"

"Don't Ask Me—Mary Is the Mother Now"

The next day, March 5, Mrs. Picard continued in her comatose state. She did not require any extra tranquilizer. Mary was now out of the hospital after a four-day stay and had come to be with her mother again. The family accepted live flute music at the bedside, particularly Mrs. Picard's favorite pieces, "Ave Maria" and Pachelbel's "Canon." Mary sang along. Mrs. Picard seemed calmer after the music. The family also used cassettes to play her favorite classical music. I got up to leave, and Mary followed me outside. As we sat in the family kitchen, Mary said,

> It's hard for my father. He is having a hard time over the last few days, since it has become apparent that Mom is dying. He can't bear not to be able to communicate with her now. It's easier for me than for my sister, and maybe also easier for me than for my father.
>
> Today is the first day that I have not seen her smile, because she can't smile. She always had a smile on her face. Everyone said, "Oh, your mother, she's the one who is always smiling." That's how they knew who she was. She likes to touch people and to be touched, so we touch her. We hold her and caress her. She likes that.
>
> Linda is having a hard time. She is afraid of death. I told her, "Linda, you have to get some help." She is so anxious. The other day Linda asked

my mother something, asked for her advice. And my mother said, "Don't ask me—Mary is the mother now." I have to be the strong one now. But my mother is there for me. Last night I felt her actual presence there beside me, so she will always be a presence for me.

I met Mr. Picard in the hallway. He was agitated. "It upset me today when I walked in and saw all those catheters," he said. The nurses had put in a urinary catheter because Mrs. Picard was too weak even to use the bedpan. There was only one catheter, but the tube and bags seemed to multiply in Mr. Picard's mind. "I don't know" he went on. "I didn't look closely, but I didn't like to see that. She is so much weaker, but she's holding on. She's gone through her birthday now." Tearfully, he went into the elevator.

The family and staff made sure that Mrs. Picard's favorite music tapes were played continually. Even though she was comatose, the music played all night. She died early the next morning. The family was not present, but they arrived soon after. Her death was described by the staff as peaceful.

"Evenings Are the Worst"

At first, Mr. Picard called Mary 20 to 40 times a day. He was crying all the time. He insisted that his children clear Mrs. Picard's things out of the house the day after the funeral—her clothes and jewelry, the mementos. Mary told me that she found this difficult, but they respected their father's wishes.

When I spoke to Mr. Picard five months after his wife's death he still seemed to be deep in his grief, though by this time he was calling Mary only five or six times per day, usually about "little things." He carried his wife's photograph with him as he wandered around the house. He put it on the dining table while he ate. "I try to avoid the house," he said, "because all the furniture and decorating was done by my wife." He was considering moving the next year, to get away from "the memories in this place." He played golf during the day, and this was a good distraction, but he found it difficult when he got back in the evenings. "Evenings are the worst," he told me. "I get so lonely." He went on:

After 53 years I was wondering if I could continue. But I spoke with her and it helped. She told me in the hospital, "I will be there for you." I go to the cemetery on the 6th of every month [the anniversary of the death], but my daughter Linda says, "Don't go so often." I don't listen to her. I listen to my heart. If I feel like talking to my wife, I talk to her. I talk to her all the time. Mary understands this, but Linda is having a hard time. When Linda comes over, she just wants to go through and look at her mother's things. She is suffering a lot.

Mr. Picard obtained a lot of comfort from being with his grandson. "I play golf with him and we talk about his grandmother and I feel better," he said. He also spoke with another grandson, who was a nurse. "His grandmother was his idol," said Mr. Picard. "I need to speak about these things. I know that some people must get bored or annoyed with me."

On what would have been their 53rd wedding anniversary, Mr. Picard went to the cemetery with his daughters and one granddaughter. He found the ritual helpful. However, he found the day of the six-month anniversary difficult, even though his daughters were there.

When I phoned him shortly after this, he sounded relaxed, calm, confident, steady, and in control. "I'm doing better," he said. He was thinking about his wife almost constantly. "She said to me before she died, 'I hope you'll continue to live.' But I can't go out with just anybody. I like to go out with my daughters. I see friends and play cards on Wednesday nights. I don't feel the need for a woman friend right now, although my friends are pushing me in that direction."

Mary, Linda, and Mark

Mary expressed disappointment in her relationship with her father at this time. She told me, "My sister and I are trying to help my father, but we are also suffering, and he doesn't see that. According to him, he's the only one who has the right to mourn. He never asks how I'm doing emotionally, only physically. My son and daughter, and Linda, I can speak to. Linda asks me a lot, how I'm doing. And I need to talk. My mother and father never really talked. She always talked with me. Maybe he feels guilty about not having communicated better with her. But I try to tell him not to feel guilty, that Mom forgave everything before she died, that she died in peace. But I think that he feels guilty about things that he didn't do in their relationship."

Mary had begun to volunteer in a palliative care program three months after her mother's death. "Even if it's just to hold someone's hand," she said, "I feel that I'm contributing something. I'm a listening ear. I love that work. She then spoke of the joy and comfort that her granddaughters brought to her in her grief.

> My granddaughter Kim is extraordinary. She is three years old. A few days ago we were walking by a pond with ducks. She said, "The ducks will die. Will Grandma feed them after they die?" She speaks incessantly of Grandma Rose. I have another granddaughter who was born on May 6— my mother died the 6th of March. I felt her presence there in the delivery room. This is a baby who is always smiling. Jade is her name. We associate her a lot with my mother. My mother used to say, "I won't see this baby born, but speak to this child about me." Kim said, "Doesn't Jade smile like Grandma?" I hope my grandchildren continue to grow like this. They're extraordinary.

Mr. Picard had also spoken to me about Jade. "This last grandchild," he told me, "born three months after her death, on the 6th—it's as if my wife sent her. She's here to guide us, this grandchild." The sixth of the month had become an important, difficult day.

Linda was doing better now than when she first learned of her mother's cancer diagnosis. She was very anxious, however, about her father's welfare, not wanting him to go far, and was worried about him dying, too. Linda was very close to her father, continuing to call him every day, as she had done even before her mother died. Mark seemed to be coping in a different way; he never spoke about his mother. Mary was never able to speak with him alone, without the children there, to see how he was feeling, and he didn't seem to encourage such discussions.

Getting On

Mr. Picard was experiencing the change of seasons differently now. As autumn came, he said to me, "I didn't want to go out. My children had to come see me here. Between the sixth and the ninth of this month, it was difficult. I felt the winter coming. Then the leaves fell, there were no leaves. The trees looked different. I was glad to have my family around."

The first Thanksgiving was difficult. They were not looking forward to Christmas. "I have to buy Christmas cards," Mr. Picard said. "My wife used to do that. So I'm trying to do that in the same way my wife did it. We're trying to carry on living, even though she's not here. Last week, I cooked dinner for the whole family. The year before she died she taught me how to cook, do the laundry, clean the house. She used to do everything. If she hadn't taught me, I would have had a hard time right now. She was understanding and practical. I could not have had the same life without her. She was wise. She was always right when she said things."

Mr. Picard found it difficult to plan vacation trips, since he had always traveled with his wife. But now he was planning to visit his grandson in Texas. When Christmas, came the family coped by celebrating in new ways. They rented a house in Vermont and had pot-luck dinners. Mr. Picard found it helpful to have done something different.

When I spoke to Mr. Picard one year after his wife's death, he was still very conscious of her presence. This was both reassuring and distressing to him. "In July, I will move to another apartment," he said. "Because she's here with me all the time. We speak often. Is this normal?" I reassured him that it was. "She tells me, 'Rest, you've had enough,' or, 'Continue with your life.' When I play with my granddaughter. I see my wife's brown eyes and that helps me.

"I'm lucky that my children are so helpful," he went on. "Like when I told them I would move, they told me not to worry. They would help. Here I see her everywhere. I know I won't forget her, but by changing surroundings, maybe it will help me get on with my life."

Authors' Comments

Mrs. Picard's oncologist gave her a very specific answer—"approximately four weeks"—in reply to her direct question regarding prognosis. Although this turned out to be accurate, we try to stay away from giving precise estimates, as we are often wrong. As the Picard family discovered, the dying process can take many days or even weeks. Families are often not prepared for this, and experience mental anguish as they keep vigil. Mrs. Picard developed terminal delirium in the last days of life, requiring sedation. This common symptom causes families much distress and divides family members—some of whom will agree to sedation and some will not, believing that it will shorten life or that it will reduce opportunity for some meaningful, final communication. Whether parenteral hydration should be used at the same time as sedation at end of life is an issue that requires careful case-by-case consideration and good communication with the family.

In the present environment of legally available medical aid in dying (MAID), the family's exhaustion and that of Mrs. Picard herself might well have encouraged them to request euthanasia. As it was, the family was asking for more sedation than was strictly necessary, producing a dilemma in the mind of the nurse. A euthanasia request in these circumstances would illustrate very well the findings on the most common reasons for these requests that we discussed in the General Introduction: it is not poorly managed pain or other symptoms that underlie most requests but the feeling that life has lost its point, that existence itself is the harm from which the individual wishes to be freed.

Mr. Picard experienced intense grief following the death of his wife of 52 years. This would in fact be categorized as normal under the circumstances. His children could not help him since they were dealing with their own reactions. It is interesting that Mary started to volunteer in a palliative care program three months after her mother's death. This brought her a sense of meaning. The meaning and joy that grandchildren can bring to those at end of life and to the bereaved is also exemplified in this narrative. Linda, however, might have benefited from some counseling, but, because of her location, she could not be linked up with the bereavement service of the PCU. There was no record of whether she had an established relationship with a family physician who might have helped her.

Finally, there is this noteworthy observation of Father Francis, the pastoral worker assigned to the PCU, regarding Mrs. Picard's religious faith: "It's surprising to me, because the more she declines physically, the stronger her faith. But it is a balanced faith, not an exuberant faith. It isn't, 'I believe in God no matter what, everything rests with Him, and you'll see—He will save me.' It isn't the kind of faith that's like a lifesaver." Mrs. Picard herself said,

> I am not afraid of dying. I am facing it with serenity. I want it to be beautiful. I want it to be me. Then, in the church, I don't want any fanfare. All I want is for the ones I love to be there. I have accepted this, but it hasn't been easy. I don't want to flinch too much, but it hurts.

Father Francis is describing, and Mrs. Picard is expressing, an experience of faith that can be affirmative and hopeful while fully recognizing the reality of loss and grief. Perhaps this is the very posture that Czesław Miłosz was invoking in the words we quoted at the end of the General Introduction: "I am not seeking an escape from dread but rather proof that dread and reverence can exist within us simultaneously."

9

Victor Sloski

"If I Had to Do It All Over Again, I Would Do It"

Narrated by Patricia Boston

Victor Sloski learned that he had lung cancer when he was 57. The news was hard to take. He had lived happily with Shirley, his live-in companion, for 20 years. Still, when experimental treatments failed, he was prepared to die, hoping the end would come soon. It didn't. His cancer metastasized from his lungs to his stomach, spleen, colon, and finally, to his brain, causing him to go blind. The palliative care team offered to arrange an admission to the inpatient unit, but Mr. Sloski insisted that he wanted home care. He wanted to die at home regardless of how ill he became. Victor Sloski did die at home. Afterward, Shirley said, "Caring for a dying husband was the biggest challenge of my life. But if I had to do it all over again, I would do it." Getting to that point had been very hard. At times Shirley felt that she was too exhausted, emotionally and physically, to go on.

Life Before: A New Beginning

Victor Sloski had never been afraid of hard labor. He was 18 years old when he first arrived in Canada to look for work. Born in Poland just before World War II, he was raised with a brother and two sisters on a farm 30 miles from the city of Warsaw. Most of what he knew about reading and writing came from 4 or 5 years of elementary school before he went to work on the farm. When times got difficult in Poland, he emigrated to Canada, where his experience in farming stood him well. He found a job on a small French-Canadian farm 20 miles north of Montreal.

This job lasted only a few months, but the farmer helped him find work at the local farmers' market, loading and unloading fruit and vegetables from the trucks that brought produce to the markets every day. When that job folded, he found work at a larger city market, unloading fruit and vegetables from rail cars and from the ships at the city's dock. He held that job for the next 20 years. He might have been able to get other work if he'd had an education, but this had not really worried him. "Work never hurt anybody," Victor said. Sometimes he worked 18–20 hours a day. The pay was not much, but it put bread on his table, and he was able to send money back to his now widowed mother and his sisters in Warsaw. Most years he'd been able to send $300–400 a year.

In the kind of work he did there was little chance to meet women. He was almost 40 years old when he met Shirley, an accounts clerk at one of the central market offices. Shirley came from a farming family in Manitoba, about 1,000 miles from Montreal. Victor wasn't one for marriage; he couldn't guarantee enough security. But he liked Shirley a lot. She was "kind" and "a good looker." She liked Victor. He was "the strong, silent type." They lived together for the next 20 years in a small, one-bedroom apartment over a grocery store in the small working-class suburb of Ste. Marie. They had no children as they couldn't afford to raise a child. "You never knew whether or not you'd be out of work and have to go on welfare," Victor said.

The guys who worked with Victor were good buddies who would help out without asking why "if you were short of a dollar." After a day's unloading at the dock, they'd had many a good night at the tavern with a few beers and a smoke. Victor had been a smoker all of his life, smoking two to three packs of cigarettes a day, sometimes lighting one cigarette with the last. He never thought about it much, for everybody had smoked. Some of the guys never had a cigarette out of their hand, Victor said to me. Besides, he added, when you were the worrying kind, a good cigarette helped you relax.

Something's Wrong

In 1993, Victor began to notice a nagging cough. He had always had a smoker's cough, but this was more persistent. It kept him up at night and made him feel tired on the job. He began getting short of breath, and even small tasks became hard to cope with. Some days, instead of stopping off for a beer at the tavern or fixing gadgets around the house after work, he needed to go straight to bed.

In October, Mr. Sloski saw James Gregory, his local general practitioner, and asked him for some cough syrup. After listening to Victor's chest, Dr. Gregory ordered chest X-rays and a computed tomography (CT) scan. The X-ray showed a large mass, and the CT scan showed a hilar mass and a small lesion in the right lung. Following a transthoracic needle aspiration to obtain a small biopsy of lung tissue, the pathology report indicated a large-cell undifferentiated carcinoma. Further tests revealed metastases to the liver and spleen.

A few months later, a surgeon at the city hospital performed a splenectomy in an attempt to arrest the spread of the cancer, but it was immediately clear that further surgical intervention would not be effective. At this point, Mr. Sloski was referred to Dr. Raymond Limberg in medical oncology. From March to August of 1994, Mr. Sloski received six courses of experimental chemotherapy. A follow-up CT scan showed there was no change in the tumor, and X-rays revealed further progression of the disease. Over the next year, the oncologists tried two more experimental drugs, but Mr. Sloski's cancer did not respond. In December 1995, Dr. Limberg consulted with Dr. Gillian Webster of the Palliative Care Service.

Around this time, Mr. Sloski began to complain of difficulty with his vision. He also began to feel unsteady on his feet. He would be walking along and then suddenly keel over to his right side. In January 1996, Dr. Limberg ordered another CT scan. The cancer was in Mr. Sloski's brain.

"I Knew the Real Story"

The best option that Gillian Webster and the palliative care team could suggest was to refer Mr. Sloski for a palliative course of external beam radiotherapy to the brain. Radiotherapy is sometimes used therapeutically in palliative care to alleviate a tumor's pressure by reducing its size. Victor agreed to undergo five radiation treatments. He knew that the radiation treatments would not make his cancer go away. In that sense, he said, he knew "the real story." He had never been one for avoiding things that needed to be faced. Still, he recalled to me later, "they said the radiation would stay with you at least for a month. So I thought it would do some good. Maybe stop the pain in my head."

While it may have helped reduce his headaches, it seemed that his sight was still worsening. As the days and weeks passed, he couldn't read the paper even with his glasses.

Despite these setbacks, his appetite was good—at least for the moment. Shirley prepared his favorite foods, even if it was an expensive piece of steak, just to get him to eat a few mouthfuls.

Eating was small comfort, however, when so many other things were going wrong in his body. He was beginning to have seizures, or "fits," as he called them. At times everything would go black for a few seconds. Gillian prescribed phenytoin, which seemed to work, and after a few days Mr. Sloski reported fewer seizures. By March, however, he was having more abdominal pain. Gillian prescribed omeprazole, which helped to alleviate the discomfort, but Mr. Sloski was in emotional turmoil. What would happen next to his body? He couldn't sleep through the night, and he had panic attacks almost every day. He also experienced periods of intense depression. Gillian prescribed nortriptyline, which helped to lift Victor's spirits, and clonazepam and rivotril to calm him and control the acute panic attacks.

By this time, Grania MacDonald, the palliative home care nurse, was following Mr. Sloski. When she visited their home in Ste. Marie, Grania found that Mr. Sloski and Shirley were very comfortable talking about the progression of his illness. Mr. Sloski talked easily of his experiences with his symptoms and what it was like "to be living like a sick person when you had worked all your life." When Grania mentioned our research project to them, they said they would be very willing to participate. They both thought it important that doctors and nurses be aware of what these experiences could be like. I visited their home for the first time in early March.

"It's Scary for Me and Scary for Her"

Ste. Marie is a community that visitors might pass through on their way to other places. It is a world of commerce and small-housing tenements that sprawls untidily along the northern end of Montreal. The stretch between Montreal and Ste. Marie includes factories and some fine 19th-century stone buildings and churches, blackened by age, and French-Canadian homes built at the turn of the 20th century that open directly onto the sidewalk. Mainly immigrant families live in these homes now, families of Italian, Polish, Greek,

Ukrainian, Russian, or Czechoslovakian descent. Many arrived at the turn of the century or immediately following the world wars.

Some of these buildings are three or four stories high, with heavy lace curtains veiling windows so that passers-by cannot easily look inside. In late summer and fall, painted window boxes are full of hardy perennials. In the spring, tulips, daffodils, and hyacinths are in bloom, the bulbs having been carefully stored in dark basements over the winter. Other stretches of the road to Ste. Marie are less well kept. Buildings with dull, uncleaned windows or frames filled in with cardboard or plywood, stand on grounds littered with old beer bottles, cans, and cigarette butts. Many shops line the route, with several *dépanneurs* (corner convenience stores) and local bakeries producing delicious smells of breads and other goods, where one can buy a dozen fresh bagels—baked on hot coals while you watch—croissants, or a fresh baguette. Fast food cafes and restaurant chains are everywhere; at lunch time workers line up for inexpensive hot dogs, souvlaki, pizza, or French fries and gravy (a popular local snack known as *poutine*).

Victor Sloski could not imagine living anywhere else. Although their apartment over the grocery store had three rooms, to me it looked no larger than two regular-sized rooms. The main room doubled as a sitting room and bedroom. A large television took up one corner. The rest of the room was dominated by a king-size bed with red, braided bedcovers and bright red and pink satin cushions. Most of their socializing took place at a tiny kitchen table at the back of the apartment, whether their guest was a friend, neighbor, nurse, doctor, or priest. Most of our conversations were at that table, too.

On my first visit, Victor appeared as a tall, lean, broad-boned man who must have looked more muscular before he got sick. He was almost bald, which, Shirley explained, was due to the radiation. Most of the time, Mr. Sloski didn't look directly at me when he spoke; he stared straight ahead, as if he were recalling some event. On this occasion, he spoke freely and easily, in carefully chosen words, about his life and the progression of his illness.

It was hard to understand, he said, how he could have become so sick, with so many things going wrong all at once. He had no illusions—he knew for sure that he was going to die. People were kind and helpful, but there was too much wrong with his body. The worst part was just having to sit and wait, with all this time on his hands, worrying that more pain would come. Here at home he still had a lot of work to do—fixing the place, painting, caring for the tomatoes and flowers on his balcony. But he could do nothing. "If I lay down,

I can't breathe," he told me. "It's like something choking me. I cannot stand up and walk. It's too much. I know that I'm getting blind, too. Every day I see less and less. I eat a little bit at a time. But even my appetite is going. I got pain in my stomach and chest. I'm scared of all this." He motioned toward Shirley. "It's scary for me and scary for her."

At this point, Mr. Sloski was receiving hydromorphone 10 mg by mouth every 4 hours for pain, phenytoin 100 mg orally three times a day for control of his seizures, and clonazepam 0.5 mg twice a day for anxiety. Dr. Webster had also prescribed Colace 100 mg taken orally twice a day to prevent constipation, and a liquid antacid whenever he needed it after eating. Victor wondered if taking so many pills contributed to his blindness. How could you know? he thought. It could be anything.

On this particular day, Shirley said, things weren't too bad. She had been able to persuade Victor to eat two soft-boiled eggs. The previous day he had eaten some Cream of Wheat and a little boiled beef with mashed-up potato, carrot, and turnip. He had liked that, and it had stayed down. He had managed to take a shower without any help and watch his favorite science fiction programs on TV.

Shirley said that the best thing for Victor right now was when his family called from Poland. In all these years, he had not been one to have much contact with his mother or his brothers and sisters. He hadn't even wanted to mention his illness. But after a lot of discussion and persuasion from Shirley, he finally called his older sister Melinka and told her about it and that he would not get better. Victor still wasn't convinced that his family needed to know so much. As he put it to me, "How you gonna call it? Boring! It's not pleasant for them. Now they're all crying about me. What can they do back there?" When Shirley and Gillian Webster wondered if some of his family might come over now to see him, Victor objected that it was just not worth it, it was too far to travel, his mother was too old at age 84, and so on.

Anxious and depressed as he was, and even though he feared more pain, Mr. Sloski did not want to die before his time, and he didn't want anyone to help him do it, either. Speaking of the possibility of suicide, he told me, "I've thought about that. But I don't believe you have the right to take your own life and no one else has the right to do it for you. When your time is come, he will decide for you, and if you have to suffer, you have to suffer."

Although as an adult he had not gone to Mass every Sunday, he had been raised Catholic in Poland, attending Mass regularly with his mother and sisters as a child and saying prayers together nightly. In many ways, his childhood faith had remained with him. Although it wavered some-times, he still believed in God, and he was sure there was a life after this one. What was happening to him was God's will; his life was in His hand. Victor believed that if one suffered, it was probably for all the wrongs one had done in this life. One had to pay for them—if not here then in the next place—and it was better to pay for them now. Even if he were to suffer more, he said, the most important thing was to die at home, in his own bed, with Shirley at his side.

"Why Don't You Two Get Married?"

Over the next several weeks, Mr. Sloski weakened rapidly, and he seemed to withdraw more into himself. "I'm just a burden to everybody," he would say. "Why bother with me? I'm finished already!" At times, both Victor and Shirley were openly angry. "He worked so hard all his life and now this!" Shirley shouted during one of my visits. "Why him? Why not some of those miserable people who never did anyone any good?"

Grania MacDonald, their home care nurse, really liked Victor and Shirley. She felt tremendous empathy for them, yet she felt helpless in shielding them from the ceaseless rain of problems. She later recalled to me,

> Everything had gone so fast. It seemed like they got hit by one blow after another. They would have liked the stomach problems to be ulcers, fixable with Maalox or another antacid. But the stomach problems were not ulcers, they were cancerous tumors. There was no radiotherapy for that because it could do more harm than good. Then a lump he felt under his arm was radiated, but it didn't get smaller, it just got hotter. And it went on and on. It seemed that from one week to the next, there was another affront to this poor man's body. They really seemed to be in a boat with no oars.

At this point, Grania was visiting twice a week. She tried to focus on the things she could do that would make a positive difference. There didn't seem to be much. Victor worried what would happen to Shirley when he passed on. There wasn't much money—a few government retirement bonds and a small pension. While they lived in a common-law marriage, they were not legally married, and he wasn't sure whether she could legally benefit from the small estate he would leave.

Grania saw an opportunity. "Why don't you two get married?" she asked during a home visit in March. "It could easily be arranged and perhaps legalize things so that you could put some of your affairs in order." Victor and Shirley liked this idea, though things would have to happen quickly. Victor's mind was still clear now, but as the disease in his brain increased, he would quite possibly become more confused and disoriented. By the time a civil service could be arranged at City Hall in Montreal it might be too late. Grania knew another nurse who was also a minister and explained the situation to her. Later that month, the minister came to the house, married Victor and Shirley with some neighbors as witnesses, laid out the refreshments on the kitchen table, and took the photographs.

Victor told Grania he wished they had thought of this earlier, so Shirley could have had a nicer wedding. But he took satisfaction from the assurance that Shirley would be provided for more securely. He still worried about her; it seemed to him that Shirley was denying things. She should realize that he was a dying man, he said. "She shouldn't go down to the stores and tell the neighbors and the store people that I'm getting better." Actually, Shirley did know her husband was dying. "But," she said, "I try to put it to the back of my mind, and look on the bright side." This did not suit Victor. As he put it, "I'm sick and I'm dying and that's it."

Grania shared some of Mr. Sloski's concerns about Shirley. Whereas Victor talked about what he felt, Shirley seemed more fragile, more isolated. She had a sister and brother in Winnipeg, but that was 1,000 miles away. Victor's family were in Poland, and he didn't want to see them. Here in Ste. Marie, Shirley had few friends. Her neighbors worked 12-hour shifts in the factories. They had their own troubles. How could she ask them to come in and look after Victor for even an hour?

Financial Problems and Other Worries

The Sloskis' finances were a more immediate problem. In Quebec, the government allows certain financial benefits to defray the cost of medication and treatment measures, but not all of these are covered by the government allowance. The most convenient option for opioid delivery for Mr. Sloski would have been a fentanyl dermal patch (changed every 3 days) But, at the time, that preparation was not on the government formulary. When Dr. Webster called the local pharmacy, she discovered that the patches would cost $250 for 2 weeks, which the Sloskis could not afford. The next most convenient option, long-acting morphine rectal suppositories given every 12 hours, cost $200 for 2 weeks. Grania suggested that the cheapest option of all would be oxycodone suppositories, which she could obtain free from the hospital. The problem was that Mr. Sloski might need two or three suppositories every 4 hours to equal the hydromorphone he was receiving now. Gillian finally decided simply to increase the dosage of oral hydromorphone for as long as he could swallow.

Gillian knew that as Mr. Sloski deteriorated there would be a risk of aspiration pneumonia if Shirley continued feeding him as she was. At this point, she chose not to dwell on this with Shirley, who was just getting used to the idea that her husband was dying. Still, Gillian did mention to her that there was a possibility that her husband could develop pneumonia, so that she could be prepared for that eventuality.

"If I Could Pull God Down from Heaven, I'd Beat Him Up!"

"Why doesn't everyone just leave me?" Victor said to me during one of my visits in the spring. "Can't they see there's nothing to be done? Everything has been tried. Nobody should bother." He would sometimes stop in the middle of a sentence, as if it hardly mattered to him whether he finished it or not. "Forget it!" he would say at last after a long pause.

Shirley had stopped praying. She was Catholic, went to church regularly, and received the sacraments of the church. But now she was angry. "This morning I cried all morning," she told me one day. "I just couldn't stop. I called out to God, 'Why are you doing this to us? To me?' After I had cried for what must have been a good 2 hours, I felt more peaceful inside. Maybe God *was* there?" If he was, she told Grania, she had some business with Him. "If I could pull God down from Heaven, I'd beat him up!" she said.

Victor was not sure that God was necessarily at fault. He had always believed in miracles, even if he was not a practicing Catholic. But perhaps the miracles were not meant for him. Some people, if they prayed hard enough, would get their prayers answered, he said, but he was resigned to the idea that maybe God was punishing him for some wrongdoing. After all, the couple had lived together unmarried for 20 years. They were married now, of course, but they had not been married in a Catholic Church, and, in the eyes of the church, that was a sin. No doubt, there were also other sins for which he was now being punished. Grania suggested a visit by the local priest, which seemed to bring some comfort. He heard Victor's confession and spoke to Shirley at length. She was relieved that Victor had been able to receive the Sacrament of the Sick. "If he has sins on his mind, now they will be forgiven before he leaves this world," she said.

Shirley was still worried about how she was going to cope, especially at the end. On one of Grania's next visits she flung question after question at her: "What shall I do? How will I know when he's gone? What have I not done that I am supposed to do? Should I find the funeral home now? Do I have to give his papers [Social Security card and ID cards] to the funeral home? How will I know what to do when the time comes? Victor just wants to be left to die, but what about *me*? What will *I* do?"

Grania actually believed that Mr. Sloski ought to be admitted to the Palliative Care Unit (PCU) for the last days of his life. Even as she tried to reassure him that his wife was a strong woman who would come through for him in whatever ways she needed to, privately she wondered whether Mrs. Sloski might break down in a crisis. At the same time she was also aware of Mr. Sloski's unshakable determination to die at home. She explained that all Shirley would need to do when the time came would be to make a telephone call to the city emergency health services. Everything would then be arranged from there. The city emergency service ambulance and a physician would come. The Palliative Care Service would have already apprised them of Mr. Sloski's situation, so everything would happen smoothly. It was possible that when Mr. Sloski died, Shirley might have to wait for an hour or so—sometimes that could happen. But the emergency services would come, she could be assured of that. Grania described how things usually worked with respect to funeral organization and planning, the papers she would need to have handy, and what would be expected of her.

Later, Grania told me,

I tried very hard to stay with what she needs to know. At some level she doesn't want to deal with the hard cold facts of funeral homes. Ideally, I think she'd like to feel he'll improve. But she knows he won't and I reiterated that, because I think it helps her deal with what she has to know. I hope I was gentle with the information. I know I must be careful to say things gently, kindly. But lies would be no better.

Nursing Victor at Home

In addition to Grania's twice-per-week visits, nurses from the local community health center came to the apartment to help Mr. Sloski with bathing and
dressing and to administer medications. More often than not, it was Shirley
who needed the most support, as there were times when she felt despair. Yet
she had to go on: "A couple of cigarettes and a good cry and I just carry on,"
she said. It didn't matter what kind of care was needed. If Victor needed a
bedpan, a back rub, or help with his bath, she would do it.

Shirley still seemed to believe that if she pushed Victor to eat more, he
would get stronger and perhaps the end could be delayed. "He's so thin and
undernourished," she said. "Perhaps a little soup or some ice cream. I keep
thinking and thinking, 'I could help him to get a bit stronger.' Maybe I'm not
being very realistic, but I can't stand the thought of him dying, of having to
see his life end. Surely there are things I can do."

"What can I do to prevent his pain?" she asked. "Can the doctors predict
ahead of time what pain he will have and prepare for it?" Grania did her best
to explain the effectiveness of the medications and to explain the potency of
hydromorphone and its equivalent in morphine. Shirley seemed to understand that Victor's pain medication was already at a very high dosage, and
that his pain was well controlled. On the other hand, he was more and more
bedbound, and he had become very thin. His thigh bones and coccyx were
barely covered by skin, and his body had little protection against bedsores.
Thin as he was, however, he was a well-built man. Even with two people it was
hard to lift him in the bed or to maintain balance when getting him out of the
bed into a chair. Grania and Gillian marveled that Mrs. Sloski could keep on
doing so much by herself.

On one visit in June, I witnessed first-hand how much Mrs. Sloski had
learned about nursing care. We went together into Mr. Sloski's room. He
seemed much less responsive, although he occasionally opened his eyes
and made eye contact. Mrs. Sloski knelt beside the bed and brought her face
very close to his. He said something to her that I could not hear, and then
she straightened up and deftly rearranged the pillows. Gently she moved
her husband's head and in no time she had placed three or four pillows in
comfortable positions beneath his head and arms. I offered to help, and Mrs.
Sloski promptly gave me instructions, undoubtedly unaware that I am a
nurse myself. Under her direction we arranged ourselves on opposite sides of

the bed, took hold of the sheet, and—on her count of three—scooted Victor up toward the head of the bed. Then she gave him his medications, holding his head forward and supporting it carefully while he drank from the cup and swallowed the pills. When all was done, Mr. Sloski opened his eyes and looked wide-eyed into his wife's face.

A Family Visit

Beyond an occasional phone call to see how Victor was doing, people didn't come around much, so Shirley Sloski often cried alone. She tried not to cry in front of her husband. She could cry with Grania there, and sometimes she cried on my visits. The team worried that there were not enough support services for not only her, but for all of the family caregivers who wanted to care for their loved ones at home. Grania contacted the community social service agency so they would visit, and she asked the priest if he could make regular visits. Shirley was willing to talk to the priest and the social worker, but, for the most part, she was taken up with caring for her husband. In such a tiny apartment it was hard to talk about things that were on her mind with any real privacy or without constantly feeling that Victor needed her.

Dr. Webster was aware of the many arguments the Sloskis had had over the possibility that his family could visit from Poland. She sparked one of these discussions during a home visit when she asked Mr. Sloski how his family was reacting to his situation. "They are upset, and they feel helpless," he replied. "They are upset because I am young to have this. But I don't think they should come over. It's too late for them to come over. I could die tomorrow."

Mrs. Sloski jumped in, "They *could* come over."

"Where would they stay?" Mr. Sloski asked her.

"They could stay here."

"What would they do?"

Mrs. Sloski thought for a moment. "Well," she said, "I think it would be good for you to see them." She turned to Gillian. "Don't you think it would be good for him if he saw his family again?"

Dr. Webster tried to be diplomatic. "It's not up to me to say," she replied.

"Well," Mrs. Sloski went on, "I tried to organize for them to phone again on Sunday—"

Mr. Sloski interrupted. "I'm having problems with my speech."

"Your speech isn't that bad today," his wife countered, with another glance at Gillian for confirmation, "is it, Doctor?" She turned back to her husband. "It's just on and off that your speech is a problem."

"Well, it's too late for them to come," Mr. Sloski said, as if to put an end to the matter. "And they are not well themselves."

Despite her husband's doubts and protests, Shirley made a point of keeping regular contact with Melinka. Meanwhile, Mr. Sloski was sleeping more and more, and at last Shirley took it upon herself to call Melinka and invite her to visit. Regardless of Victor's preferences, she wanted Melinka to come. In late June, Melinka arrived from Warsaw with her 20-year-old daughter, Miriam. Though Victor was now too ill to have much meaningful interaction, Melinka wanted to see him before he died. She had not seen her brother in 30 years.

Melinka and Miriam stayed for 1 week, during which time Grania made one of her visits. She told me that Melinka seemed horrified at her brother's appearance, even though she knew he was dying, and that Miriam looked frightened when she was with her uncle, whom she had never met before. Yet Grania also thought Mr. Sloski was able to recognize them and seemed to appreciate the fact that they had come because he was dying. As the three women nursed him together, he seemed more at peace.

A week after Melinka and Miriam returned to Poland, Mr. Sloski's breathing became more labored. Grania suggested to Mrs. Sloski that he might go soon and once again offered the option of transferring Mr. Sloski to the PCU. "I don't want you to take him to the hospital!" Mrs. Sloski cried. "I want to have him here at home. If I can't manage then I'll just have to tell someone and I'll just call." Grania reminded her that all she needed to do was pick up the telephone and a PCU admission would quickly be arranged. The next day, Mr. Sloski seemed more congested in his chest and his breathing became more labored. Shirley went to the phone and called the hospital. When she returned to the bedroom, Victor was dead.

Bereavement

Mrs. Sloski remembered everything that she needed to do. She called the city emergency health services, and the physician and ambulance arrived within minutes of her call. Even though she knew her husband was gone, she told me later, when the ambulance came and the attendants were taking the body from the apartment she asked them, "Are you sure he is dead?" and they said,

"Yes, madam, he is." She had felt bad when they had taken off Victor's watch and his cross and chain. They had also taken off his wedding ring and put it on the kitchen table. Mrs. Sloski said to them, "I didn't want you to do that." They told her. "We have to do this, but you can ask the funeral parlor to put them back on." Later she took the wedding ring and cross and chain to the funeral parlor, and a woman there helped her put them back on.

Shirley organized a big party for the funeral. Everyone whom Victor and she had ever known was invited to come back to the house after the service. She ordered food from a local catering company who gave her a special discount because they had personally known Victor. Only about a dozen people came back, but Mrs. Sloski said it didn't matter. Victor would be looking down from Heaven and he would know she had made the party for him anyway.

During the next few months, I visited Mrs. Sloski on several occasions. She told me that having to watch Victor suffer had bothered her most of all. There was very little she felt she could do. Sure, she could nurse him and do the necessary things. But as time had gone by and he got sicker and sicker, she felt more and more helpless. "I felt I did not do enough," she said. "Or maybe there was something else I could have done, even the day he died. Maybe I shouldn't have left him for that minute to make the phone call. Sometimes I think I did things wrong out of sheer desperation. Like trying to feed him and forcing him to eat, which I'm sure didn't help him."

It was odd, she said. She knew Victor would die. The odds were against a miracle happening. But she was often able to put this on the back burner and deny it to herself. Being so busy with all the nursing care, she didn't need to think about it if she didn't want to. It had been difficult when she went to the funeral home to choose the casket. She told me that she couldn't even enter the showroom at first. The man at the showroom had been very patient, and she had gone outside for a cigarette. When she came back in, she picked out a casket that seemed all right. The man began to suggest some additional items, she recalled, smiling at this memory. "Now," he had said, "would you like—" "No! I wouldn't!" Mrs. Sloski told him. "I would like to get out of here!" She was laughing now as she told me this. "And I left."

When I visited her 3 months after her husband's death, Shirley said she was often having "fits of crying." The nights were long and lonely. Twenty years was a long time to live with someone; being in the house alone still required some getting used to. She had always felt safe having a man in the house. Before he got sick, Victor was a strong man who could tackle anything. There wasn't much chance of a break-in with Victor around. She usually stayed in at night now. If she did go out and it was dark when she returned, she was very careful. "I don't just walk in and turn the lights on," she said. "I creep up the stairs. I turn the light on." She laughed again. "I check all the cupboards, and under the beds."

The bereavement team from the PCU had been very kind, Mrs. Sloski said. A social worker from the local community agency had visited regularly, and she had been able to talk about some of her fears. Gillian Webster had called to see how she was coping. And Grania still visited regularly. Reflecting on the help she had received, Mrs. Sloski said, "I could not have expected any more and I don't think my husband expected any more. He knew at the end there was nothing to be done, no cure. Things weren't ideal, but he knew we were all caring for him in the best way we knew how." Then she said, "Caring for my husband, knowing he was going to die any day and not knowing what would happen, was never easy. I would say it was probably the biggest challenge of my life, if you can call it that. But if I had to do it all over again, I would do it."

Now she planned to attend a bereavement group at the hospital, made up of other family members who had lost a loved one to cancer. "I want to try it. The neighbors have been very kind, but they have husbands who come home to them at night and someone to have supper with." The bereavement group would be good for her, Mrs. Sloski said. These were people who had gone through the same thing, "who knew what it was like to sit home alone and watch TV and feel empty."

Authors' Comments

Every Canadian province and territory in Canada offers a general social assistance program for low-income families. Given their limited financial resources the Sloskis might have qualified for extra home care. Certainly, they were unable to afford anything extra beyond what the hospital was offering on Medicare. Medication coverage was also an issue for Victor. Twenty years ago the Quebec government did allow certain benefits to defray the cost of medications and certain treatment measures. But we note that while the most convenient option for Mr. Sloski's pain relief would have been a fentanyl dermal patch (changed every 3 days) to replace the oral hydromorphone he was receiving every 4 hours, the fentanyl patch was not available on the government formulary. The Sloskis would have had to pay out of pocket and could not afford to do this, though today this option would be fully covered.

We note that Shirley had stopped praying. Now she was angry. "If I could pull God down from Heaven, I'd beat him up," she said. Compare this with Klara Bergman's anger and argument with God, which we mention in the Authors' Comments to that narrative. It is not clear whether or not Shirley might have found comfort or reconciliation through counselling from a Catholic priest at this juncture. It is also possible that both she and Victor may have been suffering from depression, in which case a psychiatric consult would have been appropriate, with the added possibility of antidepressant medication. It was helpful to Victor that Grania offered to ask for a Catholic priest. It might have helped this couple to find more peace if the priest's visits had been offered as part of the routine care at an earlier point, or even when Victor was first diagnosed. Pastoral care has always been readily available to palliative care teams and was available at the Royal Victoria at that time. It is worth noting, however, that in the past 20 years there has been considerable attention paid to spiritual distress and spiritual well-being in palliative care in both the research literature and in clinical practice and, by extension, a greater awareness of its significance by palliative care providers.

What seems to compound the challenge of family caregiving is the constant knowledge of impending loss that accompanies the physical act of caregiving. Shirley Sloski clearly had strong support from the palliative care team for the increasingly complex requirements of caring for Victor, but her grief in the knowledge of his impending death was clearly painful. She feared the moment when Victor would die. "What shall I do?" she asked. "How will I know when he's gone? Victor just wants to be left to die, but what about *me*?"

Family caregivers caring for a terminally ill loved one must deal with many kinds of losses: Loss of the future as anticipated, loss of the relationship as it once was known, loss of a loved one to share life's tasks, loss of the reassurance of ongoing love. . . . The majority of grief research to date has focused on the emotions and perspectives of people following a loss. In recent years, however, more focus is being placed on what is called *anticipatory grief*.[1,2]

Shirley tried so hard to help Victor get a little stronger. Despite the knowledge that he was dying and there was little hope of his health improving medically, she still tried to coax him to eat in the hope that it might improve his condition. Victor knew he was dying and that he was now at the end of his life. But, as Shirley put it, "I can't stand the thought of him dying or having to see his life end. Surely there are things I can do." This situation appeared to change, however, after the rapidly arranged visit of Victor's sister and niece from Poland. This was a huge event. Victor died about a week after his sister had gone home. It is possible that seeing his sister after so many years helped to give Victor some closure that enabled "letting go." Similarly, was it only a coincidence that Victor died at the very moment when Shirley went to the telephone to call the hospital? We can ask whether Shirley's anxious hovering at the bedside and trying so hard to make him stronger had kept Victor "stuck" in some way, and, when he was alone, he was able to die.

References

1. Coelho A, Barbosa A. Family anticipatory grief: An integrative literature review. Am J Hospice Palliat Care. 2017;34(8):774–785. https://doi.org/10.1177/104990911 6647960
2. Coelho A, de Brito M, Teixira P, Frade P, Barros L. Family caregivers anticipatory grief: A conceptual framework for understanding its multiple challenges. Qualitat Health Res. 2020;30(5):693–703. https://doi.org/10.1177/1049732319873330

10

Leonard Patterson

Jagged Edges

Narrated by Yanna Lambrinidou

Leonard Patterson was a 62-year-old White American man with rectal cancer. His poverty, tumultuous relationships with his family, and unmanageable pain produced a cluster of unresolved problems in the final months of his life. Despite the painstaking efforts of hospice to offer him a peaceful death and his family a smooth transition to a life without him, this case left many of its participants unsettled. One of the questions it raises is whether the best of palliative care can ease shattered lives in situations that are not only complex but also depart from the economic, social, and cultural "norm" of the families that hospice tends to serve.

"His Heart Was as Big as a Bushel Basket"

My first attempt to meet Mr. Patterson was unsuccessful. Unknowingly, I drove to the wrong apartment and knocked on the wrong door. No one answered. I called Mr. Patterson, but no one picked up the phone. I left surprised and disappointed because I had spoken to him only 20 minutes earlier, and he had sounded eager to meet me. He playfully pretended to calculate if my 20-minute ride to his place would give him enough time to put on his pants. I worried. Did he change his mind? Did he not want me to visit him after all? Was he too shy to tell me on the phone? When I returned to hospice, I mentioned the incident to Chaplain Steve Holbek. Steve knew Mr. Patterson and often had good insights about the patients with whom he worked. He told me that Mr. Patterson was "somewhat of a simple man," at the very low end of the socioeconomic ladder, who might have been intimidated by the language I used to introduce our work. The term "research project" itself might have scared him.

Steve's hypothesis was certainly not the full explanation of my failed first meeting with Mr. Patterson since, as I quickly discovered, I had not made it to Mr. Patterson's house after all. Steve's thoughts had nonetheless captured something important. Mr. Patterson had had a difficult life. He was 62 years old and very poor. He had a wife and an adult daughter who depended on him. For years he had made a living driving a truck, delivering bread to neighborhood grocery stores. When I met him, he had already left that job, but I could see that something about it fit him perfectly: the hard-working hours behind the wheel, the silence that must have accompanied his work, the delivery of bread.

Mr. Patterson was a quiet man and a self-effacing provider. Not only did he support his family, but he also worked as a handyman for neighbors. Cleaning, painting, gardening, building, and repairing were all tasks within his expertise, and everyone knew it. His physical appearance revealed both his kindness and strength. He was thin, but muscular and strong. His round brown eyes communicated a sweetness that many in the community recognized and cherished. His best customers were elderly women. Mrs. Hillary Milford, a 77-year-old Lancaster County native, had relied on his services for 12 years. She recalled,

> Mr. Patterson would do anything under the sun that you asked him to do. He would wash and wax my kitchen floor. He washed and waxed my car. He did the yard work and raked leaves. He clipped the bushes. He planted a whole row of arborvitae trees down in my back yard. His heart was as big as a bushel basket—nothing was too much. When my dog got sick one time— she got somehow into a bag of chocolate—I called Len. He said, "Hillary, just put kitty litter on it and come and get me." Now, not everybody would do that.

As a young man, Mr. Patterson left his home in Kentucky to start a new life with several "guys," as he called them. He spent much of his time on the road moving from town to town and making a living out of household projects. His skills gave him pride. But that same period brought him shame as well. He saw it as the beginning of his troubles. "I drank my way up to Pennsylvania," he once told me. When he reached Lancaster County, he decided to end his trip. He met his wife, Ruth, and got married. Ten years later, Mr. and Mrs. Patterson gave birth to their daughter Sarah. But alcohol continued to rule his life.

Mr. Patterson assumed all the responsibilities of running the household. He cooked, cleaned, looked after Sarah and his wife. He was the glue that held his family together. Mrs. Patterson required protection. Since her pregnancy 21 years earlier, she had been unable to work and was on welfare. Her husband explained her condition as "pinch nerve." Their daughter characterized it as "laziness." Mr. Patterson presented his wife's inability to work as a permanent and indisputable condition. Mrs. Patterson appeared unkempt. Her hair and clothes often looked unwashed. Several of her teeth had fallen out, and the ones that hadn't seemed in bad shape. Chewing was a challenge for her, so she limited her diet almost exclusively to liquids.

Whenever Mrs. Patterson talked about her marriage, she focused on what she called "the rumors" that Mr. Patterson's friends spread about her. These rumors said that Mrs. Patterson wasn't a good wife. She didn't know how to care for Mr. Patterson, didn't satisfy him sexually, didn't want children. Rumors also had it that Mr. Patterson had had affairs. A decade earlier, a 28-year-old woman had called the Pattersons to let them know that she was Mr. Patterson's daughter. Later the Pattersons were told that a neighbor considered Mr. Patterson to be the father of her new baby. And, in 1991, someone sent a letter to the Department of Children and Youth claiming that Mr. Patterson had molested Sarah. Mrs. Patterson asked,

> Who would be spreading around these rumors and why? What kind of sick people are they? And my mom said that Len can't have no kids. Len was fixed. How am I supposed to know if he was or wasn't? Sarah still believes that he did get somebody pregnant, and she still believes that girl who called is his daughter, and I said "no!"

Mrs. Patterson never confirmed if her husband was unfaithful to her. She always wondered. The one time she went to look for him in the middle of the night she, herself, was raped. "It seems like somebody's pickin' on me, you know?" she'd often say. She realized that her image of Mr. Patterson was different from the neighbors'. "Some people didn't see him as a heavy alcoholic," she said. "They saw him, the opposite side of him, you know, religious, stuff like that." Although the neighbors blamed Mrs. Patterson for her troubles, she blamed her husband's drinking. She believed that if it weren't for that, they would have a better life. She was also lonely. Her most dependable companions were Squeaky, her cat, and Flour, her dog. Without them she would have no close relationships at all.

Sarah had a tumultuous relationship with both her parents. She was a 21-year-old single mother of three boys. Chris, the father of her firstborn son, had fled to Nevada, and Jason, the father of her two youngest, was in jail. It was extremely hard for her to make ends meet. Although she worked full-time at a restaurant, she depended on her father for a roof over her head and on her mother for babysitting Kevin, her eldest. Her babies stayed with Jason's mother. Sarah had deep appreciation for her father. In one of our conversations, she said, "If it would not have been for my father letting me live here, I would never have been able to get my life back in gear." A few years earlier, Mr. Patterson had taken both Sarah and Chris in. But when he realized that Chris was unwilling to work, he kicked him out, and Chris left for Nevada. Sarah then fell in love with Jason. Jason was a crack cocaine user. Mr. Patterson urged her to get rid of him as well, but Sarah fought back. Although she loved her father, she resented him for the marred childhood he had given her. She said,

> He is my father, I love him. There was just a lot of stuff that my father did to me when I was younger that I can just never get rid of. That is always going to be inside me. I mean, you know, all my life he was physically abusive. He used to beat me with a belt, and he would call me names. Before, I used to weigh 200 pounds, and he would call me "porky" and make fun of me, and that hurt me. When I got older, he would also be abusive with my mother, and I wouldn't allow that. I would step in and say, "You are going to hit her, you are going to deal with me." And we would get into fights—we would get into fistfights and everything. I do love my father, but there is just that ha-tred. It stays inside of me because he has put me through a lot of stuff.

Although Sarah tried to get close to her mother, she was convinced that her mother didn't like her. Mrs. Patterson, Sarah felt, wanted her daughter to comply with conventional social rules. "My mother wanted her girl to be Miss Little Goody Two-Shoes," she once told me. Sarah never fit that role, and this brought perpetual tension between them. Through the years, Mrs. Patterson called Sarah a "slut," a "whore," and an "unfit mother," among other things. Sarah's theory was that her mother's anger stemmed from her own two miscarriages and two stillborn births years earlier. More importantly,

Sarah claimed, Mrs. Patterson was jealous. She had always wanted the two things Sarah took for granted: fertility and Mr. Patterson's attention.

"It Was a Shock to Len"

In October 1996, Mr. Patterson noticed a dramatic decline in his health. Severe abdominal pain and a lack of stamina started to disrupt his daily existence. He resorted to Maalox and soft foods, but neither helped. He felt increasingly unable to work. On October 31, he was hit with the most unbearable pain he had ever experienced. He also noticed rectal bleeding. Reluctantly, he went to the doctor. After several tests, he was told that he had cancer of the rectum with liver metastasis. Mr. Patterson heard the news in disbelief: "Are you sure you're talking about *me*?" he asked. Mrs. Patterson recalled,

> It was a shock to Len. And even though I went through rough times with him, with his drinking and stuff, I love him. Some people say, "How can you, when you went through rough times with him?" Sarah, too, you know? It bothered her.

Mr. Patterson underwent a colostomy and started chemotherapy, but he didn't stop working or helping his neighbors. Mrs. Milford recalled that he continued to help her until the last day his body allowed him to. He took the bus to her house and carried out all tasks as usual, but the work exhausted him at a much faster rate than before. At 62 and with cancer, all he asked from her was a ride back home.

Four months of nausea, vomiting, diarrhea, and dehydration had passed when Mr. Patterson was told that the chemotherapy had not worked. The side effects alone had taken a toll on his body. His medical report described him as "a disheveled, poorly kept white male with terrible hygiene" suffering from a small bowel obstruction. His treatment was terminated. One month later, in March 1997, Mr. Patterson called the Hospice of Lancaster County at the suggestion of a friend at the welfare office. To control his symptoms, he was given prochlorperazine, megestrol, loperamide, long-acting morphine tablets, and oxycodone for breakthrough pain. He also asked for chaplain visits. Although he was not a member of any specific faith community, he believed in God and wanted spiritual support.

Following his first visit to the Pattersons, George Tiles, the hospice social worker, reported, "The patient cleans the home and does all the cooking. He continues to ride his bike to the grocery store, but he fell yesterday and scraped his head." Mr. Patterson's goal was to remain as active as he possibly could. Karen Blackwell, the hospice nurse, learned to plan her weekly visits around his schedule. Mr. Patterson liked to go to McDonald's for breakfast with other regulars and visit his neighbors during the day. Even on quiet days when he stayed home, he sat on the porch and watched the traffic. Steve, the chaplain, saw him as the heart of his neighborhood.

"He Is Going to the Hospice House, He Is Very Sick"

By the middle of April, Mr. Patterson was markedly weaker and more somnolent than before. He had lost weight and, having been thin to begin with, looked bony and pale. The chills that raced through his body led him to cut down on the frequency of his baths. Just the idea of undressing became intolerable to him. As his health declined, so did the condition of his apartment. Squeaky started peeing on the rugs, possibly because her litter box had been taken over by cockroaches. The house acquired an overpowering smell of urine. Fleas hopped freely between the walls, the pets, and the furniture. Someone from hospice warned me not to carry my bag into the Pattersons' unless I intended to bring "critters" back home with me. Mr. Patterson was trying to keep things clean. In one of her visits, Karen, his nurse, found him scrubbing the bathtub.

On May 27, two months after his admission to hospice, Mr. Patterson collapsed in his neighborhood grocery store. Unresponsive, he was taken to the hospital. Because he regained consciousness with naloxone, an opioid antagonist, it was presumed that he had overdosed on narcotic analgesics. The possibility that he had taken "too many pills," as he put it, disturbed him greatly. It confronted him with the possibility that he was no longer able to take full charge of his life. Mr. Patterson was not a man of many words. But from his first meetings with Chaplain Steve, he expressed a need and appreciation for prayer. He liked to be reassured that things would be all right "in God's hands." He benefited from an affirmation of faith—a reason to trust and hope. In the hospital, Steve got the sense that Mr. Patterson feared for his family more than his own death—he wondered how they would manage when he died. Steve lifted Mr. Patterson's fears up to God. That seemed to relax him.

When Mr. Patterson returned home, things had changed forever. Mrs. Patterson and Sarah understood that the very person on whom they had depended for their well-being now needed their help to survive. Frightened by the events of the previous days, they asked a hospice nurse to tell them which medications might have caused the overdose and how to prevent another crisis. The nurse labeled all bottles clearly, set up a pill-tender for easy tracking, and reviewed the times each medication was to be administered. She also encouraged Mrs. Patterson to keep the morphine in her possession.

Two days later, Sarah called hospice to announce that her parents were overwhelmed. Mr. Patterson refused to take his medications, and Mrs. Patterson spent a sleepless night trying to look after both her husband and Sarah's crying boy. Hospice offered their 12-bed inpatient unit as a temporary respite option. Sarah and Mrs. Patterson agreed. But Mr. Patterson turned down the offer without further consideration. As the head of the household, he was not prepared to abandon his family. Word went out that the Pattersons were in crisis. Paul Hankin, a family friend and long-time volunteer at the Hospice of Lancaster County, called Mr. Patterson to find out how he could help. When he mentioned the inpatient unit, Mr. Patterson pushed back: "I am not going to the hospital." Mr. Hankin explained that hospice was not a hospital. Mr. Patterson retorted that he would not know how to get there. Mr. Hankin offered to give him a ride. Mr. Patterson declared that he was not ready to leave his home.

Things shifted the next morning. Mr. Patterson agreed to a five-day hospice stay for respite. The inpatient unit accepted patients only for symptom management, temporary respite care, and palliative care in the last days of a patient's life. Once his symptoms were controlled, Mr. Patterson would have to leave.

Mr. Hankin recalled,

Ruth called me and said Len is ready to go, and he would like it if you could come to the house. So I immediately left and went to the house, and it was a picture, you know, driving up in front of an apartment building and seeing Len's wife for the first time, on the front porch holding this little three-year-old fella, and Len sitting on the front porch step looking very sick, carrying a little plastic bag with a pair of soiled long pants, waiting for me to take him to the Hospice Center. . . . We stood and talked, and I introduced myself to his wife, and a neighbor lady came by and said, "Len, are you going away?" And Ruth responded with, "He is going to the Hospice House, he is very sick, and he may not come back home." So I got Len in the car and we had a nice talk from his house to the Hospice Center, and I refreshed his mind with what this was all about—this was *not* a nursing home, and it was *not* a hospital, and that it was brand new—and he kept saying, "Oh, thank you, oh, thank you, but I want to go back home. I want to go back home."

"Would You Look at These Fine Pajamas?"

Three days later, I met Mr. and Mrs. Patterson in the inpatient unit of the Hospice of Lancaster County. Mrs. Patterson and Kevin, Sarah's three-year-old son, were sitting in the living room, surrounded by comfortable furniture, color-coordinated wallpaper, a brand-new fireplace, a cozy alcove with a variety of toys for children, and a view of hospice's flower garden. They had walked from the bus stop, about half a mile away, and appeared fatigued. They were waiting for Mr. Patterson to wake up. Mrs. Patterson looked disheveled, with stained clothes, untied sneakers, and no socks. She was visibly distraught. She kept twirling her hair around her finger with intensity. In tears, she told the social worker, George, that she wanted her neighbors to stop spreading rumors about her. Word had it that she was to blame for Mr. Patterson's transfer to the inpatient unit. The accusation seemed to be that if she were a capable and caring wife, Mr. Patterson would have been able to stay home. George attempted to divert her attention to her family and relationship with Mr. Patterson, but to no avail. "If Len dies, I want to go, too," Mrs. Patterson cried. George asked if she intended to take her own life but got no answer.

When I entered Mr. Patterson's room, he was lying in bed quietly, his eyes half closed. No one was around him. It felt peaceful. But I had a feeling that Mr. Patterson was not in peace in his private room with wall-to-wall carpeting, hand-crafted maple furniture, a leather couch with pillows that matched the carpet, an entertainment center, a large private bath with a whirlpool, and two French doors leading to carefully landscaped gardens. The trees and bushes had only recently been planted so they weren't big enough to block the view to the highway. I saw this as a distraction from the unit's serenity. Mr. Patterson thought otherwise. "I like looking at the highway," he said. "I've always loved watching trucks and vans and big vehicles." The day he entered the unit, he received a used pair of pajamas from the nurse and new under-wear, socks, sweatpants, a pair of slippers, and a matching robe from Mr. Hankin. He expressed gratitude for hospice, but in the next breath he looked up at me and said, "If I had the choice, I'd want to be at home any time."

Mr. Patterson's unease with hospice, combined with his gratitude for every service offered to him, touched many of the nurses. Descriptions of him as a "sweet man," "a sorry little soul," and someone you would want to "take under your wing" were offered freely at every mention of his name. As difficult as it was for him, Mr. Patterson gradually began to accept the care of others. He took all his medications and reached a level of physical comfort he had missed for several weeks. One nurse recalled, "I'd go in his room, and he'd say, 'Would you look at these fine pajamas?' You know, they were just typical, eve-ryday pajamas. And his slippers, he's like, 'Look at those slippers!' And he'd show them to me, he'd show me the bottom and the soles, and these are just the greatest things that he ever saw. And I thought, this is so neat. You know, I've never looked at a pair of pajamas and thought, 'This is the greatest thing.' And that's how he was."

The most tangible sign of Mr. Patterson's transformation was his relation-ship to baths. Mr. Patterson had resisted the whirlpool for fear of taking his clothes off and freezing. But soon he was convinced to give it a try. The heat was turned up for an hour prior to his arrival, so when it came time for him to undress, he was able to do so without discomfort. He loved the water, loved the warmth. "It was so great to see him enjoy that bath," said one of the nurses. "He needed a bath because he had not been taking them at home be-cause they gave him chills. He really did need one." Another nurse recalled that "you could scrape off a layer of old skin, dirt, that kind of thing. He ac-tually had little black specks in the bed when he was laying in there before we got him in the tub. He was unshaven. Mouth was pretty disgusting. He smelled like urine. His colostomy, I'm sure, hadn't been changed for quite some time. So, he was just in a real bad state."

For Mr. Patterson, the whirlpool became a cleansing ritual—both physi-cally and emotionally. Wrapped in warm water, hot steam, and the nurturance of his nurses, he found his baths conducive to vulnerable reflections about his life and imminent death. He expressed constant worry about his family. The Chaplain, Steve, focused on these fears. He reminded Mr. Patterson often that, "You've done a lot for others and maybe, speaking theologically, this is a time when Jesus wants to wash *your* feet—that you need to be cared for and loved in certain ways, and it can happen through the hospice and through others." In a matter of days, Mr. Patterson left a lasting mark on the inpatient unit staff. Again and again, nurses told me that he was one of those patients they would never forget. Reserved as he was, he developed friendships not only with staff but also with other patients. There was one elderly woman in particular, Mrs. Myers, with whom Mr. Patterson liked to share meals and loved to make laugh. The friendship between them was mentioned by several nurses. I heard numerous times about one warm day when the two decided to go for a stroll in the gardens. Both were in wheelchairs, both were pushed by nurses. At some point, Mrs. Myers's wheelchair got stuck in the ground. Mr. Patterson shot up to help get it unstuck. He lifted the front of her wheelchair while the nurses pushed from the back. It didn't matter that the exertion exhausted him.

Evelyn, a nurse, told me that Mr. Patterson helped her as much as she helped him. She said,

> I am only 25, and when I think of older people and having such a drastic illness as this, I relate them with my grandparents. They are so conservative and so private, and they don't talk about anything, and they certainly don't talk about their private life. Len was just different. He would talk with you and he would relate things, and it was like, "Wow, not everybody is so hush, hush." He was one of the first patients I really talked with, and he treated me like an equal, not like a little child. When I came here, I knew I liked hospice, I knew I liked the concept and what it meant, and I liked everything behind it, yet I did not know if I was going to be good at it. Len showed me that I *could* be, and that I could give anything I wanted, and I could give my heart, and it would be all right. I don't know how else to put it.

Once his condition stabilized, Mr. Patterson's stay at the inpatient unit had to come to a close. Since his Medical Assistance did not cover private-duty nursing at home, George, the social worker, and Karen, the home care nurse, assessed that his only reasonable option was to move to a nursing home. George found one that accepted patients on Medical Assistance, as Mr. Patterson's meager earnings would cover only a portion of the cost. He also worked on locating support systems for Mrs. Patterson. To hospice it was clear that Mrs. Patterson's well-being was going to require careful attention for Mr. Patterson to die peacefully. In the beginning, Mrs. Patterson rejected all of George's efforts to help. In turn, George suspected that she did have the ability to take care of her basic needs, but that her parent–child relationship with her husband had deprived her of the opportunity to exercise her in-dependence. With her reluctant permission, George eventually connected her to the Mental Health/Mental Retardation Office for an evaluation. If she were diagnosed with a disability, he thought, she would be eligible for Supplemental Security Income (SSI). Without the support of welfare, George worried that Mrs. Patterson would lack the means to survive.

I visited Mr. Patterson in the inpatient unit on the day of his transfer to the nursing home. Again, he has lying in bed with his eyes half closed. He seemed withdrawn. The day before, he had had a conversation with the hospice's medical director, which revealed how hard he was taking this new development. According to a nurse who witnessed the exchange, the doctor said, "Tomorrow is the big day!"

"Yes," replied Mr. Patterson, "I'm going home."

Surprised, the doctor asked rhetorically, "Now, where are you going tomorrow?"

"I'm going home."

"Don't you remember where we were talking about Len?" the nurse asked gently.

"Oh, yeah, I'm gonna go over to the nursing home for a little bit," Mr. Patterson replied.

Although George and Karen seemed relieved to have found a place that would offer Mr. Patterson 24-hour care, some inpatient unit staff felt ambiva-lent about this transfer. One nurse asked, "Who are we to go in and say, 'This house is too dirty and your wife doesn't take good care of you, therefore, you know, you've served the community well all of your life, so we want to do something 'nice' for you' "?

"It's an Awful Thing When You Tell
Yourself You're Gonna Die"

The next time I saw Mr. Patterson, he was lying in a four-bed ward at the nursing home. His slow-release morphine had been increased from 30 mg to 100 mg twice a day. He looked comfortable but felt lonely. "It isn't like the Hospice Center," he had told his friend Mr. Hankin. The first thing he men-tioned to me was that he wanted a television. His roommate spat, cursed, and hollered obscenities at all hours of the day. Mr. Patterson remarked that his cancer exhausted him. His pain was often excruciating. His daily activi-ties had been reduced to looking out the window, taking pills, cleaning his colostomy, drinking the liquid supplement he could digest, and sleeping. He blamed himself for his condition. He was convinced that it was his alcoholism that made him sick. "The doctor told me *that* was what ended my life . . .," he said, "that's what ended my life, drinking and drinking. Drinking this wine and whiskey—too strong. I thought I'd have a little more time with my family, a little more living . . ., but I don't think so. But it's an awful thing when you tell yourself you're gonna die." Soon, our conversation shifted to Mrs. Patterson. "I don't have nobody to watch my wife," Mr. Patterson continued. "Nobody at all to watch my wife. She's a very nice woman though. Me and her have been married 20 some years. And she's always been right there by me. She's always been right there."

Mr. Patterson grew weaker and thinner. He reported increasing pain. Three days after his admission to the nursing home, he was accidentally overmedicated. In the morning, he was given the 100 mg slow-release morphine. A few hours later, he said he was still in pain. Helen, a substitute nurse from hospice who was present at the time, asked one of the attending nurses to administer a short-acting medication for breakthrough pain. Accidentally, the attending nurse gave him the 100 mg tablet that he was to take 10 hours later. Helen recalled her shouting, "Oh my God! Gross med error! Oh my God, oh my God, I made a terrible medication error!" Terrified by her mistake, she called the nursing home's medical director who instructed her to keep a close eye on Mr. Patterson. Extreme sedation or respiratory depression would be signs for worry. But Mr. Patterson slept his medication off.

When he wasn't in pain, Mr. Patterson displayed a perpetual state of lethargy. He slept a lot, and, when he had visitors, he had a hard time keeping his eyes open. I remember him trying to keep up with conversations while his eyes rolled back into his head.

Sarah hadn't seen her father since the day he entered the hospice inpatient unit. In our conversations, she sounded ambivalent toward him. Mr. Patterson had abused her in the past, but in her adult years he insisted on protecting her from romantic relationships that were destructive. Sarah resented his advice, but she recognized—then and now—that he cared for her deeply. His admonitions haunted her. "My father was right," she would say. "My father was right." Mr. Patterson's voice seemed to be with her all the time. It was a voice she would miss:

When my father dies, it is going to hurt, and I know that day is going to come soon. Right now, I pray every night that he lives, I pray that they find a cure. That is mostly what I pray for. I had told one lady at hospice, "If anybody hurts my dad out in the nursing home, I am going to beat their butt," you know, being protective. I mean, that is my father and if anyone hurts him, then they deal with me. That is the way I am. But, of course, my father has hurt me, which don't make sense, but I still feel like that.

Sarah was concerned that her mother had not come to terms with the seriousness of her father's condition: "She always claims, 'He's coming home, he's coming home.' And he is *not* coming home. You know, she claims that he told her he was coming home, and from what the lady at hospice said, he wasn't coming home. He is staying in there." Squeaky, the cat, and Flour, the dog, seemed to be Mrs. Patterson's only source of comfort. Flour accompanied her everywhere she went. Squeaky represented stability inside the house. Mrs. Patterson was as worried about the pets' well-being after Mr. Patterson's death as she was about her own. She didn't want to lose them. This was one of the reasons she rejected George's proposal that she move to low-income housing. In the high-rises, she said, "you're not allowed pets."

"I Wanna See Them Happy Before I Go Anywhere"

I saw Mr. Patterson again three weeks after his admission to the nursing home. He was eager to tell me about his wife's visit a few days before. She looked calmer than usual, and he was able to reach out to her in a way he had never done before. He said,

> People are trying to help her out, and evidently, they must be doing pretty good. All they got to do is talk to her. When she left here, she was in a great mood. We was watching my roommate's television. And I said, "Ruth, I wanna tell you. . . . Sit down there now." I said, "Sit down there and take it easy. I just wanna tell you: if I have *any* time, *any* time whatsoever that I could spend it with *anybody* in this world, it would be with you." Well, she gets up and she goes back in the kitchen. You could tell she was crying a little. And about an hour after that, she started to laugh and shakin' my hand and kissin' me. That's what I've gotta keep on doing—being nice to her. Got to. I wanna see them happy before I go anywhere.

Mr. Patterson kept asking when he'd be able to go home. "I want to sit around the house, watch television, go to the store, get a soft drink, drink it. Just like normal people. We're not different than normal people. I'm normal," he told

Steve and me. Steve affirmed his goal, but also asked him what he was going to do if getting well and going home wasn't in the cards. Mr. Patterson paused. "That's a super-duper big question," he replied.

With Steve's help, Mr. Patterson acknowledged that his wife had grown. She was not as helpless as he thought. Steve was heartened by this admission. He felt that Mr. Patterson's recognition of his family's ability to survive without him would be necessary for his own ability to let go. At the end of our visit, Steve asked Mr. Patterson if he wanted prayer. Mr. Patterson always did. Steve knelt. He took hold of Mr. Patterson's right hand and started to stroke it. Mr. Patterson turned his gaze toward me and gave me his left hand. I held it with both of mine. Together, we tuned out the noises on the floor and joined in prayer. Steve asked God to hear Mr. Patterson's wishes—to receive his desire to go home. He said that we knew that things might not end up the way Mr. Patterson wanted, but asked God to help him receive and grow from whatever he was given. He closed with a plea for God's blessing. Mr. Patterson said he felt better. He looked better. His skin and eyes seemed energized. He had perked up. "God bless you," he said to both of us as we left.

The hospice staff had mixed feelings about Mr. Patterson's desire to go home. An employee who was familiar with the case but not directly involved in it told me that she couldn't understand why a patient who was receiving 24-hour care in a nursing home would want to return to an unhealthy environment and risk his safety. George and Karen feared that Mr. Patterson's pain would escalate in an unsupervised environment. Mr. Patterson could not afford private-duty nursing. Keeping his pain under control would require close supervision and a strict medication schedule. Steve, on the other hand, found his colleagues overprotective. Mr. Patterson had promised that if he were to return to his family, he would not do any work. But even if he broke his promise, Steve argued, hospice could not control the choices of its patients. Steve stressed that the prospect of going back home had given new meaning to Mr. Patterson's life—a significant development to which hospice needed to pay attention.

"You feel ready to go home?" I asked Mr. Patterson a few days later. "Sure do!" he replied. "I think I feel ready now. I feel a little better. It's not up to me though." "Whom is it up to?" I asked. "I don't know," he said, "some big wheel in here. I don't know who that is. I don't know. They decide whether you're ready to go home for a week, whether you're ready to go home for a month, or whether you're ready to go home for good." The decision in Mr. Patterson's case was made jointly by hospice and nursing home staff. Mr. Patterson was given permission to go home for four hours.

"Our Boy Is Going Home Today"

"Our boy is going home today," announced Karen with a big smile when she greeted me one morning at the hospice. Karen, George, and Steve had arranged for a volunteer to drive Mr. Patterson to his apartment at 1 P.M. and take him back to the nursing home at 5 P.M. Within that time window, Karen scheduled a home nursing visit as well. The volunteer, Robert Gardner, dropped Mr. Patterson off as scheduled. He was surprised to see that neither Ruth nor Sarah were home. Mr. Patterson ambled into his house through the unlocked door. He assured Robert he was going to be okay and encouraged him to leave.

Karen and I arrived a couple of hours later. We expected to see father, mother, daughter, and grandchildren together, but found ourselves in an entirely different scene. Sarah had not been informed about her father's visit and was apparently at work. Ruth and young Kevin were outdoors, playing on the sidewalk. They had left Mr. Patterson alone to sleep. Mr. Patterson was inside, lying on his bed with his eyes half closed. Karen and I tiptoed into his bedroom and sat on the two kitchen chairs next to him. His room was small and dark. It was hot. The smell of cat urine was overwhelming. Mr. Patterson seemed blissful. Turning his head slowly, he looked around and said, "This is my life." He paused for a second and continued: "I'm proud of it."

Two hours later Mr. Patterson was taken back to the nursing home. Everyone there noticed a decline. He was weaker, slept more, had increasing difficulty cleaning his colostomy, and was unable to keep up with conversations. Periodically, he would lift his arms up in the air while opening and closing his fists as if he were trying to reach something—a relatively frequent sign of drug toxicity or metabolic complications. Several of his caregivers got the impression that he had entered a liminal space between the world of the living and that of the dead.

Money Worries

When Mrs. Patterson's welfare status came up for review, she was denied the minimal support she was receiving. The reason was a doctor's note asserting that she was able to work. Hoping that she would apply for SSI, George encouraged her again to get a health evaluation. Although SSI is designed for persons with extremely low income, he explained, one still needs a physical or emotional disability diagnosis to qualify for it. On her behalf, he scheduled a meeting with the Mental Health/Mental Retardation Office and accompanied her to her appointment. Mrs. Patterson's welfare was extended for a month. In that interval, it was agreed that a doctor would reconsider her capacity to work.

Money was a private matter in the Patterson household. There wasn't much of it, and everyone protected what they had. Mr. Patterson was afraid that his wife would use up his limited savings, so he hid the $160 that he had. Sarah spent her salary carefully and demanded that her mother babysit Kevin to compensate for not contributing to the household's expenses. Mrs. Patterson feared that if Sarah knew that she had any money at all, she would take it from her to pay the rent.

In the Nursing Home

After six weeks in the nursing home, Mr. Patterson was lonely and depressed. He couldn't sleep at night. He couldn't understand why friends and relatives didn't visit. "I do not mean that much to them," he said softly. "It's hard to tell who might show up. So, all you can do in a situation like that is just wait." "Waiting" meant dozing off, staring out the window, or looking at the bare walls surrounding him. Mr. Patterson's complexion had acquired a yellowish tone. He looked even thinner than before—"emaciated" might be a better word. I could see his skull. His skin was tight around his bones, and his eyes looked sunken in. His voice had lost its strength, and his words had started to run into each other. I struggled to understand him. Our conversations were slow and labored. I repeated almost everything he said, to make sure I heard him right. He corrected me, again and again, until I understood. Hospice staff offered him a second trip home. Initially, he responded affirmatively, but soon his pain started to overwhelm him. His abdomen had grown distended and hard with tumor.

In early August, I visited Mr. Patterson with Karen. He was lying in bed as usual. He told us that his pain had gotten worse, running from the left to the right side of his abdomen. It was unbearable. Karen left the room to ask the ward nurse for a short-acting painkiller. The nurse looked harried and, although she agreed to administer the medication, quickly disappeared into someone else's room. Forty minutes later she still hadn't given Mr. Patterson his pill. It was clear that Mr. Patterson was in severe pain. He was quiet but pale and tense. In the few sentences he was able to utter, he expressed worry for Flour. He didn't think Mrs. Patterson or Sarah would be able to care for the dog without him. Then came his lunch. He couldn't touch it.

Karen was distressed. Although she was confident that there were medications that could alleviate Mr. Patterson's pain, her hands were tied. As a hospice nurse, she had almost no authority in the nursing home setting, and, even worse, she posed a threat to the ward's overworked and underpaid staff. In contrast to nursing home staff, Karen worked for an agency known in the area for its luxury and comfort. She didn't have to wear a uniform, she had only a handful of patients to look after, and she worked on a flexible schedule. More importantly, she was an expert in palliative care. She explained to me that even the slightest criticism of nursing home staff could turn them against her.

Frustrated and unwilling to make further appeals, Karen advised Mr. Patterson to become his own advocate. She told him that he had to place demands on his nurses by asking for painkillers when he needed them. Mr. Patterson nodded. "I've got to say something," he concurred. He told us that he wanted more help cleaning his colostomy as well. Several times it had filled up and no one was there to empty it. That humiliated him. It was possible that if Mr. Patterson were to start speaking up, his care would improve. As it was, he just laid in bed waiting to be noticed. To complicate matters further, when he felt pain, he often didn't look uncomfortable. The discrepancy between his experience and his appearance required that he be asked about his pain on a regular basis, which nursing home staff had neither the time nor the energy to do.

Karen came up with a new idea. As it was, Mr. Patterson was scheduled to take 100 mg of slow-release morphine twice a day and an additional 30 mg of short-acting morphine syrup at regular intervals. The frequent administration of the liquid morphine, however, placed an overwhelming burden on nursing home staff. Karen decided to suggest eliminating the syrup and increasing the dose of the slow-release pills. This way, she figured, Mr. Patterson's pain would be managed better without need for round-the-clock attention. An additional advantage to this approach could be decreased drowsiness. Karen's proposal was not received well by the nursing home. She recalled,

> When I suggested the change, I kind of think that the nursing home's medical director interpreted that I was trying to increase the morphine, when in fact I was trying to move the major portion of the morphine dose from

the rapid-acting to the time-release—which would be a better delivery for the patient and the staff also, but I don't think they ever listened to me. I don't think they really understood, and the doctor's response was. "Well, what we are doing is working, so there is no reason to change it." Once he said that, the staff really became defensive and did not want to hear any more about it.

Another hospice nurse remarked,

I don't like to question somebody's authority on their grounds. That is *their* game over there. Two or three visits ago, I asked a nurse what they were doing for breakthrough pain, and she said they would give it to him when he asked for it. I said, "Well, he is complaining of pain now, so he should probably have it now." She said, "It is interesting that he only complains about pain when you guys from hospice are here."

A few days later, when Steve and I visited the nursing home together, Mr. Patterson reported that the pain from his abdominal and rectal tumors kept him up at night. Steve asked what he wanted God to do for him. Mr. Patterson replied faintly, "To take away the pain." One could hardly hear his voice anymore. As he was losing his strength, he wondered if God was really with him. The previous day, he told us, he had prayed to not be given a bath, but he got one anyway. It was too cold for him. He suffered. He confessed that although he did feel God by his side, he felt him only "a little," adding, "I would be ready to go if it is the time."

"I Wish Len Would Come Back Home"

The smell of cat urine had started to seep out of the Pattersons' apartment and up to the second floor. Angry neighbors called the landlord demanding an immediate solution. The landlord delivered an ultimatum: Sarah and Mrs. Patterson had until September 1 to get rid of Squeaky and Flour. It they failed to do so, they would all be kicked out. Mrs. Patterson declared that she would rather live on the street than part with her pets. Sarah argued that only Squeaky caused the problem. She pleaded for permission to keep Flour, but the landlord was adamant: both animals had to go.

Not only did Mrs. Patterson not have the money to move, she was also told that she would be taken off welfare. A second doctor had confirmed that she was fit to work. When I spoke with her on the phone, she sounded de-spondent. "I wish Len was here," she cried. "The doctor said I can work, but I can't. I'm tired and weak, my ankle and foot hurt from arthritis, I get bad headaches from my teeth, my neck and back hurt. People are not going to hire you if you don't have good shoes and nice clothes. I wish Len would come back home."

"Let's Hope This Will Not Be It"

It was the morning of August 29, and it was hot. When I arrived at the nursing home, Ann Marie, a personal care nurse from hospice, was giving Mr. Patterson a sponge bath. For the first time in her work with him, she noted that he refused to close his eyes. He was afraid, he said, that if he were to fall asleep, he would die. Ann Marie had drawn a curtain around him, so even though I couldn't see his expressions, I could tell he enjoyed the bath. Long silences and a few faint words of appreciation revealed contentment. Then the curtain opened, and Mr. Patterson turned to greet me. Two red, un-blinking eyes stared straight at me.

Mr. Patterson had grown worried not only about his family but also about himself. He was alarmed by the fact that he seemed unable to tolerate solid foods. His diet had been reduced to a few cans of liquid supplements a day. Ann Marie assured him that each one was like an entire meal. "Your body doesn't know the difference," she asserted. "Just like I told you with Jesus. It might not feel like He's here, but He is, and everything will be all right." On her way out, she called Steve, George, and Karen to let them know that Mr. Patterson was declining. "I would not be shocked if he died tonight," she said. Steve appeared minutes later. "You're sick and tired of being sick and tired, aren't you?" he asked softly. Mr. Patterson nodded. He said he wanted to see Sarah. There was a sense of urgency about him that convinced us he was getting ready to let go. Steve left to pick up Sarah from work. I sat next to Mr. Patterson and waited. I remember not knowing what to say. Soon, I found myself repeating the comforting words of Ann Marie: "Everything will be okay, and Sarah will be okay, too." To my surprise, Mr. Patterson pushed back: "No she won't. I know she won't be okay. Everyone says she will, but I am her father, and I know."

Sarah arrived, looking composed but scared. Nervously, she sat in the chair by her father's bedside. Mr. Patterson turned his head slowly toward her and asked her questions. Was she still working? Was she making enough money?

Did Jason get a job? Sarah assured him that everything was okay. The last thing he asked of her was to promise to take care of her mother. Sarah agreed. "I have flashes that I'm going to die in a day or two," he told her. His eyes remained wide open, while his head sank back into the pillow. He seemed to withdraw into himself as if in a state of meditation. An awkward silence filled the room. Then Mrs. Patterson came in. Someone from hospice had called her to notify her of her husband's condition. Her walk from the bus stop made her look sweaty and disheveled. She stopped at the foot of the bed, staring at her husband from a distance. Mr. Patterson seemed disconnected from his surroundings. With a glazed look in his eyes, his gaze was fixed at the ceiling. It wasn't clear if he knew that his wife had arrived. I assumed he wasn't listening at all until Mrs. Patterson made a reference to a bill. "What bill?" he suddenly exclaimed. Mrs. Patterson would have proceeded to answer his question if Steve hadn't cut the conversation short.

Both hospice and nursing home staff feared that Mr. Patterson would suffer a torturous death if he didn't stop worrying about his family. He was seen as defying nature by holding onto life in a body that was almost dead. Everyone felt that his spirit needed soothing so that he could leave this world in peace. With Steve's redirection, Mrs. Patterson walked closer to her husband, looked him in the eyes, and said, "I love you." "I love you, too," he responded, still looking up. But quickly, Mrs. Patterson's tone changed. "What do you want me to do with your clothes?" "What do you want me to do with your tools?" "What do you want me to do with all your things?" she cried in desperation. Mr. Patterson gave no response.

Once Mrs. Patterson and Sarah left, Steve sat quietly by Mr. Patterson's side. "Having Ruth and Sarah over was the best thing," said Mr. Patterson after a brief period of silence. "It would be a lie not to say I love them." He then asked for a pill that would put him to sleep. I could sense a heaviness in the air. The interaction between Steve and Mr. Patterson seemed to unfold in slow motion. There was silence and a set of burning, unblinking eyes crying out for help. Steve seemed like he was at a loss for words. Finally, he told Mr. Patterson that he wouldn't want to give him such a pill because doing so would prevent him from experiencing the good things that can happen during one's dying. Later, I asked Steve what he was thinking at the time. He replied.

Inside myself I am thinking, "Holy shit! We are not going down that road." It is not appropriate and, of course, [I] remember[ed] that he was afraid to close his eyes, because he did not want to go to sleep and not wake up, and [him] thinking about being put away now—and [I] recognize[d] that he was in that tension. What I have seen is that there are still miracles and blessings that can occur with people of faith in their understanding of who God wants to be for them, experiencing God in some very powerful ways that are awesomely reassuring and, of course, sharing their struggle with their family members. So, I think euthanasia would be inappropriate because he was not clear at that point. He was still struggling and trying to negotiate that and come to some kind of resolution.

When I said goodbye to Mr. Patterson that day, he gave me a short response: "Let's hope this will not be it."

Squeaky and Flour

On August 31, Squeaky and Flour were still in the Patterson apartment. Mrs. Patterson had spent days calling friends and neighbors to ask if they would be willing to take in her and her pets. One night, Sarah deliberately locked her mother and Flour outside in the rain. On September 1, the tension at the Patterson household climaxed. Fearing eviction, Sarah insisted that the animals leave. Mrs. Patterson refused. A screaming fight ensued, and Mrs. Patterson's parents arrived with an invitation to take their daughter into their home. They were not going to have Squeaky and Flour, however, so Mrs. Patterson turned the offer down. Then arrived the police, who were apparently called by the neighbors. When the altercation stopped, Mrs. Patterson and the animals disappeared. They were gone all night. To try and resolve the conflict, George offered to take cat and dog to an animal shelter. Sarah consented, but Mrs. Patterson did not. In desperation, Sarah kicked Squeaky out of the house and made arrangements, without involving her mother, for George to take Flour to the Humane League.

"There Is Just No Way I Can Make Myself Believe That They Are Going to Be Fine"

Mr. Patterson had lost almost all the energy it took to speak. Most of his interactions were reduced to faint nods and shakes of his head. He indicated to Steve that he was no longer worried about his wife, but he wanted to see his sister from Kentucky to seek her forgiveness. His sister had been so disapproving of his alcoholism that she haunted him. Steve knew that this part of Mr. Patterson's history disturbed him. In response to Mr. Patterson's request, he asked, "Do you know that God has forgiven you for that and the mistakes you made as a result of your drinking?" "No," Mr. Patterson replied. "So that opened a whole new territory to explore," Steve told me later. "I reassured him that God is with him and is compassionate, merciful, and will take care of him, and that God is also forgiving." At the end of Steve's visit, Mr. Patterson announced that he was ready to let go. Karen put in a request for round-the-clock hospice care. She had a strong feeling that Mr. Patterson would die within the next three days. In a worried tone, she said to me, "You see most of our families through this difficult time, and you know they are going to be all right, eventually—once they allow themselves time to grieve. You know they are going to do fine. This family, there is just no way I can make myself believe that they are going to be fine, and that is frustrating."

One week later, Mr. Patterson's medical records indicated significant periods of unresponsiveness, sleep with intermittent apnea, and no urine output. His pulse was too weak to be taken at the wrist, so the attending nurse measured it with a stethoscope. Steve believed Mr. Patterson's last day had come. He decided to go to the nursing home, and I went with him. The hospice chaplain spoke to Mr. Patterson about the love of God. He told him what a good person he thought Mr. Patterson was, how much he loved him, and how thankful he felt for having gotten to know him and walk with him on this journey. Mr. Patterson was unresponsive. When Steve asked him if he was going to go with the Lord, if the Lord reached out to him, Mr. Patterson nodded.

Sarah, too, visited her father that day. She recalled,

I thought, "Oh my God, he is dying." I was there and I touched him, and I told him I was there, I said, "I love you, I am here," but it was like touching nothing. I know he is going to go, but it hurts me. I had a lot of anger and a lot of hurt. My anger and my hurt are towards my dad, but I mean now that he's on his death bed, I mean you really can't have that towards him because he is dying. And then I feel guilty for having that towards him.

When everyone left, Mr. Patterson suddenly sat up and lifted his hand as if he were reaching out to someone at the foot of the bed.

By September 10, Mr. Patterson was unresponsive to almost all verbal and tactile stimuli, markedly jaundiced, with no bowel sounds. "Every day he looks ten times worse than he did the day before," Karen remarked. Both hospice and nursing home staff were convinced that Mr. Patterson was holding onto life out of concern for his family. George asked Mrs. Patterson to reassure her husband that everything was going to be okay. Instead, and within Mr. Patterson's hearing range, she exclaimed, "Well, he knows I won't be okay!" For the first time, Mr. Patterson's caregivers started seeing Mrs. Patterson as a liability that had to be contained. They instructed each other to try and control Mrs. Patterson's interactions with her husband because, they decided, her need for his support kept him from letting go.

"In God's Hands All Is Well"

Steve returned to the nursing home on the morning of September 11. He was astounded to find Mr. Patterson still alive. Mrs. Patterson was with him, worrying aloud about her future. Steve got close to Mr. Patterson and said, "If Jesus comes for you to take you home, it is okay to go with Him." He proceeded to reassure him that "in God's hands all is well—even when it does not look, seem, or feel that way." "At that point," Steve recalled, "came a tear at the corner of Mr. Patterson's eye that welled up enough that it trickled down his cheek. I was rubbing Mr. Patterson's arm, making contact with him and trying to be comforting, and Ruth on the other side started doing the same thing. You know, kind of modeling a little bit as it turned out, and she even eventually said, 'I love you.' I said, 'Len, did you hear that? Ruth said she loves you and she really cares about you.' That was short lived. But it did happen!"

On September 12, with prompting from a hospice nurse, Mrs. Patterson told her husband that it was okay to let go. That night Mr. Patterson died.

"If You See George, Tell Him Thanks for All His Help"

Following Mr. Patterson's death, Mrs. Patterson moved in with her parents. Sarah and Jason had another child, against Sarah's wish to limit their family to three. Flour was adopted by a new family. Squeaky was killed by a car. Hospice expected Ruth to need intensive support from its bereavement counselors, but she did not. After seeing her at the memorial service, both

George and Steve confirmed that she was more independent than she had seemed. Mrs. Patterson had appeared with a new haircut, clean clothes, and the determination to introduce her family to each and every hospice employee who was there to pay their final respects. I remember her confidently taking me, too, by the hand to her sister and explaining the purpose of our research project.

A few months later, I got the chance to speak with her again. Excitedly, she announced that her SSI had been approved. In only a few more weeks she was going to be back on welfare. "If you see George," she said, "tell him thanks for all his help, and tell him that I'm getting SSI for sure." And she quickly added, "I just don't want Sarah to know about it."

Authors' Comments

Mr. Patterson suffered greatly from poor management of his pain and other distressing symptoms throughout his illness. There were two main reasons for this, both of which would likely not be as much of a problem today. During his four months of chemotherapy, and before his enrolment in hospice, Mr. Patterson was dependent on his oncologists to control the nausea, vomiting, diarrhea, and dehydration that were the side effects of his treatment. While oncologists typically believe they are capable of managing these symptoms, often they are not, and unless the patient has pain, they may not think of referring them to palliative care until very late in the course of the disease. Today, at least in locales with robust palliative care expertise, integration of palliative care specialist consultation is much more likely to follow closely on a patient's diagnosis of cancer and to accompany patients through their anti-cancer therapy.

In the nursing home, Mr. Patterson's pain management was grossly inadequate—even to the point of a potentially serious medication overdose—mainly because hospice nurses had little clarity about their role and authority when visiting Mr. Patterson there. Management of his pain was largely in the hands of understaffed, inexperienced nursing home personnel. Today, it is much more common for hospice organizations to have formal contractual relationships with nursing homes that clarify their roles, responsibilities, and authority in patient care. Combined with the strong specialist palliative care resources of the present-day Hospice and Community Care, a patient in Mr. Patterson's situation would undoubtedly fare much better today—though we must reiterate the caveat that the availability of these resources is subject to great regional variation in both the United States and Canada.

If we compare Mr. Patterson's narrative to those of Frances Legendre, Richard Johnson, Martin Roy, and Jenny Doyle, a noteworthy difference stands out. Each of the other four patients—and their families—were very assertive about their needs and preferences. Each acted as if they were accustomed to exercising autonomy and control. Compare their attitudes to Mr. Patterson's answer when I asked him who was responsible for deciding whether, and for how long, he could make a visit from the nursing home to his own house: "I don't know," he said, "some big wheel in here. I don't know who that is. I don't know. They decide whether you're ready to go home for a week, whether you're ready to go home for a month, or whether you're ready to go home for good." In the event, he was allowed to visit his home for four hours.

Mr. Patterson's lack of a sense of personal agency, and the ease with which both the hospice and nursing home staff assumed almost parental control (even referring to him as "a sorry little soul" whom you would want "to take under your wing") is reminiscent of Shamira Cook's experience—though without the terms of endearment—and may well be similarly class-based. It is hard to envision such attitudes and behaviors, no matter how well-intentioned, being applied to patients and families who were manifestly used to wielding executive control.

In his last days and hours of life, Mr. Patterson's hospice team despaired of orienting his wife to letting go of her own anxieties about her future so that Mr. Patterson could be easier in his mind about letting go of life. In addition to fears of pain, shortness of breath, and being left alone, concern for those left behind is one of the most common worries among dying people. Mrs. Patterson's inability to give her husband reassurance was one more of the jagged edges we are left with in this narrative.

Contemplating these jagged edges, we might wonder whether hospice could have done more to smooth things out for Mr. Patterson and his family. A similar question occurs in the case of Richard Johnson. In both of these instances, however, the conflicts that arose during the care of these men, and which were left unresolved after their deaths, were rooted in relationships and personalities with long histories. In Mr. Patterson's case in particular, the difficulties arising from the family history were aggravated by inter-institutional issues within the health and social welfare systems. Mr. Patterson was also a man of very limited financial means, which further restricted his options for care and support at the end of life[1]—an issue we also encountered in the narrative of Albert Hoffer. These cases are therefore excellent examples of the unavoidable interdependence of individual, family, team, and societal factors in the overall effectiveness of hospice and palliative care. To expect the hospice team alone to solve all the difficulties associated with dying would be unrealistic and unfair.

Reference

1. Wachterman MW, Sommers BD. Dying poor in the US-Disparities in end-of-life care. JAMA. 2021;325(5):423–424.

11

Miriam Lambert

Total Pain and the Despair of an Unlived Life

Narrated by Anna Towers

It happens on occasion in palliative care that a person's pain remains uncontrolled despite the best efforts of the team. Miriam Lambert was referred to our study because of the difficulty of her case. She had not had an easy life, and emotional issues compounded her situation. The palliative care team tried to control her pain with a full spectrum of medications, as well as with anesthetic blocks. They tried supportive nonmedical and psychological interventions, such as art therapy, music therapy, and massage, to reach her in any way they could. Nonetheless, the pain persisted.

"I'm Not a Very Open Person, You Know"

Miriam Lambert was 68 years old when I met her in the Palliative Care Unit (PCU) on October 1, 1996. Pale, with blond, neatly combed shoulder-length hair, she sat rather stiffly in her hospital bed. She looked proud and dignified, and she was soft-spoken. She had just recently been diagnosed with melanoma, which had started in her foot and had now spread to her pelvis and spine. She had been in almost constant pain for three months. Her affect seemed flat, even as she spoke of her discomfort, and she avoided my gaze as we spoke, her face masklike. I wondered: Was this demeanor a result of the pain? Although she did not look like she was in pain, when asked directly, she would say the pain was unbearable. It was always there, especially in her back and her left leg, and it was excruciating when she moved.

In her room I noticed tasteful art posters on the walls, with books about music on her bedside table. Judging from the books and the way she spoke, I thought that she must be well-educated. I was surprised to learn that she had done odd jobs all her life; most recently she had been a supermarket cashier. There was something that didn't fit. Over several visits, I tried to engage her in conversation about herself. "I'm not a very open person, you know," she said. Slowly, through my conversations with her, but mostly through conversations with her brothers, nieces, and the caregivers on the PCU, a portrait of her life emerged.

"She Got Lost Somewhere Along the Way"

Mrs. Lambert was of working-class, French-Canadian origin, born and raised in a small town, the tenth of 12 children. Two siblings had died in infancy. According to her older brother Peter, Miriam was the "glue" for the family. Her brothers felt that Miriam had not realized her potential. She was very bright and was always top of her class at school, but then she settled for menial jobs. Peter said of her,

> As a person she is closed, isolated, and does not speak of emotions. She is a pleasant person in company, but she isn't open. She is very reserved. She doesn't speak much. She never had a life with a rhythm of her own. She is very generous and did a lot for her husband. He demanded all of her time. She couldn't live a full life. She went from one small job to another. She tried to look after other people's problems, but not her own. What a waste of potential! She did very well in school, but she didn't socialize well. She had always been alone before she got married. Maybe it's because of the relationship with my parents.

She had a few friends but no intimate friends. When she spoke of her mother, she said that she didn't feel loved; she felt left aside when she was growing up. She saw a psychiatrist for depression when she was an adolescent and periodically later in life. She felt as if she had done something wrong, though she didn't know what it was, and that she had not been forgiven. As an adult, she continued to live with her parents. When her father died, she looked after her mother through a long illness. Her mother died when Mrs. Lambert was 37 years old.

Mrs. Lambert had never been involved with men until she met Roger, a man who was thirty years older and about to get divorced. Miriam Lambert was not the reason for the divorce—she was clear that her values would not have allowed that. She and Roger started to live together, but after six months Mrs. Lambert realized that she did not love him. Nonetheless, they had stayed together 30 years in a common-law relationship, out of convenience.

They were able to enjoy life for a few years, but after that one hardship after another occurred. Mrs. Lambert had to spend a lot of time looking after her ill sister, who died within a couple of years. Roger, who had been a young-spirited, active person when she met him, developed heart and lung disease, making him more dependent on her. Now he was 98 years old and had been in a nursing home for six months, ever since Mrs. Lambert had become ill. Mrs. Lambert felt guilty about this. Although she did not readily share her feelings, she spoke frequently about Roger and her concerns regarding his comfort. According to her brother, she was not emotionally close to Roger; rather, she felt a great sense of duty toward him.

Before Roger got ill, she had gone through a series of temporary jobs. She did not feel fulfilled in these jobs, and she expressed a lack of personal realization: "I have always been in the service of others," she said to me. "I don't know who I am." She and Roger had no children of their own. Roger had children from his first marriage, but they were not close and were not involved in his care.

Her one relaxation was listening to classical music. She had played the violin briefly as a child and would have liked very much to have studied more, but she had had no opportunity to do so. She hadn't gone out much for the last four or five years, as Roger demanded all of her time. She panicked now, thinking Roger would die, for it was as if she didn't exist without him.

Mrs. Lambert's nieces were the most significant people in her life, particularly her niece Carole, who was in her mid-40s. Another niece, Sandra, was a successful lawyer, and Mrs. Lambert was very proud of her. A third niece had been murdered by her boyfriend. Mrs. Lambert occasionally spoke about this, but without emotion. Although Mrs. Lambert was close to her nieces, she did not confide in them.

Mrs. Lambert came from a religious Roman Catholic family, but she had lost her faith early in adult life. She had felt betrayed and deceived by the church: There was so much ritual and dogma, but where was the truth? She was looking for answers within herself, but she had not reached a state of peace. As Carole put it, "She does not love herself, she is extremely hard on herself, and she is hard on others. I have the impression that life was difficult for her. She got lost somewhere along the way."

Beginning of the Illness

In October 1995, Mrs. Lambert developed swelling and pain in her big toe. At the time she was busy looking after her husband. He was needing more and more care, and Mrs. Lambert was getting tired. When she finally took the time to see her doctor, he told her that she had an infection or an ingrown toenail and gave her antibiotics. It seemed to get better for a few weeks, but then the swelling returned, and Mrs. Lambert could hardly walk because of the pain in her foot. After Christmas she went back to the doctor for a biopsy, which confirmed that she had melanoma. The tumor did not seem to have spread, but the surgeon told her that she needed to have the toe amputated.

Mrs. Lambert had mixed feelings about this. She had been having so much difficulty coping with Roger. She had promised him that she would never place him in a nursing home, but he was now chair-bound because of his ill-ness and had started to become forgetful and demanding. His vision was also very bad. So she was almost happy that she needed to go into the hospital to have the amputation. It meant that Roger would have to go into the nursing home after all.

In the hospital she at last had time to consider her own situation. She had not had to deal with doctors before, except for psychiatrists. Could the doctors not have diagnosed the melanoma sooner? She was angry and felt that she could not trust physicians, losing faith in them just as she had lost faith in the church.

Following the surgery, she convalesced at her brother Peter's house for three weeks. While she was there, she spoke non-stop about her life and people she had known, but said little about her feelings, except for remarks like, "I've always been in the service of others. I feel like a servant." Although she spoke a lot about Roger and the constant care he had needed for the past three years, during the weeks she was in Peter's home, not once did she call her husband. Later Peter said to me, "It's as if she felt totally liberated."

In May 1996, a few months after her surgery, she went to see the surgeon again. He had bad news: the melanoma had spread to her groin. She was dev-astated, but she wanted to fight for her life. She agreed to have surgery to re-move the lymph nodes in her groin. The oncologist offered her experimental chemotherapy. Though the chance that it would help was not great, Mrs. Lambert wanted to go through with it.

"How Can My Life Be Ending? It Hasn't Started Yet"

In July, Mrs. Lambert began to have pain in her left leg. During July and August she spent up to ten hours each day in the bathtub, trying to get some relief. One day she spent twenty hours there. By August she had developed tumor in her pelvis and severe pain in her left lower abdomen; the pain in her leg got worse. A scan showed tumor in her lumbar spine with nerve root entrapment.

Things were happening so fast that Mrs. Lambert didn't know what to do. When the surgeon offered her radiotherapy, she refused. So far everything had failed, so why have more treatments? But when the pain got worse in late August, she was admitted to a general surgical ward for pain control. She now accepted a course of radiotherapy to try to reduce her pain and started taking small doses of the opioid analgesic hydromorphone.

At this time, her attending surgeon told her that she had a prognosis of a few weeks. Mrs. Lambert became despondent, saying to her brother Peter, "How can my life be ending? It hasn't started yet."

Nerve Pain

Her pain was out of control. She rated it 10 on a scale of 0 to 10—the worst pain possible. When pain is due to tumor invasion of nerves, opioids alone are often not sufficient to control it. The surgeon consulted Dr. Julie Bonin of the Palliative Care Service, who suggested an increase in hydromorphone and the addition of carbamazepine (an antiepileptic agent) and amitriptyline (an antidepressant) as co-analgesics.

The oncologist also considered offering her palliative chemotherapy to try to control the pain. However, within two or three days, Mrs. Lambert was feeling better. She was walking around and in better spirits. The oncologist, seeing that she was more comfortable, said that he would not favor more chemotherapy unless the pain could not be controlled by other means. The medical team felt that she might be able to go home. A few days later, however, burning pain was back in her left leg and groin. She rated its intensity as *15* out of 10. Any movement made the pain much worse. Dr. Bonin transferred her to the Palliative Care Unit on an urgent basis.

On August 30, 1996, she was admitted to the unit, receiving a room with a private bath so she could have hot baths as often as she wanted to ease her pain. One of the nurses described her as "stoical, friendly, open but afraid to bother others for help." Her nieces brought her gifts and things she needed. They related to each other in practical ways. Mrs. Lambert did not discuss her more serious concerns with them.

Within a few days, her pain medications seemed to be working, as the pain was less, and she was able to walk. The staff began planning her discharge home, and she began to look forward to resuming her normal life. But the relief was short-lived. Mrs. Lambert began to have hallucinations, which Dr. Bonin believed were from the high doses of hydromorphone. She switched medication and asked the anesthetist for help. Perhaps an epidural or a nerve block would reduce the need for medication. On September 11, Mrs. Lambert tried the epidural analgesia, but it did not help. She was unable to move her legs when she received the epidural medication, and the pain was still there.

It is rare that epidurals do not work in this context. Mrs. Lambert was so discouraged that she cried. Dr. Bonin was surprised and disappointed. Once or twice a year they had a patient like Mrs. Lambert on the unit—a patient whose pain persisted despite their best efforts. Julie continued to try different kinds of medication, but she was rapidly running out of options.

In mid-September, Mrs. Lambert's older sister died, also of cancer. Her family tried to include her in the funeral at a distance, sharing their plans for the rituals and prayers. She was touched by this, but her sister's death, along with her worry over her own tumors growing, provoked feelings of despair. She asked the psychologist, "Why live when death seems to be the way out for all of us?"

Trying to Get Closer

In the nursing home, Roger would occasionally remark to his niece or nephew, "It's not going well for Miriam, is it?" Once in a while he telephoned Mrs. Lambert. Commenting to me about these calls, she said, "I feel so helpless. He calls and says things like 'I need help. No one is here to get me to the toilet.' What can I do? This is what happens when you don't have children." In fact, her husband did have children from a previous marriage, but they did not visit him.

The nurses found it difficult to communicate with Mrs. Lambert at a deeper level. Linda, her primary nurse, told me, "Her conversation is superficial—difficult to pierce. She will barely skim the depths. I couldn't get down in there, like I can with other patients. She is bright, and loves to play with words, but somehow it is difficult to get close to her." Though she had very little to work with, Linda tried to interpret Mrs. Lambert's reserve. "She could not use her potential," she speculated to me. "She did not have a career. She has a sense of failure about this. She feels a great sense of responsibility toward her husband. I think that her emotional pain is linked to the fact that she can no longer look after her husband."

Patients are selective in the caregivers with whom they will share their feelings—if they choose to open up at all. In Mrs. Lambert's case, it was Gloria, the art therapist. She told Gloria that she saw her life as a failure. In an art therapy session Mrs. Lambert made a painting of a swirling bluish cloud, bordered by a blue square, and wrote the word "fiasco" underneath, in large blue letters. "I don't do anything well," she explained. "My life is a fiasco." Of the painting she said, "This is bad. It doesn't look good. It's horrible, but that's how I feel." She wanted to put the painting on the wall of her room, along with others that were more cheerful and comforting to her. Despite these moments of self-disclosure, Gloria felt that Mrs. Lambert was "hiding."

Mrs. Lambert developed a new burning pain, this time in her right leg. Crying with pain, she stayed in bed and did not move. X-rays confirmed that the tumor had spread. She was scheduled for more radiotherapy, but sometimes she was in so much pain and was so tired that she did not go down for the treatments. Dr. Bonin continued to increase the opioid and co-analgesic medications, adding new ones to replace those that seemed ineffective.

During this time, Mrs. Lambert met with the psychologist. She kept away from serious subjects, expressing the desire to talk only about light things. After about half an hour she told the psychologist that what she really needed to talk about would make her break into tears and, she said, "If I cry, I will feel more physical pain." The serious talk would have to wait.

Mrs. Lambert also received music therapy. During a relaxation session in her room, Mrs. Lambert reported no pain when she listened to the sound of ocean waves. In early October, she began to attend a creative arts group. She collaborated with another patient on certain images of a house. At the next session she asked Gloria, the art therapist, to make some drawings for her. Gloria recalled this session to me: "She spoke a great deal about 'feeling sad or angry inside but smiling on the outside.' She created an image of a woman smiling but holding a more somber woman inside of herself. She reacted favorably [to it] but did not want to place it in her room." Gloria wondered aloud, "Perhaps it's a little close to home?"

Mrs. Lambert's conversation was becoming more superficial, even with Gloria. Gloria wanted to see if she could explore Mrs. Lambert's world more deeply by using visualization techniques. "I brought her a peaceful picture," Gloria said, "seeing if she could imagine herself in it. She always blocked me when I tried to image with her. She is playing 'hostess with the mostest,' wanting to please me by *trying* to image." Subsequently, however, Mrs. Lambert became more involved with these techniques. One day, Gloria reported, Mrs. Lambert and one of her nieces visualized together that they were entering into one of the drawings that Gloria had made for her—a peaceful, happy city scene. Mrs. Lambert imagined a rooftop restaurant in the scene, and she and her niece went in to have a meal there together. Another day Gloria brought a number of magazine photos, and Mrs. Lambert chose one that showed two small children kissing.

Total Pain

On October 10, Mrs. Lambert had another pain crisis. Dr. Bonin realized that her regular medications for neuropathic pain were not working. Believing that this was a case of "total pain," in which physical, emotional, mental, and spiritual elements are combined, she had already asked the psychologist to help. Now she also consulted the anesthetist and the psychiatrist. Mrs. Lambert did not react well to the latter referral, saying to her brother, "The doctors don't believe that I have all this pain. They even got me to see a psychiatrist." In fact, Dr. Bonin knew very well that Mrs. Lambert was experiencing intense physical suffering. But because of the interrelation of the various elements in Mrs. Lambert's suffering, the team was trying to adopt a holistic approach, an approach that Mrs. Lambert either did not understand or did not want to accept. She did appreciate massage therapy, however; the nurse, occupational therapist, or volunteer took turns at massaging her legs and back. She also continued to use music and imagery techniques, even though she worried that she was taking up too much of the therapists' time.

By this time I was visiting Mrs. Lambert regularly as part of our project. During my visits, Mrs. Lambert would usually stare straight ahead, looking vague and distant. When she spoke of her pain, her affect stayed flat, even when she used expressions such as "It's like my bones will break." She accepted my silent presence but would not allow me into her world. Yet she did say, "The only thing that helps my pain is if someone sits with me." One morning, when she was having a particularly bad pain crisis, she could not keep from crying out loud: "It's not humane. It hurts when I cry. I can't even cry!"

When the pain was this bad, she preferred to be alone. She said to Linda afterward, "When the pain is really bad, nothing helps. It's better if you leave me alone then. I hope I'm not offending you. I don't want you or anyone else to take it personally. I need to be angry or cry without having to explain myself each time." Mrs. Lambert had begun to feel frustrated and even angry with Dr. Bonin. Her brother reassured her, "Dr. Bonin is doing her best." She replied, "I know that she's doing her best, but even if she controls the pain I'm going to die anyway."

Mrs. Lambert was totally desperate. She had feared pain all her life, and now here it was, with no relief in sight. Although she had some spiritual beliefs, she could find no meaning in her suffering. She did not think that God had inflicted this pain on her; she had no concept of God.

To the staff there seemed so much more that Mrs. Lambert could not express. They felt shut out. Linda commented that Mrs. Lambert was "not accessible." Gloria was still trying to use the art sessions to help Mrs. Lambert become more open about her feelings, but she did not have much success. She told me:

> There is something that blocks her from investing in other people. She must have been very hurt. Any artwork that is more probing, more personal, she shuts away. Or maybe there was something basically missing in the mother–child relationship. But it's really sad.

Toward the end of October, Mrs. Lambert was completely bedbound because of her pain. She had periods of confusion and seemed to be giving up. "I am dying," she told Dr. Bonin. "I am losing everything. It's not that I'm accepting of it." She phoned her lawyer and arranged for him to come to the hospital to help her get her affairs in order.

Julie wanted the advice of the other physicians and members of the team, so she presented Mrs. Lambert's case at the weekly multidisciplinary ward rounds. At the meeting she offered her opinion that "the pain is not only physical—she had a total pain syndrome." She mentioned that Mrs. Lambert was a classic example of what Michael Kearney, a palliative care specialist in California, called "soul pain," a deep-set anguish due to unexpressed unconscious conflicts. But the various methods that Dr. Kearney used in such cases, often with some success—visualization, guided imagery, deep relaxation—had all failed for Mrs. Lambert.

What was the team to do? The anesthetist, having reassessed her that day and found that she continued to have back pain, believed that an intrathecal block would be possible, but Mrs. Lambert was not keen on that option. Julie was considering using more sedative medication so Mrs. Lambert could sleep through these periods; however, this was not an easy decision to make. She knew that when sedation was used for pain it could shorten the person's life because the person would be asleep and not able to eat. Parenteral nutrition was not an option for her because it does not significantly prolong life in cancer patients who are losing weight because of the effect of the cancer on their metabolism. The other physicians on the team agreed that sedation was the only option left.

When Julie mentioned this possibility to Mrs. Lambert, she was receptive, but she hesitated because the lawyer was coming to help her sort out her affairs. She met the lawyer on two occasions, and Dr. Bonin tried to ensure that she was as lucid as possible during those times. Then, with Mrs. Lambert's consent, Julie ordered more sedative medication—ketamine and midazolam. Ketamine is an anesthetic agent that, in lower doses, produces a dissociative reaction, whereby a person may still have pain but will experience it as if it were happening to someone else. The person may therefore feel less distressed. Because ketamine has side effects, however, it is usually administered with a sedative drug such as midazolam to try to minimize the frightening hallucinations or other so-called emergence phenomena that can occur with this drug.

"When the Pain Gets Better Is When I Feel Worse"

Within two days of starting the ketamine, Mrs. Lambert was pain-free. She was neither confused nor hallucinating. As Dr. Bonin expected, Mrs. Lambert entered a dissociative state. "I feel drunk, but I don't care!" she said to Julie. Later, she said, "I feel like I'm not myself. I don't know what to do without the pain. The pain was so present before, and now I feel lost."

She was able to enjoy visits and was particularly pleased to see her youngest brother who had come from out of town. She was beaming when I entered the room, and introduced me to a strapping, fit-looking blond man. She said, "This is my baby brother. Isn't he handsome?" She found his visit stimulating and entertaining as they joked around, keeping the conversation light. I wondered if she was actually connecting with anyone.

At this point, I began to understand how difficult she was to reach. I had seen her at least fifteen times by now, and although these were relatively brief visits, I still felt that it was taking so long for us to connect! My previous visit was the first time I felt any human connection at all. She had cried and cried, like a small, abandoned child, but she did not respond to me as a person. She needed a warm body at her side; it could have been any warm body. When she spoke of her pain (now usually in her right leg), she looked straight ahead of her, eyes unfocused, as if in a trance. Her voice was almost expressionless, even before the ketamine was started. I wondered whether she would be labeled as having a borderline personality disorder on a formal psychiatric evaluation.

I reflected on what I knew of her family constellation. She came from a very large family, the first three children being girls, then four boys, then Miriam, then two more boys. "I was sandwiched between brothers," she once said with a vague smile on her face. Was this a sexual reference? I wondered if there was a history of incest or abuse. Mrs. Lambert also said something at this time that sounded paradoxical: "When the pain gets better is when I feel worse." I wondered what terrible inner anguish emerged when she no longer needed to focus on her physical pain.

By October 23, she was sleeping most of the time because of the ketamine and midazolam. The staff felt that she was suffering less now and agreed that it was better to keep her sedated. The ketamine dose was reduced, however, because Mrs. Lambert began to have bizarre and vivid dreams of fire or boiling water rushing into her room. Such distressing visions are a possible side effect of ketamine.

During one of the periods when she was more wakeful, I visited her. As I walked into the room, she was drinking water from a glass, trying to get her pills down. For the first time, she looked angry to me. Though I was visiting her in the context of our research, I tried to listen as actively and as therapeutically as I could. She motioned with her glass of water and medications cup. "I could throw this at someone," she said.

I responded, "You're angry."

"Last night," she continued, "I would have killed myself if I could, because of the pain in my legs and in my abdomen." She started to cry. "Nothing they try works and the syringe driver hurts my arm, or wherever they put it. Wherever they put the needle, it hurts. They have to change it every day. Before, I wanted to be alone, but now I always want someone with me—over the last couple of weeks." She was still crying. "Before, I was too proud."

"Are you afraid?" I asked.

"No, I'm not afraid. I'm only afraid of having pain. I have pain, that's all. If only this could be all over." She was silent for a while. "Everyone brings me biscuits or candy. But I'm not hungry. If I listened to them, I would have a roomful of biscuits and candy. It's not that I'm not grateful for their good will."

"Nothing helps."

"No. I always like to have someone with me. I don't know why. I have less pain somehow. I feel less alone." She started to cry again.

"That's it," I offered. "You feel alone."

"One has pain, pain, pain," she replied, "and there's nothing that can be done about it." She cried. "[The psychiatrist] came. He said to me, 'There is nothing I can do here.' I don't think he is coming back."

"What about our psychologist?"

Mrs. Lambert paused. "She came a few times. I don't know if she'll come back. I guess it depends on me."

In fact, the psychologist did try to see her on several occasions in the weeks that followed. Usually Mrs. Lambert was asleep, or tired, or in too much pain to have lengthy discussions with her.

Glimmers of Trust

After this conversation, I felt that there were so many things that she did not know how to talk about. But she was able to open up in art therapy, where she did not need to be verbal. The next day, at the art therapy session, the pain was better. She was in a recliner in the solarium, joking and talking. She did not want to paint or draw herself, but she wanted Gloria to draw and paint in her presence. She found this a safe way to express herself—to respond to the drawings Gloria made. Her response to a picture of a tree was, "It looks like a peaceful place." Her response to a painting of flowers was, "That's beautiful. You keep it somewhere for me." It was as though she did not feel ready or able to own the beautiful object, to keep it in her room. Yet, in a previous session, she had found a particular picture beautiful—one of children playing in a natural setting—and had asked Gloria's permission to keep it in her room. Now she said to Gloria, referring to that picture, "I had to throw it in the garbage." Then, "If I didn't like you, I wouldn't have told you. I like you and I know you will understand."

As she became more open with Gloria she spoke of a brother and a sister who had died when they were young and of mothers loving small children. "We're always related to somebody," she said. "And we're always somebody's baby." She thought a lot about her mother and occasionally spoke of her husband with fondness and sadness. Mostly, though, she thought about the distant past. When Mrs. Lambert's nurse Linda asked Peter, Mrs. Lambert's brother, what Mrs. Lambert had been like when she was young, he replied, "She was an unhappy child. You shouldn't go deeper in discussing it. It might hurt her."

The staff understood that they had to tread softly. While they did not want to abandon her, given her troubled past, their goals in Mrs. Lambert's case had to be very limited. They would try to control her symptoms and help her achieve some quality of life in the short time left to her, but they could not resolve her deep-seated psychological problems.

Slowly, the kindness of the staff began to touch her. One morning, when she was more wakeful, I visited her as Linda was finishing putting Mrs. Lambert's hair in rollers. Mrs. Lambert looked happier than I had ever seen her. She said, "People are so kind here. They don't have to do this," referring to Linda who was doing her hair. I admired the artwork on her walls. "Gloria leaves me this artwork and she says to me, 'It warms my heart to give them to you,'" Mrs. Lambert said. Her eyes opened wide, as if she were marveling at love freely given.

"The Angels Are Telling Me to Die Peacefully"

Only a few times a year did the staff have patients as challenging as Mrs. Lambert. These patients always made everyone distraught, for palliative care staff like to feel that they can relieve suffering in all cases. They had known other patients who, like Mrs. Lambert, had symptoms that were difficult to control. Sometimes they saw the patient undergo a shift of perception: the pain would still be there, but it would be experienced differently and the suffering reduced. The patient would reach a deeper level of understanding, almost as if the suffering had been given new meaning. Unfortunately, this transformation had not occurred in Mrs. Lambert's case.

Mrs. Lambert had developed more tumors in her pelvis. None of the medical solutions they had tried so far had relieved the pain for any length of time, and the pain was increasing again. Julie Bonin and the nursing staff found it difficult to tolerate her dissociated state. She was not herself and seemed detached and distant as she spoke, but she said that she still had pain. She expressed guilt about not being able to be with Roger but said she did not want him to visit—she'd been exhausted after the one time they had tried it.

Julie was running out of ideas. On November 7, she again presented Mrs. Lambert's case at ward rounds. Just before this meeting, the anesthetist had tried to perform a spinal block at the L2–L3 level, but the attempt was unsuccessful. Julie decided to try another co-analgesic drug, gabapentin. The other physicians considered the case carefully but could not come up with anything else. Mrs. Lambert said that she did not mind being more completely sedated—she was preparing to die.

On November 18, Dr. Bonin reported,

> She feels that she is getting weaker, especially over the past week. She is very sad about this. She was hoping to make it to Christmas. She was so glad when people put up the holiday decorations in her room. She especially likes the little white angels, but now she says, "The angels are telling me to die peacefully." She asked me questions about how and when she would die.

The next time Gloria saw her, Mrs. Lambert was too sick to do art therapy. When Gloria said to her, "I'll see you Wednesday" (in two days' time), Mrs. Lambert replied, "Yes, if I'm here." This was the first time she had spoken to Gloria about dying.

But she did not die. She continued to suffer. She developed dizziness that she attributed to the gabapentin, so she asked that the drug be discontinued. She stopped eating and drank very little. Her brother reported that she was more closed in on herself now, not speaking to family members when they visited. She slept most of the time, and, when Gloria came back two days later, Mrs. Lambert was barely responsive. Gloria sat with her, holding her hand. When Mrs. Lambert opened her eyes, she seemed to recognize Gloria, then closed her eyes again.

Linda

Around this time, Mrs. Lambert's nurse Linda sought me out. She wanted to speak with me because Mrs. Lambert had aroused strong feelings in her. Linda saw that Mrs. Lambert was deteriorating and thought that she might die soon. She told me how patients often affected her as a nurse, how she tried to empathize, and the repercussions of this.

I'd like to speak now, because after they die, I forget. That's how I protect myself, I guess. I'm remembering everything that she said now, but when they die, I forget. I have to forget so that I can carry on with the next patient.

In the beginning, her pain was uncontrollable. One day she had severe electric shock-like pains that made her scream. She knew that her screaming wouldn't upset me, and that knowledge reassured her. She appreciated getting consistent nursing care. She leaned on her two primary nurses quite heavily.

I entered her pain at one point. I was in pain, too. We had tried absolutely everything, and nothing was working. On that day, my neck went into spasm from stress, and I had to go home early because of the pain. I had had neck pain in the past, but when I feel that people need me all at once, my neck pain comes back. I knew then that I had overstepped my boundary and that I couldn't get so involved. She greeted me crying, saying she'd never get out of bed again because of the pain, and she never did. She told me that her emotional pain is more than her physical pain.

She has learned to express her needs, which she had difficulty doing before. She is able to ask the volunteers for help. She makes volunteers feel special. However, she realized that some people may come for their own comfort and not hers. Sometimes we need to feel that we are doing something, but it doesn't help.

Inducing Sleep

On November 25, the pain became unbearable; the ketamine was no longer having an effect. Dr. Bonin came to see her and found her lying in bed, "asking for something to be done." Julie interpreted this as a possible request for euthanasia. Since euthanasia was morally unacceptable to her and was not a legal option in any event, she offered Mrs. Lambert deep sedation, to which Mrs. Lambert agreed. Julie stopped the ketamine and started methotrimeprazine, a medication that is both analgesic and sedative. It would give Mrs. Lambert some respite, and the sleep induced by this medication could be reversed at any time.

Mrs. Lambert's family and friends organized a visiting schedule to ensure that there would be someone with her most of the time. Mrs. Lambert slept quietly over the next few days. Dr. Bonin felt that she had probably developed septicemia, a bacterial infection in the bloodstream. She decided under the circumstances not to investigate this further, nor to treat it with antibiotics. Although Mrs. Lambert could no longer speak with the members of her family, she was able to have important, albeit brief, exchanges with Dr. Bonin about the sedation. She was still in pain. She said, "The physical pain is now worse than the mental pain. I can't bear this anymore." Julie asked her if she wanted the sedative increased. She said yes.

The next day, Mrs. Lambert slept continuously. She was not responding when people spoke with her. The music therapist continued to see her every day and to play for her even though she seemed to be in a coma. On the evening of December 5, Mrs. Lambert was sleeping peacefully in her room, her niece Carole beside her. The light was subdued—only the Christmas lights were on—and soft, relaxing music played. Carole lit some incense and read silently from a Catholic prayer book. Mrs. Lambert died later that evening, with two of her nieces present.

Roger

Roger had not planned that his wife would die before him. At the funeral, he cried as he touched his wife's body. But he never spoke of her after that. One of Mrs. Lambert's nieces and her husband, who were now the closest people to Roger, told me that he never showed any emotion if someone mentioned his wife by name. If someone reminded him that she had died, he would say calmly, "Oh, yes."

It seemed that Roger had reached a certain tranquility. He died in July 1998, 18 months after his wife's death and 4 months after his 100th birthday. He had hoped to reach that milestone.

Medication and Pain Control Record

August 23 Admitted to surgical ward for pain control. CT scan showed destruction of the right side of the sacrum, with tumor extending into the S1–S2 neural foramina, possibly into the spinal canals. She received radiotherapy to this area. Started on hydromorphone 4 mg SC q4h.

August 25 Pain intensity 10/10. Palliative care consulted. Started 24 h. continuous subcutaneous (SC) infusions of hydromorphone 36 mg, and haloperiodol 3 mg to prevent nausea.

August 27 Seen by oncologist who is considering palliative chemotherapy. Patient walking around and in better spirits. Pain 5/10.

August 28 On hydromorphone 16 mg PO q4h, naproxen 250 mg twice daily, carbamazepine 150 mg twice daily, lorazepam at bedtime. SC medication discontinued to prepare her to go home.

August 29 Patient says that most helpful pill is the anxiolytic lorazepam. Pain 10/10. Amitriptyline 25 mg added at bedtime, with plan to titrate upwards.

August 30 Mrs. Lambert did not go home; she was transferred to PCU on an urgent basis because of left leg and groin pain that she described as 15 on a scale of 1 to 10. Carbamazepine increased to 200 mg PO bid, and amitriptyline 50 mg PO at bedtime.

September 3 Switched to a room with a tub, since hot baths help the pain.

September 5 The pain was better; she was walking. The staff again considered planning discharge home.

September 9 She started to have hallucinations and myoclonus; Dr. Bonin believed this was from the hydromorphone. She rotated the opioid to fentanyl patch 125 mcg/h and increased the carbamazepine to 200 mg three times daily and the bedtime amitriptyline to 75 mg. Naproxen discontinued. Dexamethasone 80 mg IV given over 1 h, tapering doses over 5 days.

With this, she was totally pain-free.

September 11   48 h trial of epidural bupivacaine and hydromorphone, aiming to decrease the systemic medication. Pain in groin 7/10 after epidural. Paralyzed legs but no effect on the pain. Anesthesist: Epidural catheter well placed.

As she was also getting weaker and was bedbound, the oncologist decided not to offer her any chemotherapy. Dr. Bonin: "Long discussion about where we are at in terms of pain control, disease progression, past history. Understands disease is progressing, with tumor along S1-S2 nerve roots."

September 14   Mexiletene added.

September 16   Epidural discontinued because not helping. Not moving at all because of the pain, 10/10 on movement, 8/10 at rest.

September 22   Mexiletene titrated up to 200 mg PO three times daily. Increased amitriptyline 100 mg PO at bedtime.

September 24   Trial of transcutaneous electrical nerve stimulation (TENS) for 3 days, prior to mobilization. No relief with repeated trials of up to 50 minutes.

September 30   New burning pain R leg. Received radiotherapy to the sacrum. Increased fentanyl patch to 150 mcg/h q3 days.

October 4   Increased pain. On fentanyl 200 mcg/h q3 days, lorazepam 1 mg twice daily. Increased mexiletene 300 mg q AM and 400 mg at bedtime.

October 9   Music therapy. Patient reported no pain during relaxation session.

October 10   Pain crisis. Received pamidronate 90 mg IV. On fentanyl patch 250 mcg/h with hydromorphone breakthrough, carbamazepine 600 mg PO daily, amitriptyline 100 mg PO at bedtime and mexiletene 700 mg PO daily.

October 12   Amitriptyline discontinued since it was deemed ineffective. On clonazepam 0.5 mg PO bid and 0.5 mg PO at bedtime. She continued to complain of back pain. Anesthetist was re-consulted. Ketamine 240 mg and midazolam 24 mg q24h were started via SC infusion. Mrs. Lambert experienced dissociation symptoms but she still complained of pain. Anesthetist: An intrathecal block would be possible, but the patient was not keen on this option.

October 19	Pain-free at this time but has blurred vision and slowed language. Not confused or hallucinating. "Feels drunk, but does not care!" Dr. Bonin's plan: gradually decrease medication other than ketamine: Decreased clonazepam 0.5 mg bid, mexiletene 300 mg bid, fentanyl patch 200 mcg/h q3 days.
October 23	Severe pains again in legs and abdomen. Despairing. Expresses suicidal thoughts.
October 25	Pain better. Enjoyed solarium and art therapy session.
October 28	Sleeping most of the time with the ketamine and midazolam combination. Ketamine dose was reduced because she began to have vivid dreams. She started to have myoclonus, so fentanyl was reduced. Consult with psychiatrist and psychologist. Psychiatrist reports: "There is nothing I can do here."
October 30	Discontinued mexiletine since it was ineffective. Gabapentin 100 mg three times daily started, to be titrated up. Hydromorphone 6–12 mg PO q3h breakthrough.
November 5	Mrs. Lambert said that keeping the radio on all night helped keep her mind off the pain. Spinal block failed at L2–L3 level—no CSF [cerebrospinal fluid] obtained. Anesthetist feels there is tumor there.
November 7	Team tried massage, no help. Anesthesia: Epidural was ineffective; will try caudal block this week.
November 13	Variable pain; variable mood. Continues ketamine 200 mg, midazolam 24 mg SC over 24 h and gabapentin 400 mg PO three times daily.
November 15	Bad pain. "I'm suffering. I'm suffering."
November 18	Pain 10/10. Still on ketamine. Gabapentin to be tapered over the next few days since patient developed generalized muscle weakness of unknown etiology, but she asked to stop this medication.
November 22	Ketamine 240 mg SC over 24 h.
November 25	Fentanyl increased to 300 mcg/h.
November 26	Ketamine discontinued since no longer effective, and methotrimeprazine sedation was started at 30 mg SC over 24 h. This helped her pain, but she was now sedated.

December 3   Mrs. Lambert still had "a bit" of pain. Following discussion with her, sedation was increased to methotrimeprazine 50 mg SC over 24 h.

Case presented to visiting professor. Her commentary: "This was a case of mixed neuropathic and somatic pain—conus medullaris syndrome, which started with L2 radiculopathy. She probably also had vertebral body involvement and spinal instability, and thalamic neuronal involvement and its concomitant brain neurophysiological changes. This is the reason why the epidural analgesia did not work. Although melanoma is not a very radiosensitive tumor, radiotherapy is indicated for pain control in these cases. The team could have tried a neurolytic epidural block earlier in the course of this patient's pain. Methadone might have helped but sedation is a possible side effect."

December 4   Mrs. Lambert is comatose, unresponsive to verbal commands.

December 5   Comatose. Still seemed in pain when she was moved. She died later that evening.

Authors' Comments

Although the palliative care staff had tried their best to help Mrs. Lambert, they were frustrated by the inadequate pain control and by their inability to get in touch with her inner world. Over a period of almost three months, they tried everything they could in their approach to Mrs. Lambert's total pain. On the biomedical side, they tried every drug and anesthetic intervention that was appropriate. On the psychosocial side, they tried to get her to open up to others, to learn the meaning of trust and love, even this late in life. Yet the great tragedy of her life became evident—the tragedy of a life unlived because she was unable to trust herself or others.

Pain had become her identity, and, with its removal, she was left with the hollowness at the center of her sense of self. It is also likely that what pain relief she did achieve left her open to be more conscious of the existential and psychological aspects of her lifetime of unhappiness.

At various points during her time on the unit, Mrs. Lambert showed signs of beginning to share her inner life. Once during the final period of her sedation, she awoke when the music therapist came and asked her to play some music on her flute. She cried, which was a big step for her. She started to come alive in her contacts with some of the staff, especially with Gloria and Linda. She could not fully express herself to them, however; the journey had just begun. Perhaps she understood that she was to get no further in this lifetime. Would the outcome have been different had the staff had more time to work with her? On this we can only speculate.

Add to this complexity the fact that these cases are very intense, even draining, for the staff. The quote from nurse Linda is an example of the kind of profound staff reaction that is not infrequent. More hidden and insidious is that staff may be experience anger and resentment at the frustration of their unconscious rescue fantasies and the lack of gratitude for their efforts. These issues are why, embedded within palliative care philosophy, it is important to provide breathing space, debriefing, and reflection opportunities for staff. The ever-present potential for counter-transference reactions makes it vital that administrators formally provide staff support services. Led by psychologists, psychiatrists, social workers, or other highly and specifically trained personnel, such services provide safe and confidential spaces for either group or individual staff debriefing. Some units provide weekly staff support rounds, while others might call for meetings when there has been a particularly difficult case. Where staff would otherwise become too emotionally drained to carry on, staff support may reduce turnover and enable palliative care providers to dedicate their careers to this difficult yet rewarding field.

As we have discussed in the General Introduction, medical aid in dying (MAID), or voluntary active euthanasia, is now legal in Canada. Today Mrs. Lambert would possibly have made a direct and specific request for MAID. In the event, she was maintained in a state of sedation over the last few days of her life, and she was comatose when she died. In the Authors' Comments for the narrative of Frances Legendre, where these issues were also prominent, we explore some of the ramifications of these requests. That discussion is also relevant here.

12

Sadie Fineman

A Question of Denial?

Narrated by Patricia Boston

Sadie Fineman was 80 years old when her doctors discovered that she had a large cancerous mass in her pancreas. Despite a course of experimental therapy, the tumor continued to grow, and the best option that Mrs. Fineman's doctors could offer was palliative care. Mrs. Fineman and her family made it clear to the palliative care team that she wanted to be cared for at home, even though there were many times when the nursing care she required exceeded the knowledge and skills of her family. This was not her caregivers' only challenge; the Fineman family insisted that the word "cancer" be avoided in all dealings with the patient, to keep the truth from her at all costs.

A Family Meeting Without the Patient

Sadie Fineman lived with her 54-year-old daughter, Rachel, in a middle-class neighborhood in suburban Montreal. Widowed 40 years ago, she had raised two children. Rachel was now an executive business secretary, and Henry, 57 years old, was a lawyer. Rachel had never married and had always lived with her mother. She had received many opportunities to marry but, as she told me when I met her, she "enjoyed her freedom" and felt most comfortable with her mother in the home where she had been born and raised. Rachel shared the housework, cooking, and financial expenses. When her mother became ill, she became the main family caregiver.

Henry lived with his wife, Julia, about two miles from his mother's home. Henry was always available, "on call 24 hours a day," as he put it to me. Both Rachel and Henry loved their mother and felt close to her. Rachel in particular said she felt "very bound and connected emotionally." It was impossible for her to imagine what life would be like without her mother in the world.

At the time Mrs. Fineman was diagnosed with pancreatic cancer in the spring of 1991, the tumor could be only partially resected. By August 1995, the tumor in the body of her pancreas had enlarged. Mrs. Fineman was now beginning to complain of mid-back pain and pain in her shoulder. The tumor had spread. Although no further surgical treatment was available, she did have the options of experimental chemotherapy, palliative chemotherapy, or supportive care. Mrs. Fineman's oncologist, Dr. Isaac Levitan, suggested a family meeting to discuss the possibilities.

Mrs. Fineman did not attend. She did not care much for these kinds of meetings. They involved a lot of medical talk. In Dr. Levitan's previous conversations with Mrs. Fineman, it had become clear to him that she was not ready to talk about her illness. Her major worry, and all that she was willing to deal with, was her back pain and the nagging pain in her shoulder. As she explained to Dr. Levitan, "the main problem is my arthritis." If that could be looked after everything would be okay. She was a busy woman and needed to get on with things.

Dr. Levitan met with Henry, Julia, and Rachel. Mrs. Fineman was especially comfortable having Henry involved. He had a "good mind," as she put it to me, and she was used to relying on him when there were decisions to make. Dr. Levitan assured the Fineman family that pain control would not be a problem. But how should they proceed with treatment? It was difficult to know, Henry said. Yes, there was the possibility of offering his mother experimental treatment, but why do it when it would make her very sick and prolong suffering? On the other hand, his mother still enjoyed her life, even loved life, so why not provide her with whatever could be made available?

Dr. Levitan felt that his patient had the right to decide for herself what to do. But to make this kind of decision she needed to know the seriousness of her condition. He told Henry that, in his opinion, it was always best to tell the patient the truth. Dr. Levitan preferred to tell people the gravity of their condition so that they could take care of their affairs, complete unfinished business, and perhaps even do some of the things in life that they hadn't done up to now. It was possible that Mrs. Fineman might only live for a few more weeks. Surely, she needed to be prepared for that possibility.

Henry and Rachel implored Dr. Levitan not to tell their mother how ill she was. Henry said that his mother was already 80 years old, had taken care of her affairs, and had already done all that she wanted to in life. She was happy and content with her life at home with Rachel. "Besides," Henry said, as far as he and Rachel were concerned, "what if her affairs are left in a mess?" When the time came to deal with them, they would do it. For the most part, Henry said, he "preferred to avoid those kinds of realities." As he explained to me later, "My attitude is, everything one has to know about death, one will find out when the time comes."

At this point, Henry preferred to focus his energies on how his mother was living, not how she was dying. After all, the only thing that was of any real concern to her just then was her "arthritis." Henry and Rachel told Dr. Levitan that they would explain to their mother that there were drugs available to help her condition, but that the drugs might not work. Dr. Levitan agreed to give her the option of the experimental therapy.

The Ability to Hear What She Wanted to Hear

With Rachel's agreement, Henry explained to his mother that Dr. Levitan had told him that her illness was serious—she had a recurrence of her tumor—but that some experimental drugs were available for her to take. Henry decided not to use the word "cancer" in any of his discussions with his mother because the word was too frightening. When people hear that word, he believed, they think of it as a death sentence.

Mrs. Fineman readily agreed to the experimental therapy. Henry and Julia accompanied her to the oncology department and sat with her while she underwent the treatments. Henry told me that it was hard to see all those people down there in the chemotherapy clinic. They looked so ill, and yet some of them seemed braver than the people accompanying them.

Mrs. Fineman's therapy did not work; her cancer was rapidly metastasizing. Dr. Levitan continued to worry that Mrs. Fineman did not realize how very ill she was. He emphasized to the family again that Mrs. Fineman really ought to know the full extent of her condition. Dr. Levitan feared that she might survive only two more weeks. Henry agreed to talk again with his mother. Together with Julia, he explained to Mrs. Fineman that the treatments had not worked, but quickly added that the doctors would be trying to do all that they could for her. Henry realized that he was not being as direct about his mother's situation as he could be. But that was how he preferred to handle things. "Besides," he told me, "even when you told my mother what the reality was, it wouldn't necessarily be a reality for her." He continued, "My mother is a tough, courageous woman. There was never a problem in telling her about her illness. But she also had the ability to hear what she wanted to hear."

Henry and Rachel rationalized their approach with the belief that "hope should not be taken away." As Rachel asked aloud to me, what if there were family events planned for the next year or the year after that? Their mother loved a good family wedding and all the gossip and planning that went with it. Why should she miss out on that hope? "Why," Henry chimed in, "should I say, 'No, you are not going to live to make that wedding'? Why would I be so stupid, so blunt? Even if there was not much time, better to let my mother think, at least, that she had some future to look forward to."

"In the Realm of Miracles"

Mrs. Fineman's tumor progressed. She began to lose weight and looked ill and pale. But she did not die. Dr. Levitan was amazed. Five months had passed since the experimental treatments. He said to Henry. "You know, we're not dealing in the realm of medicine now, we are dealing in the realm of miracles. I have no medical explanation for why she is still alive."

Meanwhile, Mrs. Fineman was continuing to live as fully as she knew how. She boasted to me of winning at cards, going for car rides with her friends, and "talking too much on the phone." Henry and Julia felt confirmed that it was a very good thing that Mrs. Fineman had not known or realized "the truth." Henry later recalled to me,

> She lived better, as things turned out, than if we had over realistically told her. She knew the tumor was growing. She saw the symptoms progressing. Her legs were swollen, and her stomach was protruding. Still, she enjoyed her life in the fullest sense of the word.

When Dr. Levitan requested a consultation from Dr. Gillian Webster of the Palliative Care Service, Gillian noted that Mrs. Fineman has lost 35 pounds during the preceding six months. Mrs. Fineman was still complaining of pain in the middle of her back, and in her left shoulder.

The back pain, she explained to Gillian, was "from gas," the shoulder pain "from arthritis."

Palliative Care

It was at this point, in February of 1996, that Sadie Fineman entered our study. My first meeting with her was at the small apartment she shared with Rachel. Gillian Webster had explained our project to her, and she was very open to participating in it. Gillian described Mrs. Fineman to me as a "strong, stoic lady" who expressed her own views on her illness. She asked few questions about her prognosis and had not even inquired whether her illness was serious. As Gillian noted at the time, "I am not really sure what she knows. No one in the family is actually discussing it. When the subject [of her illness] is broached, she offers her own explanations."

When I met Sadie Fineman, she certainly didn't strike me as a woman who was concerned that she might be dying. She was tiny and frail, and slightly stooped, yet she stood up as straight as she was able. She had a tremendous aura of authority, her voice clear, loud, and purposeful. I had the feeling she was a tremendously strong lady in spirit. She wore a green and yellow floral housecoat and comfortable, fluffy yellow slippers. Yet her greeting to us (I made my first visit with Dr. Webster) was almost formal. As she shook our hands in welcome, I noticed how pale she looked. There was a hint of jaundice around her eyes, which were otherwise dark, clear, and sharp.

We sat around the dining table in one corner of her large living room. The table was covered with a dark brown wool cloth protected by yellow plastic place mats. The room felt cozy. There were a few pieces of well-worn furniture; the sofa was decorated with large, plumped-up, green pillows, and a crocheted floral blanket. The walls were painted a shiny cream and were decorated with family photographs, some of which were faded and taken perhaps 30 years earlier. Many marked special family events: a large photograph showed a young man in graduation attire, and another showed a young woman holding what might have been a diploma. There were also photographs of family weddings, couples, and children. At one end of the room, several small coffee tables were piled up with papers, envelopes, and magazines.

Mrs. Fineman didn't look directly at us when she spoke. Sometimes I wondered if she was paying attention, but she was quick to correct us on the date or time of an event. She could recall not only those events leading up to her illness, but also life events that had occurred 40 years before. Sometimes as she spoke, I thought, "How ill she looks!" But it was also easy to forget her cancer and its prognosis. She spoke with energy and vitality about her life, and spoke about the future as if there could be no doubt about its coming.

Mrs. Fineman's abdominal tumors were easily palpable—it was difficult not to be aware of her large, protruding abdomen. Yet Mrs. Fineman did not seem concerned, and she didn't ask Dr. Webster any questions about it. Instead, she chatted easily and amiably about how she felt inconvenienced by diarrhea because it interfered with her lifestyle and her outings. She liked to go to the senior citizens' organization across the street to play cards. She confirmed that she was being visited frequently by the palliative care nurses from the home care service, but all that was really needed, she said, was "something to stop the diarrhea" and some ointment to stop her skin from itching. It was annoying, she said, to have to keep scratching her hands and arms.

"She's Not Going to Die from an Overdose of Ice Cream"

A few days after my visit, I heard from the home care nurse that Mrs. Fineman had been admitted to the hospital with biliary obstruction caused by her growing tumors. John Brant, her surgeon, inserted a biliary tube to help relieve the obstruction. Although she now had a tube draining through her abdominal wall, Mrs. Fineman didn't seem at all concerned about this procedure. Another of the palliative care physicians, Mary Thompson, recalled that Mrs. Fineman's major concern at this time was being able to get her hair washed. "It has been three days and they haven't washed my hair," she told the nurse and Mary. Later, the nurses washed her hair.

Once the tube was inserted, Mrs. Fineman went back home. When Anita, the palliative home care nurse, came to see her, Mrs. Fineman's major concerns were "to get something for my diarrhea," and "to get some foods that I'll feel like eating so I can put some weight on." She also wanted Anita to see if she could obtain some more comfortable undergarments to take care of her itchiness and skin rash. Anita suggested some special underwear from a medical and nursing supplies store and arranged for these to be delivered directly to Mrs. Fineman's home. Dr. Webster also continued to make home visits. She would always allow time for Mrs. Fineman to talk at length about how she was feeling and any concerns she might have. But Mrs. Fineman wanted only to discuss practical nursing issues, such as making sure her biliary tube was draining properly and getting medicine for pain.

Rachel worried whether her mother was eating enough or whether she was taking enough vitamins. She worried about the quality of the food her mother ate. "She doesn't get enough protein in her diet, and she shouldn't really be eating so much dairy foods," Rachel said to me.

"I shouldn't really eat so much ice cream," Mrs. Fineman said on one of my visits. "Rachel says it's not very good for my digestion. It never was. I always loved ice cream, but it didn't love me!"

Sometimes Rachel would call Henry to share her worries. This irritated him. These were such small things! If their mother liked ice cream, and wanted to take a chance and try to eat some, why shouldn't she? He explained to me:

> Sometimes [Rachel] will call me with the smallest things and she'll worry about some food that Mother is having—maybe too much sugar. So what? Let her do whatever makes her happy. I say, "Why are you worrying about things? She's not going to die from an overdose of ice cream. Let her do what she wants."

The Tube

Biliary tubes are shaped something like a letter T. One end of the cross of the T passes into the liver and the other end passes into the patient's duodenum. Routinely, it is necessary to clamp the external part of the tube, the long stem of the T that protrudes out onto the patient's abdomen. Clamping the tube ensures that the internal part of the tube is draining. Health professionals with surgical training have detailed knowledge of the various ways a biliary tube drains and have little difficulty with its management, which is a common practice for them. But for people who are not specially trained in surgical techniques, management of a biliary tube can be daunting. Mrs. Fineman's biliary tube needed care daily, perhaps even hourly. It would have been easy to manage her care if she were in the hospital or on the Palliative Care Unit (PCU). But Mrs. Fineman and her family felt that staying at home was best.

The community agency nurses visited Mrs. Fineman twice a week, and Anita, the palliative care nurse, visited once a week, sometimes once every two weeks. But management of the drainage tube nonetheless posed a real challenge for the nurses and the family. As Anita put it, the tube drainage could be a "messy business" when the biliary fluid leaked out onto Mrs. Fineman's abdomen. Not everyone felt comfortable handling a tube that seemed simply to protrude from a gap in the patient's stomach. Often the biliary fluid would drain copiously and soak the dressings around the drainage tube, and sometimes Mrs. Fineman felt pain at the site of the tube insertion. Or the tube would appear to be loosening and seem to slip. Rachel would get worried and wonder if she was doing something wrong when she changed the dressings around the tube. Henry would then telephone Dr. Brant or Anita. On one of these occasions, Mrs. Fineman was readmitted to the surgical unit to have Dr. Brant reinsert the tube. Once Mrs. Fineman was back at home, the tube drained effectively into a large plastic bag taped to her abdomen, but then the stitches at the site of the tube insertion gave way. The copious amounts of biliary drainage may have weakened the suturing. Dr. Brant resutured the area, and, for a while, the tube seemed to work satisfactorily again, but despite his efforts, it worked only sporadically from then on. The spread of the tumor was the principal cause of the problem.

These events were frustrating and somewhat of an ordeal for the nurses, doctors, and the Fineman family. Mrs. Fineman began to complain of pain in the area where the tube had been inserted and in her back. Dr. Brant had prescribed oxycodone and acetaminophen, but it didn't seem to work. Rachel didn't know what to do. Mrs. Fineman was frightened and called Henry.

Henry tried to leave most of the day-to-day caregiving to Rachel, since she was the one who was at home with their mother. Rachel oversaw the medication regime, the tube drainage, the meals, and the general duties of the household. But if things didn't go smoothly, Rachel became upset and nervous, and both she and her mother wanted Henry to intervene. Now was such a time.

Henry decided to take his mother directly to the hospital's emergency department, where Mrs. Fineman was examined by Dr. Marc Boileau, the on-call palliative care physician. He prescribed morphine, which was immediately effective. He gave Mrs. Fineman a prescription for morphine to be taken every four hours.

"I'm Looking Forward to Going to the Casino"

On one of my visits to her home, Mrs. Fineman greeted me at the top of the three flights of stairs to her apartment. It was a long climb. She called out laughingly, "I came up those stairs myself the other day. You have to take them slowly!"

It was extraordinary to me that although Mrs. Fineman looked ill and frail, most of our conversation was completely unrelated to any of the symptoms of her illness. She would talk about her illness, but only when prompted. She told me she knew she had had a tumor four years before and that the tumor had been removed. "I felt fine after that," she explained. "Now I have another small tumor."

On this particular day she was busy sewing extra straps onto a pair of pants so that they would be easier to manage when she had to use the toilet. She wanted to wear the pants when she went out to play cards and Mah Jong at the seniors' center, which she was planning to do the following week. But it was not only games at the senior' center that interested Mrs. Fineman. "I'm looking forward to going to the casino," she told me. "I'm going this summer with my son Henry." She also loved horse racing. "I don't have much money." she said, "but I like to put a bit of money on the horses, and when you win you've had a bit of fun." Sometimes it was frustrating for her to have to wait for Henry or Rachel. "They don't want me to go out alone," Mrs. Fineman said, "but I like to be independent."

As I looked at Mrs. Fineman, it was hard to visualize such a tiny, frail, underweight woman doing any of these things. Six months earlier her doctors had suggested that she might have only a few weeks to live. She looked to me as though she were dying.

"Do you know where I can buy something that is waterproof other than plastic underpants?" she asked me. She was having some problems with diarrhea. "I know that the nurses can get me some plastic underpants, but I need to go to a store where I can find another kind." When I suggested that she speak with Anita, she responded, "Oh, well, if I can just find out the store where they sell them, I can go on the bus, or, if not, my son will take me."

Rachel and Anita

Rachel described herself to me as a "nervous person" even in "normal times." It had been difficult after her mother was first diagnosed to get used to the idea that she was so ill. All her life she had lived with her mother. She had never left home, and they were very close. She couldn't imagine life alone. She did have a man friend at one point, but she had ended the relationship because it had meant traveling 60 miles or so out of town to his home. She just didn't see how she could keep it up after her mother became ill. In any case, the relationship hadn't been that important. "I know I'm 54 years old," Rachel told me, "but I like living at home with my mother. I've never wanted to marry and be on my own. We're a good team. She has her opinions about things, and I have mine. But we get along just great."

Rachel continued with her full-time job even after her mother became seriously ill. The job was demanding. Sometimes she had to stay late at the office until six or seven o'clock in the evening. She would then come home to prepare meals and do the housework. There was no doubt that Rachel got tired and "worn out." But having her mother at home and living for a bit longer was worth it, Rachel said. She continued:

> I really want to stress that I feel privileged to have this extra time with my mother. It's a gift. She carries on and I feel we've been given a reprieve so many times. My brother and myself, we're amazed that she carries on. We've thought so many times over the months and now years that she was going to die. I want to take advantage of the fact that we have the extra time.

Rachel said she could manage her mother at home as long as she could have some nursing help, such as with the biliary tube. The procedure of clamping the tube for periods of time according to the community nurse's instructions made her feel very nervous. Henry would call or send a fax to Anita and ask if there couldn't be more intense and frequent home nursing care. But full-time nursing care at home was expensive and difficult to find. Of course, there was always the option of being admitted to the PCU. But Henry and Rachel felt that Mrs. Fineman was far from ready to go to a place for dying people, no matter how kind the people were. Henry wanted more skilled nursing help to support the care that Rachel was giving.

In many ways, the biliary tube constituted an active form of treatment. To care for the tube was really the job of the community agency nurses. "It's difficult," the palliative care nurse Anita said to me. "Mr. Fineman [Henry] will ask for a faster intervention when things don't go well. He will send a fax or telephone anyone and everyone—myself, Dr. Brant, Dr. Webster—and ask for faster service. I don't really blame him—he's wanting to get the best care for his mother—but we are constantly working between an active role and a palliative care role."

Mrs. Fineman might be terminally ill, Anita continued, but, at the moment, she was being cared for as if she were not. Anita was accustomed to nursing people at home who were dying and who, along with their family, were trying to come to terms with the process of dying. Sometimes, Anita said, she felt guilty about making these distinctions. She explained,

> I realize that this is a very sick patient, and I shouldn't feel this way, because she is an old lady who is going to die. She's got a huge tumor. She's got this big bag hanging down strapped to her abdomen and all these horrible symptoms—pain, diarrhea. . . . My life is great compared to hers. But when I go there, somehow it is not for palliative care. Somehow, I am second in line to the community agency nurse, and that's how the family sees me.

It was hard to nurse someone who was so ill and who would ultimately die from their illness and not be able to deal with them on that level, Anita said. Perhaps it would be possible to talk openly about some of these issues when Mrs. Fineman came to the point where she would need to be admitted to the PCU.

But the Fineman family did not plan to encourage Mrs. Fineman to be admitted to the hospital unless it became absolutely necessary. From what Henry had seen of the PCU, "it was immensely impressive." He would certainly encourage his mother to go, if and when the time came. In the meantime, he wanted time to try and cope with her illness in his own mind. He said, "I guess for the next little while, my sense is that I have to try and cope with this myself, to face reality."

For her part, Rachel hoped that her mother would never have to go to the PCU—that she would always be able to care for her at home. She was encouraging her mother to embrace life and do as much as she could. Sadie Fineman was a strong-minded, determined woman, she said. This was the way she wanted to manage things. She wasn't thinking about dying. She was busy with her life, and, ill as she was, she still did her share of the household chores. "She's thin and ill, yes," Rachel continued, "and maybe she's even dying. And she just keeps walking around, regardless of that. Just yesterday, she cleaned out the fridge—cleaned it all out—and I had told her I would do that. But when I came home from work, there she was, stooping down like the little skeleton that she is, and she'd cleaned it out."

"Cancer Was Cancer"

By July, Mrs. Fineman's abdomen seemed much more extended, as she was developing ascites. When Dr. Webster made a home visit Mrs. Fineman told Gillian that she and Rachel were managing quite nicely. Her pain was reduced by the morphine, and her diarrhea was being controlled. Although the biliary tube could be "troublesome sometimes," Mrs. Fineman didn't see the need for any specific medical intervention. She did worry, however, about the expansion of the abdomen. "But, well, what could you do?" she said; that was the way it was.

Gillian wondered: Was Mrs. Fineman not pursuing questions about her enlarged abdomen because of what she might hear? Was there a part of her that knew she had cancer? It was hard to tell whether Mrs. Fineman was anxious not to know how ill she really was, or if she was simply too busy getting on with her life to worry about it.

Anita was also concerned about what she described to me as the family's "general avoidance," especially their absolute refusal to utter the word "cancer." She worried that perhaps the Fineman family was in some kind of denial and that when the truth did come, it would be hard to take. And it would come, no matter how determined Mrs. Fineman was to carry on. After all, Anita said, "cancer was cancer."

Yet Rachel kept reminding the team that her mother had always been aware of her "growing tumor." Maybe the family had not used the word "cancer," Rachel said, but she knows how ill she is. It had just never been her mother's way to talk about defeat. Even if she was going to die, Rachel went on, "she'll keep doing it for herself until she drops. She knows she's sick, but if she can do it, she will. She gets up, makes her food, takes her medications, and as long as she can walk and move her hands, she'll do it."

One day in early October, Dr. Webster made another home visit. Mrs. Fineman mentioned that she still liked to go out once or twice a week. "Every day I try to just get out of the door for a breath of fresh air." she said. Then she commented, "I'm losing more and more weight. I've stopped weighing myself now." She paused briefly. "There's no point." Gillian listened very attentively now. Was Mrs. Fineman ready to speak more openly? She had lost 60 pounds by this time and had begun to ask what it would be like to get more and more pain. She was feeling sharp shooting pains in the upper part of her neck. Gillian thought this might be related to the cancer or to degenerative disc disease. She decided not to mention the possibility of a neck tumor, since there was no firm medical evidence to support this. However, it now seemed possible to talk more openly. She reassured Mrs. Fineman that many people, even those with her kind of tumor, manage to avoid increasing pain and that, in any event, the team would be able to control it.

Before Gillian left that day Mrs. Fineman told her, "My telephone never stops ringing. My friends call me a lot with their stories." She loved a good bit of gossip, she said. She had plans to go to the casino and the horse races "when the weather gets better." And there was a family wedding coming up next year. "I might go to that," she said.

A Blood Transfusion

One Saturday evening in mid-December, Rachel telephoned Richard Stevens, the palliative care physician on call, to say that her mother had fallen. The day before, Mrs. Fineman had gone out for pancakes with a friend but had started to feel dizzy. Now she had fallen and injured her eye and may have broken her left arm. Dr. Stevens suggested that Mrs. Fineman come to the PCU for immediate care and for reassessment of her overall condition. When Mrs. Fineman arrived, she said the room was comfortable enough, but she would not be staying long. "No use getting more things from home." she said. "My son and daughter would only have to carry everything back home when I go."

Blood tests revealed that Mrs. Fineman had a hemoglobin of 48. This explained why she had felt dizzy and fell over. She had probably suffered from an internal gastrointestinal bleed; it was very possible that she was still bleeding. Dr. Webster decided to offer Mrs. Fineman a blood transfusion, which is not a routine practice in palliative care. On this particular palliative care service, patients receive a blood transfusion only if it will help them be strong enough to get out of bed and walk around. In Sadie Fineman's case, her physicians believed that a transfusion would allow her to go home again, if only for a short while. Mrs. Fineman certainly expected to be allowed to go home. She was still busy living life!

Giving the transfusion was not easy. It was hard to find a good vein that would sustain a few hours of intravenous therapy. Marc Boileau tried to insert a small butterfly needle into the larger vein of her left arm, but this did not work. The nurses began to wrap Mrs. Fineman's arms in warm towels for several minutes at a time. Mrs. Fineman did not mind. The doctors could "poke" her all they wanted. What was important was to "get some blood inside her" so she could get back home. The fall had been "such a nuisance."

Mrs. Fineman received her transfusion. I visited her just a few hours afterward. The room seemed less cozy and inviting now, the atmosphere feeling clinical, sterile, somber. The easy chairs that normally surround the patient's bed on the unit were pushed aside to allow the nurses easier access to their patient. As I stood near, the nurses came in, looking efficient in their white uniforms, purposefully checking the flow of the intravenous tube. Mrs. Fineman looked tiny in the bed, her pale, frail form propped up by pillows in the semi-darkness. The lights in the room had been dimmed so that there was just enough to see her face and see a wristwatch to check her pulse. She gave me a big smile and leaned forward to squeeze my hand with her "good arm," as she put it. I stared at her in amazement as she called out laughingly, "You see! I've pulled through again. I'll be home by the weekend!"

But Sadie Fineman did not go home again. As the days passed, she got visibly weaker, despite the blood transfusions and the intravenous fluids that she received for improved hydration. She was not getting better, and now she spoke as if she realized this herself.

"I'm Not Up to It Anymore"

"Don't send me home for good behavior," she laughingly told one of the staff physicians. Even though she was feeling better, she said, "I'm weak and I can't take care of myself. Besides, I like it here." This was a change. Despite the continuing flashes of humor, Mrs. Fineman was showing many signs that she was aware of how sick she was. She began to talk openly about things that were on her mind in relation to her life and unfinished business. Her children had been good to her, she told me. She felt very proud of them both. She told Rachel that no daughter could have been better to her.

She was worried about Rachel. "She doesn't realize I'm so sick," she told me. She had to try to prepare Rachel for the worst. She wouldn't be able to live forever. Rachel would have to take care of things from now on. Before, during all these months, she had recovered very well. She had been busy with her life. But now, "I'm suffering from things I didn't have before," she said. Rachel would have to manage on her own. "I'm not up to it anymore," she said. But how would Rachel manage? Mrs. Fineman explained:

You see, I'm all she's got. She never married, she always relied on me. My daughter has a job, but she's not a young woman. She's at an age now where she's too old to get a job and too young to get a pension. If I'd been a wealthy woman . . . she would have no worries.

Mrs. Fineman's expressions of concern for Rachel seemed to illustrate the subtle, delicate ways people have of moving in and out of awareness of their impending death. For months the team and I had wondered whether Mrs. Fineman had been in denial. Had she been? Could it be so simple or black and white—then she was in denial, now she is not?

The nurses were also concerned about Rachel. Anita recalled how difficult it had been to approach the subject of her mother's dying with her, even though Rachel and Henry had always spoken as if it were their mother who was afraid of the topic. "When I tried to discuss her mother's possible death," Anita said, "you could see the tears and the anxiety come into her eyes. And it was like she was asking me, 'Please don't say that. Please don't talk.' So, I did little at the time. Because if you confront it too much, or if you say or do too much, ironically, you may lose the relationship and the trust that you have built."

As the time of her death approached, it was Sadie Fineman who confronted this reality with her daughter. She began to talk about the household business that needed attention. There were bills to be paid. Rachel would need to fill in certain forms to cancel her pension money. "I don't want you to go to pieces over this," she told Rachel. "But you must take care of things." Then she added, "Don't pay the gas bill—there is a credit coming!"

To me, Mrs. Fineman said that she was prepared. "I know when I am so sick that I won't make it," she said. "I won't recover now. I know it. Who lives forever, anyway?" She continued, "The time has come. And I'm ready for it. I've lived my life span. I'm 80 years old. And that's a long time. There'll never be a time when I'll go and my children don't need me. But I'm not leaving babies."

Now, four weeks after she had been admitted to the PCU, Sadie Fineman began to talk less and sleep a lot more. She had more pain, experiencing it "like something I never had before," she said. She began to have difficulty breathing, so the nurses gave her oxygen. She received morphine for pain. I could no longer have a conversation with her. "She sleeps most of the time now," her nurse Ena said. "She is dying." Rachel now visited more often. She would sit for long hours beside her mother's bed. She looked calm, and

I thought that she and her mother must have been able to talk about some of the things, at least, that they had wanted to talk about. On one of my visits when I found Mrs. Fineman sleeping, she looked gray and listless, yet peaceful. The nurses went in and out of the room to bathe her and turn her gently, talking in soft whispers.

One day in early January, Sadie Fineman stopped breathing. Ena and Barbara, another nurse, were with her. She looked happy and peaceful, Ena said. Henry arrived 15 minutes later. "I would like to have been with her," he said to me. "But she had been preparing us for the inevitable." Then he said, "My mother was in control right up to the end. She was with it. She was open and she knew what was happening. She wanted us to know it, too. And when she felt convinced that we were prepared for it, she gave in."

Authors' Comments

As we describe in the General Introduction, the years since we carried out our research have witnessed great emphasis on the importance of advance care planning near the end of life (e.g., the patient's wishes regarding resuscitation, medical representation, and financial planning, as well as any other forms of treatment that may be offered). We also noted that while Canadians feel advance care planning is important, a large majority do not regularly have this kind of discussion with their doctor. The attitudes of Henry and Rachel regarding communication with their mother suggests one reason why this may be so. They implored Dr. Levitan not to tell their mother how ill she was. Henry argued that his mother was "already eighty years old, had taken care of her own affairs and she had already done all she wanted in her life." ' Besides, Henry said, "What if her affairs are left in a mess?" Indeed, Henry decided not to use the word "cancer" in any of his discussions because he thought it was too frightening. He believed that if his mother were "told the truth," she would lose hope for any future life. Henry thought it "stupid" to let his mother know she had no future to look forward to.

Since 1995, North American palliative care literature increasingly argues in support of truthful disclosure of the diagnosis and prognostic outlook. However, in many countries outside North America, a different position prevails. This latter position asserts that "the truth" runs the risk of interfering with the patient's coping strategies as determined by his or her personality and cultural background and as understood by the patient's family. As we witnessed in this case, these contrasting viewpoints may present a dilemma for the care provider. There seems to be a conflict between our obligation to be truthful with patients and our obligation to avoid causing them harm. The obligation to be truthful—including being explicit about a patient's diagnosis and prognosis—is usually justified as respect for the patient's autonomy. But perhaps it is *more* respectful of a patient's autonomy first to inquire what sort of information about their illness they desire. This underscores the importance of skilled attentiveness to verbal and nonverbal communication. One possible approach is to say to the patient at the beginning of the relationship, "some people like to know all the details of their illness and plans for care; other people prefer only to get the big picture and don't want to get into any details. They might even want us to discuss these things with someone else in the family. What kind of person are you?" The bioethicist Benjamin Freedman described this approach as "offering truth," as opposed to unilaterally imposing truth.[1]

As family caregivers, both Henry and Rachel tried to care for their mother within their respective sibling roles. Of note is the apparent gendered division of labor whereby Rachel provided the practical everyday nursing care, while Henry made the decisions as to how things should proceed, such as the kind of information that should be communicated to his mother or whether or not she should be encouraged to continue her everyday activities. Sadie Fineman belonged to a generation when gendered division of labor was the norm. We might also consider that Sadie had her own expectations for her two children, and the roles they had undertaken may have been present from an early age.

Family caregiving has been described as "the backbone of our healthcare system saving millions of healthcare dollars."[2] As we have witnessed in other narratives, there is a need for home care support beyond what Rachel was able to give at that time. Rachel was torn between her own exhaustion and the feeling that "having her mother at home and living for a bit longer was worth it." Although a sense of competence is valued by caregivers, there are many health risks associated with the burden of caregiving which may result in poor outcomes.[3] Stresses on the caregiver's health may be due to the need to take time off work, financial strain, and out-of-pocket expenses, as well by the physical and emotional demands of providing care at the end of their family member's life.[4]

In May 2015, the government of Canada increased financial benefits for caregivers of family members suffering from an illness at the end of life who needed to take time off from work. Effective January 2016, Compassionate Care benefits allowed for claims for up to 26 weeks, which was an increase from the previous 6 weeks.[5] In September 2020, due to the COVID-19 pandemic, these benefits were extended to allow for claims for up to 52 weeks. Despite legislative initiatives to financially assist caregivers who need to take time away from work to care for a terminally ill relative, there are few opportunities for financial support for family caregivers who do not work or who are not actively pursuing work outside the home.

References

1. Freedman B. Offering truth: One ethical approach to the uninformed cancer patient. Arch Intern Med 1993;153(5):572–576.
2. Williams A. Education, training and mentorship of caregivers of Canadians experiencing a life limiting illness. J Palliat Med. 2018;21(S1):S45–S49.
3. Alam S, Hannon B, Zimmermann C. Palliative care for family caregivers. J Clin Oncol. 2020;38(9):926–936.
4. Williams AM, Wang L, Kitchen P. Differential impacts of care-giving across three care-giver groups in Canada: End-of-life care, long-term care and short-term care. Health Soc Care Community. 2014;22(2):187–196.
5. Government of Canada Employment and Social Developments. Catalogue number Em20-135/2019E-PDF. ISBN 9780660318370. Page numbers 1–12.

13

Stanley Gray

"Like Lazarus, He Came Back from the Dead"

Narrated by Yanna Lambrinidou

When Stanley Gray was admitted to the home care program of hospice, he appeared to be dying from congestive heart failure (CHF) and end-stage chronic obstructive pulmonary disease (COPD). To everyone's surprise, his condition improved. Although dependent on oxygen, morphine, and eight bronchodilator treatments a day, Mr. Gray started to lead a relatively independent and deeply religious life. A year and a half after his admission to hospice, his social worker believed he was no longer "terminal." His nurse, on the other hand, argued that although he was functional, he could die at any time. Mr. Gray was the only patient in our study who was still alive when we completed the writing of this book. His case demonstrates the unpredictability of diseases like CHF and COPD and the challenge they present to the current system of hospice care in the United States. It unfolds on the borderland between palliative and long-term care, even as it illustrates the immense personal and relational transformations that can take place near the end of life. It is also a portrait of a certain type of religious faith. Though Mr. Gray's consuming relationship with God made some members of his hospice team uncomfortable, and the nurse and chaplain even suspected that it compromised his health, Mr. Gray was convinced that it was God who had caused him to outlive his terminal prognosis.

"He Is Dying, He Has No Lungs Left, Nothing!"

Even for South Carolina, the first week of May 1996 was unusually muggy. Stanley Gray, a 57-year-old White American man with congestive heart failure (CHF) and chronic obstructive pulmonary disease (COPD), confined himself to his small Charleston apartment—he couldn't imagine surviving outdoors without his rickety air conditioner. Cool temperature was a necessity, just like his oxygen tank and bronchodilator treatments. A short time into the heat wave, the air conditioner broke. Mr. Gray sat quietly in his bedroom and concentrated on his breathing. He could feel the heat creeping into his apartment like a noxious gas. He could also feel the stiff resistance of his lungs. Two days later, his skin looked blue. Gasping for breath, he drove himself to the hospital. It was his third admission in five months.

Mr. Gray was placed in the intensive care unit right away. He was given intravenous steroids, a bronchodilator, and two antibiotics. But he continued to deteriorate. His oxygen saturation level dropped, and he got confused and combative. He didn't want to die. The thought that God had not forgiven him tormented him. The hospital called his only sibling, Mrs. Florence Laxton, to tell her that her brother's health was rapidly declining. Mrs. Laxton, a 53-year-old packaging company worker, lived in Lancaster County, Pennsylvania. She took the next plane to Charleston.

Mrs. Laxton found her brother unresponsive. She noticed that he was not getting any nutritional support. Didn't Stanley need food to survive? His physician answered impatiently that he was in no position to eat. "He is dying, he has no lungs left, nothing!" he exclaimed. Upset but undeterred, Mrs. Laxton began giving her brother small amounts of juice, then spoonfuls of ice cream and pudding. Mr. Gray responded well, but remained somnolent. After a week, Mrs. Laxton began to lose hope. Although she wasn't pious, she remembered vividly leaving her brother's room to pray. She recalled telling God that she knew she didn't have the power to cure Mr. Gray and that she realized his health was in his hands. If he wanted to take him, she was ready to let him go. But she hoped that he would cure him.

The next morning, Mr. Gray opened his eyes. Although extremely weak, he recognized his sister for the first time since her arrival. His physician told him that he had two choices: he could die in the hospital or receive hospice services at home. Mrs. Laxton wanted to take her brother back to Lancaster County. The physician argued that a long trip in Mr. Gray's condition was entirely inappropriate. Mrs. Laxton retorted that if her brother had only a short time to live, he would be happier with family in Pennsylvania than without family in South Carolina. Though he could only utter a few words, Mr. Gray seemed to agree. He accepted the idea of hospice, gave Mrs. Laxton the responsibility of signing a do-not-resuscitate order on his behalf, and said he was prepared to risk the flight to Pennsylvania by air ambulance. The hospital made arrangements with the Hospice of Lancaster County to equip Mrs. Laxton's house with oxygen tanks and a hospital bed.

In Lancaster, an ambulance met the two siblings at the airport and transferred them to Mrs. Laxton's house. Mr. Gray was unconscious. Hospice staff informed Mrs. Laxton that her brother was actively dying. To help him through his final moments, they put in place a continuous home care team.

"Bless the Lord"

I met Mr. Gray at his sister's farmhouse 15 months later, on a warm August day of 1997. He was sitting in the living room, with shorts and an unbuttoned shirt. He was a strapping man with expressive blue eyes, a full head of graying brown hair, and bushy eyebrows. His arm bore a tattoo that said, "Born to Lose." An oxygen cannula was blowing air into his nose. His walker, with two oxygen tanks hanging on its sides, was standing directly in front of him. Mrs. Laxton, a rotund woman with big blue eyes and rosy cheeks, smiled sweetly as she asked me what I wanted to drink. Tiffany Hadley, Mr. Gray's vivacious hospice nurse, had arrived only a few minutes before me and was already sitting comfortably on the living room couch with a cup of coffee. I asked for iced tea. On her way back from the kitchen, Mrs. Laxton instructed her three barking Irish Setters to quiet down and sat in an armchair across from her brother.

Mr. Gray looked drowsy. He told Tiffany that he felt sluggish—he was having a bad day. With embarrassment, he confessed that the previous night he had smoked two packs of cigarettes. He saw smoking as a careless act that destroyed the human body and insulted God. The thought that he had consciously compromised his health when God had given him a second chance at life had tortured him all night. Still, he was eager to talk. Tiffany encouraged him to give me a short version of the story about his reunification with Mrs. Laxton. It was a story he loved to tell.

Mr. Gray was born and raised in Lancaster County, he recounted. From the age of 9 to 12, he was confined to bed with rheumatic fever. His only stimulation was a small, battery-operated radio and his daydreams. In his fantasy world, he and Superman were the strongest people on earth. But when he finally recovered and was able to return to school, he realized that he wasn't strong at all. Because he had missed three years of classes, he was set back to third grade. Older and taller than his classmates, he was teased ruthlessly. So he quit school, and, when he turned 17, he joined the Army.

In 1969, following the death of his father, the end of his third marriage, and a jail sentence, Mr. Gray moved to Georgia. For 16 years he kept no contact with his relatives. Then, homesick, he made an appearance at his sister's farm. Mrs. Laxton, her husband, and their two children were very happy to see him. But when Mrs. Laxton broke the news to him that their mother had passed away a few years earlier, he was shocked. He left without telling anyone where he was going.

In December 1995, his housemate in Charleston tried to convince him to send Mrs. Laxton a Christmas card. Mr. Gray resisted. "I have been a black sheep in this family," he argued. "I have been kind of dragging the name through the dirt pretty bad." It had been 10 years since his last visit with his sister, and 27 years since he had seen his own daughter, Cynthia. "So this is how I got separated from my family," Mr. Gray said to me, "through embarrassment."

His housemate insisted that he at least send his sister a card. And he did. Around 6:00 P.M. on New Year's Day 1996, his life took a new turn. "I had a phone in my room," he recounted, "and I was lying down sleeping, and the telephone rings. I picked up the phone, and this woman's voice says, 'I am not sure if I've got the right number, but I am looking for Stanley Gray.' I am laying there and thinking that I've got a few bills down there; I figured it was just the bill collector. I said, 'Well, you've got him. This is Stanley Gray.' And right away she said—I can't remember her exact words—but I think she said, 'Oh my Lord! This is Flo!' " Mrs. Laxton had traced her brother's telephone number from the return address on the envelope. She did not know that her brother was suffering from emphysema.

"I am going to cry," Mrs. Laxton interjected as she listened to Mr. Gray tell the story. "Yeah, right," Mr. Gray said, "I got a knot in my throat, too." And he continued, "When she said that, my whole world just lit right up. What a New Year's! I knew then that God was with us." "Bless the Lord," he interjected again and again as he told me his story. He asserted that God had healed him to give him the opportunity to repair the wrongs he had committed. "I get sick just thinking about my life," he said. He stressed that he had spent most of his adult years in disgrace.

Mr. Gray had talked for half an hour. Toward the end of his story, he struggled to catch his breath. He pursed his lips and leaned forward, resting his elbows on his knees, clearly struggling to inhale. He clasped his oxygen mask to his face, but it didn't seem to help. His sister offered him a glass of water to keep his mouth from drying out. Tiffany encouraged him to make use of his short-acting morphine to ease his breathing. She also advised him to take a nap. I thanked him for allowing me to visit and arranged to return soon.

"I Just Wish All the Patients of Hospice Could Feel as Good as I Feel"

The next time I saw Mr. Gray, he was sitting alone at the kitchen table reading the Bible. Mrs. Laxton was at the doctor. She had injured her back at work and had been placed on temporary disability. At the time, I didn't realize how unusual Mrs. Laxton's absence was. Because of her own health problems and her protectiveness toward her brother, she spent much of the time at home. Most of my interviews with Mr. Gray were three-way conversations. When Mr. Gray ran out of breath, Mrs. Laxton spoke for him. And when he regained his strength, he elaborated on her statements. Mrs. Laxton, he explained to me, had done everything for him. Although she struggled financially herself, she had not hesitated to pay the $3,500 fee for the air ambulance that brought him back to Lancaster County. And, for over a year, she had devoted her entire life to his well-being. "I feel like Flo is my wife, not my sister," he said tearfully. Then he chuckled, recalling the day when a server at a restaurant assumed that he and Mrs. Laxton were a couple. "We need to start going out separately," he said. "Flo ruins the possibility of me ever getting a date!"

Mr. Gray looked strong on this second visit. "I just wish all the patients of hospice could feel as good as I feel," he said, and thanked the Lord. He quickly added that although he had accepted God into his life only in the previous 20 months, God had always been there for him. That was a point he wanted to make sure I understood and a message he wanted to communicate clearly to the readers of his story. Remembering his childhood, he described the time when he got run over by a tractor at the age of five or six:

I was in just such a position that the tractor ran over my body, the wheel ran across my body and ran across my belly—it did not run over my chest now. The wheel of the tractor ran across me and the two wheels on the trailer ran across me with a loaded trailer and the ground was just soft enough, I guess, the imprint of my body was being pushed down into the ground just enough that the full weight of the tractor never—

He stopped to catch his breath. He closed his eyes, pursed his lips, and concentrated on his breathing. A few minutes later he continued,

Praise God. Now this is God again. This is the Lord, which at that time I did not even realize. But with God and His angels—and I say this with a lump in my throat now—but the Lord sure got me out of that because the tractor and trailer ran over me.

God had saved him many times, Mr. Gray asserted. The rheumatic fever, which had given him three heart attacks before the age of 12, had left him with only a mild heart murmur. And now, 44 years later, God had gifted him hospice. His only criticism he directed at himself. "I know that I still do things that are not of the righteous man," he said. "I have not given myself fully to the Lord. I want to. I tell myself I want to, and yet I realize by my actions that I have not totally made that commitment to Him. I am still smoking cigarettes from time to time, even when I don't terribly have a bad craving, and I know I can do better."

Hellfire and Brimstone

Mr. Gray's medication regimen consisted of steroids, a bronchodilator, a tranquilizer, and short-acting morphine. He received regular hospice visits from his nurse, personal care nurse, chaplain, and social worker. The social worker, Thelma Barron, referred to his recovery as a miracle. "Like Lazarus," she said laughingly, "he came back from the dead." Thelma had come to see Mr. Gray's illness as more of a chronic than a terminal condition. Any specific prognosis, she asserted, would likely be grossly inaccurate.

"Stanley was supposed to have died a couple of times now, and he has just bounced back," Tiffany, the nurse, concurred. But she worried that Mr. Gray's religious beliefs were detrimental to his health. Because he feared eternal punishment, she argued, he was anxious. So his two main symptoms fed each other—his anxiety exacerbated his respiratory distress, which in turn increased his anxiety.

Hospice chaplain Carl Flynn agreed. A friendly and unassuming man in his forties, he told me that Mr. Gray operated out of a conservative, evangelical paradigm. His religiosity, according to Carl, was rooted more in fear than in love for God. "I am sure he came out of a hellfire-and-brimstone kind of upbringing," Carl said. He found Mr. Gray to be extraordinarily self-critical and attributed this not only to his background but also to the teachings of Pastor Lowel, a Southern evangelical minister Mr. Gray had recently started to watch on TV. In Carl's opinion, this show had given Mr. Gray the impression that there was only one way to understand God—through the Bible. Carl, a practitioner of a theological movement that views reality as a process of growth and change with infinite possibilities, found himself offering Mr. Gray counterpoints to what he viewed as the absolutist statements of the television preacher.

As a chaplain, Carl wanted to loosen the tightness he perceived in Mr. Gray's religious life. He was committed to trying to show Mr. Gray that Bible study could be enriched with actions that breathed life into his relationship with God. He believed that Mr. Gray would benefit from a nurturing connection with the divine that transcended Scripture. On one late August day, when Mr. Gray accused himself again of having sinned because he smoked a cigarette, Carl devised an exercise. He sought Mr. Gray's permission "to invite Jesus into his home." Reluctantly, Mr. Gray agreed. Carl, acting as if he could see Jesus, asked him to sit at the head of the kitchen table. He then instructed Mr. Gray to share his worries with his guest. Mr. Gray started talking, but he faced Carl instead of the empty seat. Carl redirected him to Jesus. Nervously, Mr. Gray turned his gaze sideways. When he finished talking, Carl invited him to a few minutes of silence. It was time, he said, to see if God had a response. Mr. Gray sat quietly but didn't sense any divine message.

Carl did. "I got that Jesus loves you very much," he told Mr. Gray. "That you are His own child and in fact your name is written in the palms of His Hands." Extending his own palms toward Mr. Gray, he asked him to place his worries in them. He would, in turn, offer them to Jesus. "Jesus," said Mr. Gray as he positioned his hands over Carl's, "I am placing my struggles, my concern about smoking, in your hands, and I know that when I am tempted or when I am bothered by this, I will know it is in your hands, and I don't have to worry about it anymore." As if he had taken hold of Mr. Gray's concerns,

Carl turned to the empty seat and gestured passing them gently on to Jesus. More silence. Carl chuckled. He got a mental image of Jesus holding a lit cigarette and laughing. "And I shared that with Stanley," he told me later. "I said, 'I don't know what it means, but I have a sense that Jesus is saying, 'I can hold this for you. It is no big deal.'"

Carl was happy with the exercise. He felt confident that he had helped Mr. Gray relinquish some control over his struggles and accept a force greater than himself to guide him to the righteous life that he desired. Mr. Gray felt differently. He told me later that he was less comfortable with the experience. He was relieved by the opportunity to unburden his worries, yet he saw his interaction with Jesus as a convenient but indecent way of abdicating his responsibilities. He argued that God expected His followers to take charge of their own lives. And he stopped smoking.

"Everything I Do in My Life Is Either Illegal or Immoral"

A month had passed since my first meeting with Mr. Gray, and I still didn't know what he meant when he referred to his "sinful" life in the South or what had prompted him to leave that life behind. When he made yet another reference to his sins, I asked him if he could elaborate. For a moment, he hedged. And then he told me that he had been an alcoholic. He had let prostitutes and drug dealers into his house. For years, he had felt bad about his lifestyle. But, one day, he decided to change. "I suddenly got to a place where I did not like who I was or what I was," he said. He told his friends that they were no longer allowed to carry out illicit activities under his roof. Most of them never visited again.

"What led you to that change, do you think?" I interjected.

"Although I was not thinking of it at the time that way," he replied, "I know it was the Lord. I knew that He had a purpose for me, and I truly believe that the Lord was actually touching me and trying to nudge me: 'This is not what I want for you, and you know this is not what you want.' And deep down inside, I believe it was my knowledge of the Lord and what was right and wrong."

"I have done everything in my life, short of kidnap or murder," he added. "I have stolen things that I knew were not mine. I have forged signatures on checks. I have been guilty of lying and cheating. I have been guilty of adultery. I suppose I have broken a lot of God's commandments." Glancing at

Mrs. Laxton, he suddenly paused. "While we are being taped," he said as he tried to take a few deep breaths, "I might as well tell my sister something, because I looked at her, and I don't know if she is thinking about this or not." Did she remember, he wondered, his engagement to a young woman 39 years earlier? At the time, he was stationed in a military base in the Southwest. Mrs. Laxton nodded, recalling the photograph he had mailed her of his fiancée. "That was in my imagination," Mr. Gray said apologetically. To elevate his status in the Army, he had lied about his personal life not only to his military commander but also to her. The woman in the photograph was a waitress he hardly knew. Eventually he was caught and court-martialed. "I used to say, 'Everything I do in my life is either illegal or immoral,'" he stated, "and most of the time it was both."

"I Don't Know How to Bring It Out—That It Is Okay for Him to Cry"

Although an enlarged photograph of Mr. Gray's daughter hung prominently on Mrs. Laxton's living room wall, Mr. Gray didn't talk about Cynthia often. His first marriage ended just about the time Cynthia was born, and his wife had insisted that he never see their child again. When Cynthia was little, he missed her so much that he waited on streets she frequented to catch glimpses of her from a distance. One time, he even sat in the house of her next-door neighbor hoping to see her return from school.

I met Cynthia in September 1997. She was 37. She lived in a Lancaster County apartment complex with her husband and one daughter from a previous marriage. Cynthia was a social worker. She worked in a nursing home. Her workdays were long. She looked exhausted. "It is kind of strange that I did not know my dad until a year and a half ago," she told me. "I knew who he was, I was given a name, and I was told he was my father. At one point—in fact I think twice—I had been told that he was already dead." Cynthia had spent her entire childhood wondering why her father had left her. "I wanted to know what was wrong with me," she said.

Sixteen months earlier, Cynthia recalled, she got a call from Mrs. Laxton's daughter, whom she had never met. Would Cynthia be open to meeting her father, her cousin asked. She was shocked. She felt defensive. "Dad can never get those 36 years back no matter what he does. They are gone," she thought to herself. "But," she told me, "there was no sense in holding a grudge and denying myself the chance to get to know the man who helped my being come into existence. So I said that I would talk to him, but he would have to call me." Mr. Gray called her a week later. He asked to see her before he died. "So I came to him with an open mind," Cynthia said, "and very honestly told him that there was no way he was going to make up for the last 36 years, so do not bother trying and let's start from here."

In the previous year and a half, Cynthia had visited her father weekly. "Sometimes we seem like polite strangers," she remarked. "I get the feeling that he does not trust himself or he is afraid that I am going to walk out if I learn too much." At the same time, her fear that her father did not love her had started to dissipate. Only weeks before I met her, she had found a letter that Mr. Gray had written to her mother. In it, he admitted that he was not fit for parenthood, confessed that he was in trouble with the law, expressed his love for baby Cynthia, and promised to stay away from his little girl until he became a better person. "That is an act of love," she asserted.

Upon reflection, Cynthia told me that she had come to love her father and admire him for his transformation. But she also felt sorry for him. She found him too alone. "Sometimes I think he hides his fear," she said. "He is so upbeat, and he watches what he says, and he tries to be so positive, and yet there are times I know he is having problems breathing. And he is taking morphine, and he is cramping, and his fingers are contracting, and it is like he will still put on that happy face, and he is like, 'It is fine.' And I don't know how to bring it out—that it is okay for him to cry." A tone of disappointment entered her voice. "Sometimes I feel like I am still on the outside, that they are protecting me. If I am going to be there for the good, I need to be there for the bad. And Dad is going to die. I am not afraid of death. But I am afraid of not being able to give to him."

"I Want to Get Deeper into the True Word of Christ"

As I continued my visits, I began to see what Carl meant when he told me that Mr. Gray's religiosity was rooted in fear. Mr. Gray struck me as so hard on himself that he left no room for missteps. His wrongs, in his view, had the capacity to bring him eternal damnation. "I want to learn God's word as it is meant to be," he asserted, "and I want to follow those who are more learned about it, such as a minister, who wants to teach it as it is supposed to be taught—as God wants it taught—verse by verse, book by book. Not trying to change it to suit man as he would like to have it."

One day Mr. Gray told me about a dream he had had in Charleston. He had been hesitant to share it because he wasn't sure he could relay it without distorting its divine message.

> I had a dream where I saw a vision of fire falling from the sky—just balls of fire coming out of the sky. The sky was all red, all around. People were running and screaming, fire falling on them, more or less like Armageddon, and out of all this fire a figure came through the fire or came out that was Christ or Christ Jesus. At least that is the way it looked to me. I immediately fell down and began to worship and say how much of a sinner I was, which was really the truth, begging for forgiveness.

Mr. Gray's initial interpretation was that Jesus had given him the opportunity to confess his sins and had finally granted him eternal life. But with the help of Pastor Lowel, he realized that the imposing figure was not Christ at all. Christ, he learned, would have immediately turned him into a spirit. The fact that this entity didn't transform him, but watched him beg for forgiveness, meant that he was the Antichrist. It was thanks to God, Mr. Gray went on, that he had come across Pastor Lowel, and it was thanks to Pastor Lowel that he had learned that one needs to know the Bible to be saved. "God was telling me," he said, 'Hey, you need to pay a little closer attention to my word.' I would have been truly lost. My salvation would have been just thrown right out the window, but knowing the difference now, I want to get deeper into the true word of Christ."

Mr. Gray's voice started to shake. "It is so important that people who are where I was at know that no matter how lost they think they are out there, whatever they have done, there is nothing that God won't forgive."

With pride, Mr. Gray announced that he had not smoked for three weeks. Tiffany was impressed, he reported with a smile. He had been able to cut down on his morphine, too, and, only a few days earlier, he had managed to go with Mrs. Laxton to the mall. "I used to pray for healing, yes," he said. "I thought how nice it would be to be completely healed. But under the circumstances I don't pray that way anymore. Each year that I have got this disease, I am supposed to be getting less and less. Instead of that, I am doing more and more and more. So you tell me, what is it? Well, in a sense as far as

I am concerned, I am healed. So why keep praying for healing? I am alive, so as far as I am concerned, I am as good as cured."

When Mr. Gray entered his sixteenth month of hospice, I asked Tiffany if she had considered discharging him. "He is still really a sick guy," she said. "We have been discussing him in our team meeting, and he is still really symptomatic, and he still has a lot of the criteria that justify us staying involved." Katherine Marsh, Mr. Gray's pulmonary specialist, acknowledged her patient's physical improvement, but asserted that, from a medical standpoint, his level of functioning remained low. "Even the smallest infection or a change in fluid status, if his heart did not function well, could tip him over into a bad situation where he could not recover even with medications," she explained. She had spoken with Mr. Gray about a living will. Good palliative care and the occasional checkups she gave him kept her patient alive, she observed, and then continued. "His prognosis for three years survival is probably zero. His prognosis for a one-year survival is probably 15% to 20%, as best I can give you. We don't have good statistics in pulmonary medicine, because there is so much variability in chronic lung disease. We see people who, if they don't get an infection, may remain stable for a year or two. But his disease is very severe, and I am actually surprised that he has done well this long."

"Needed Reassurance"

When a family emergency forced Carl Flynn to leave hospice, Tiffany offered Mr. Gray a new spiritual counselor. He declined. "If I find myself needing any real strong spiritual help, so to speak, I can pretty much just take it straight to Christ Himself," he said. Mr. Gray's main worry was that he had not had time to watch Pastor Lowel's television show. He missed his Bible study.

On October 8, personal care nurse Naomi Barnes found Mr. Gray in bed. He was wearing his oxygen mask and struggling to speak. Having spent the previous day picking tomatoes in his sister's yard, he had strained his muscles. He reported that the sharp, grabbing pain in his chest, back, shoulders, and scapula was so severe that he couldn't breathe. Two doses of short-acting morphine had not helped. Naomi applied warm, moist heat on the affected areas. When Tiffany arrived, she could hear no air entry at the base of his lungs. Breath sounds in his upper lobes had decreased as well. It took Mr. Gray a few days to start walking again. Tiffany suspected that he was sicker than he showed. "When he knows you are coming at 11," she remarked, "he will be sure to be out in the kitchen, have the coffee ready, and he will be there, and you see him sitting there completely comfortable." To check how he fared when transporting himself from his bedroom to the kitchen, Tiffany started appearing early for her visits. She noted that, even with his oxygen mask on, his shortness of breath came sooner and seemed more persistent. When he sat down, it took him two minutes before he could speak.

In late October, Tiffany congratulated Mr. Gray for completing his second smoke-free month. He looked embarrassed. He did not deserve congratulations, he said, because he had had another cigarette the previous day. Tiffany encouraged him to be forgiving, explaining that backslides were normal. Mr. Gray didn't seem convinced. "Needed reassurance," wrote Tiffany in her nursing notes that day. She left Mr. Gray wishing that Carl was still available to help him. She worried that even if Mr. Gray were to accept hospice's new spiritual counselor, he would not connect with her. Jane Madder was more formal than Carl. "She is not as laid back and as easy-going," Tiffany remarked, "which I know Stanley really liked about Carl. Carl would sit there and tell you a dirty joke, you know. And Stanley liked that. Because, you know, Stanley is rough around the edges."

Jane Madder

Jane Madder left her first meeting with Mr. Gray puzzled. What he had said about Pastor Lowel disturbed her. She disagreed with the philosophy that there is only one truth in the world and that the Bible has an explanation for everything. But she sat quietly and listened. Later she learned that Mr. Gray felt bad about monopolizing the conversation.

On her next visit, Jane invited Mr. Gray to talk more about his life. Mr. Gray went back to the Bible. Jane asked if there were particular passages he found especially meaningful. He could not come up with any. Jane shared with him a prayer asking for gratefulness "for new things that happen and a kind of acknowledgment that while we celebrate what we have received in the past, we also look forward to new gifts from God and from the spirit." Jane told me that she hoped to help Mr. Gray move beyond what she called the "closed system" that Pastor Lowel promoted. Such systems, she argued, made people disinterested in new ideas, gave them a false sense of security, and prevented growth.

Thelma and Tiffany

By November, Thelma, the hospice social worker, found herself also trying to direct conversations with Mr. Gray away from his faith—to no avail. "He is more consumed with the spiritual aspect than he is with the illness," she remarked. Although she had grown tired of Mr. Gray's preoccupation, she conceded that his religious life and ability to share it gave him happiness. "I think it is really helping him," she said. "I think it is a real source of strength for him, and I think it is as important as his medications." She even reluctantly agreed to borrow two of Mr. Gray's videotapes of Pastor Lowel's show.

Tiffany felt more comfortable with Mr. Gray's religiosity because, unlike the other members of the team, she found him open to differing perspectives. She also shared some of his convictions. She told me that God had given him his illness for a reason: his COPD had allowed him to make amends with his family, reestablish a connection with his daughter, and bring Mrs. Laxton closer to God, too.

"Every Day I Thank God for Bringing You Back into My Life"

On December 7, Mr. Gray celebrated his 58th birthday. Cynthia gave him a framed photograph of himself at the kitchen table with her standing behind him. Her arms were wrapped around him. They were both smiling. On the frame were the words, "Every day I thank God for bringing you back into my life. Love, Cynthia."

Naomi Barnes

By the middle of the month, Mr. Gray had gone back to smoking regularly. Increased weakness sometimes confined him to his bed. On one of her visits, Tiffany watched him stop three times on his way to the kitchen, even though he was wearing his oxygen mask and holding onto his walker. He then leaned against the kitchen doorway. When he caught his breath, he shuffled to his chair and leaned over it. Once he sat down, he dropped his head, closed his eyes, and tried to take even breaths. Three to four minutes later, he turned to Tiffany and said, "I am doing really good, all things considered." Tiffany worried. She offered to ask Mr. Gray's primary care physician to increase the frequency of his sustained-release morphine from twice to three times a day. She also encouraged Mr. Gray to consider pills or patches that could help him stop smoking. Mr. Gray resisted. "Right now, this is between me and God," he said. Tiffany was perplexed. "He is feeling like he needs to punish himself," she told me later. "Some of him is starting to get a little weird, I think."

I saw Mr. Gray the next day. He was sitting at the kitchen table as usual. Mrs. Laxton had made a fresh batch of coffee, which was steaming in the middle of the room. She had just offered me a cup of tea when Naomi, the personal care nurse, arrived. It was three o'clock. "He is my last one!" Naomi exclaimed. "I told you I save the best for last!" Naomi was an outgoing and good-humored woman. She had grown close to Mr. Gray. She told me that she liked to visit him late in the day in order to have the freedom to extend her stays beyond the time required for his hygiene. She had gained Mr. Gray's trust, helping him take showers, massaging his back and neck to relax his muscles, emptying his bedside commode, and conversing with him about his life and hers.

Naomi's family background was socioeconomically similar to Mr. Gray's. She was also a devout Christian. When she told Mr. Gray that she had worked in a prison, his guard dropped. He began opening up about his past. Every now and then, he even told her dirty jokes. He would cry with her and laugh. "With Naomi there is always this joke," he said, "and I can do most things, but one problem I do have is emptying the portable toilet." Mrs. Laxton interjected, "There are times when he doesn't get it down, and when Naomi comes, he says, 'I have a little present back [in my bedroom] for you,' and it is kind of like a joke."

"He is the type of guy that you have to let your hair down with and not be offended at anything he says," Naomi observed. "He is a sweetheart."

"I Don't Want to Go Back Again and Have 10 More Tapes Waiting for Me"

By the end of December, Thelma felt worn out by Mr. Gray's religiosity. Without realizing it, she had borrowed eight videotapes of Pastor Lowel, but had neither the time nor the desire to watch them all. Uncomfortable with the intensity of her meetings with Mr. Gray, she found herself postponing her next visit. "Maybe we are going to have to set some limits," she said with a perplexed look on her face. "I don't want to go back again and have 10 more tapes waiting for me."

"Whatever It Is, It's Working, You Know?

In January 1998, Mr. Gray had a respiratory crisis that he overcame with antibiotics and a new prescription of 100 mg sustained-release morphine capsules. Naomi increased her visits from two to three times a week. Mr. Gray requested bed baths. He told her that he was not ready to die. She sat next to him on his bed and cried.

One month later, Mr. Gray's condition had improved. The morphine capsules, together with the fact that he had stayed away from cigarettes, had reduced his need for short-acting morphine from eight times a day to three times a week. "[Dr. Marsh] was tickled to death when she saw me," he said as he started to describe a recent appointment with his pulmonary specialist. "She just could not believe how well I am doing." I asked him if Katherine had an explanation for his recovery. "Let's face it," he responded, "the doctors are not going to just come right out and say, 'Yeah, it is God doing it. It is not us.' But in a manner of speaking, they are also saying that they have done everything that they can, and they don't understand how I am doing as well as I am doing. But they are glad that whatever it is, it's working, you know?"

"Sometimes I Think I Get Strength from Him"

"I think his faith is 80% of it," said Naomi when I asked her how she explained Mr. Gray's unexpected stabilization. We were in her living room. She was nursing a broken ankle, her leg propped up with pillows. Enthusiastically, she told me that Mr. Gray and Mrs. Laxton had paid her a surprise visit the previous week. She was having lunch with a friend when she heard Mr. Gray shouting, "Hey! Hey!" She looked out the window and saw Mrs. Laxton imploring him to quiet down. She could not believe her eyes. Mr. Gray, with his cannula and mask, made it into her house with the help of his walker. When he caught his breath, he told her that he wanted to see how she was doing. He then joked that a little "present" was waiting for her in the car. Naomi laughed as she recounted the incident:

He just seems so much better. I even said to my husband, "If I lose Stanley right now, that is going to be it." That is going to tear me apart, because I just think the world of him. For him to come in here—he is terminal, God bless him—he trucks into my house because I cannot come see him! Nobody could have done anything that would have made me feel better. That was really neat. He is a such a neat man. In fact, sometimes I think I get strength from him.

Although impressed with his perseverance, Naomi affirmed that Mr. Gray was still very sick. She suspected that he didn't realize this. Drawing from his faith, he put on a happy front, but she had noticed that this dissipated at times of crisis. When he couldn't breathe, he got angry for losing control. Naomi believed that he was someone who would require a lot of emotional support when he started to actively die. She missed him. She couldn't wait to start working with him again.

Hospice's nurse supervisor corroborated Naomi's view. Even if Mr. Gray teetered between "chronic" and "terminal" illness, she argued, he clearly belonged in hospice. His medications increased steadily. When he skipped a dose, his symptoms worsened. "If we would ever get questioned on this case, which may happen," she explained, "I think we have enough documentation of what is going on. We are continually doing things for him. It is not as if we are not doing anything, socializing when we go in. We are readjusting the medications. So, this is a very comfortable case for me." Nurses and administrators were united in seeing hospice's services—emotional and spiritual support, nursing care, symptom monitoring, and urgent intervention in moments of crisis—as beneficial not only to Mr. Gray but also to his sister. They had grown concerned about Mrs. Laxton's health. Flo had brought Stanley into her home expecting him to die imminently. Instead, she had spent two years monitoring her brother's every breath. Thelma advocated for helping Mrs. Laxton switch her mindset from short-term, intensive care to long-term care, but the team resisted that very distinction. If some had grown uncomfortable with the length of Mr. Gray's enrollment in the program, it was because bureaucratic definitions of "hospice appropriateness" in the United States created what they viewed as an artificial dichotomy between chronic and terminal care.

"I Know We May Seem Like Fanatics"

In May, Mr. Gray announced that he was curious about other people's religious beliefs. He asked Tiffany if he could meet another patient of hers who, Tiffany had told him, was a retired minister. Tiffany relayed to this patient,

Mr. Peter Stone, Mr. Gray's interest. Mr. Stone called Mr. Gray and visited him three times.

Tiffany was pleased to see that Stanley and Peter enjoyed each other's company. But in early August, their relationship broke off. Mr. Stone had borrowed a videotape of Pastor Lowel and, instead of returning it himself as he had promised, mailed it back with a note. He wrote that he disagreed with some of Pastor Lowel's statements and that, for a while, he was going to be too busy to continue his visits. Mr. Gray seemed hurt. Protectively, Mrs. Laxton reminded him that Peter was a busy man. Stanley wasn't convinced. He suspected that it was differences in their religious views that had pushed him away. Mrs. Laxton turned to me and said, "I know we may seem like fanatics to an extent. But it is excitement, and I do feel that we have learned the right path."

"I Do Not Have to Be Ashamed to Say I Am a Gray"

When I saw Mr. Gray in July, he was sitting in the kitchen with Mrs. Laxton and Cynthia. He had been smoke-free for six months, but he looked pale and exhausted. For two weeks he had had difficulty urinating. His skin felt so tight that he thought it was going to break. He struggled to breathe. A few days earlier, his primary care physician had increased his diuretic from 60 to 80 mg a day, which had given him relief. "I am quite sure that [the diuretic] is going to be the key to this whole thing," he said with a smile. "And, praise the Lord, in a day or two from now maybe I will be feeling quite a bit better and ready to get out there and dance again." "That's right!" Cynthia interjected. "We have got a baby to get ready for, so you have got to get yourself feeling better."

Cynthia told me that she was three months pregnant. It was clear that everyone was thrilled. They saw the baby as an opportunity to experience together precious moments that they had missed. Mr. Gray had not held Cynthia as a baby. And for 16 years, he did not know that his only child had become a mom. "I will be there this time the best I can," he said, reaching out to hold Cynthia's hand.

In private, Cynthia told me that the most healing time of her father's life was probably yet to come. It was going to be in his final days, she thought, which were bound to rob him of his cheery façade and open room for his loved ones to give back to him. Only then, Cynthia believed, would he be able to let go. Cynthia vowed to "bully" her way into her father's world. In the brief time she had known him, she said, she had changed. She felt more complete, and confident, and more loving toward Mr. Gray. "The man I know now, I can be proud of," she asserted. "It is not like I have this terrible black cloud on that side of the family. I do not have to be ashamed to say I am a Gray. Before, I was not quite sure."

Two months later, Cynthia's baby died in the womb. She had an emergency induction of labor, with her father at her side. She was the first to hold the fetus. She then handed it to Mr. Gray. He placed it on his lap. He stared at it quietly. Tears rolled down his cheeks.

Authors' Comments

The question, "When is a patient appropriate for hospice?" is a leitmotif of this book. It is hard to give a definitive answer. Much of it depends on who is asking whom, and why. Especially in the United States, the answer is complicated by financing schemes for hospice care that require unrealistic and frequently off-putting predictions of a patient's imminent death. Physicians are understandably reluctant to make these "gloomy prognostications," as Thomas Percival described them in his *Medical Ethics* of 1803.[1] Their probabilistic nature makes them hard for medical professionals to phrase helpfully to patients and hard for patients to interpret.[2] Hospice programs also fear the financial and regulatory consequences of caring for too many patients like Stanley Gray, who far outlived his expected time of death. Their willingness to do so may depend in part on their overall financial stability and the mix of patients on their roster at any given time.

Non-cancer diagnoses, such as Mr. Gray's cardiopulmonary disease as well as renal disease and many neurodegenerative diseases, pose particular challenges in end-of-life care because of their frequently erratic course. Today, there are a number of prognostic aids available for this universe of conditions to help clinicians—and hospice providers—with such estimates (e.g., ePrognosis, developed at the University of California at San Francisco[3] and the Seattle Heart Failure Model developed at the University of Washington).[4,*] Despite efforts to standardize prognostication, however,

---

* The authors thank Brianna Ketterer, a palliative medicine specialist at Oregon Health & Science University, for references to these prognostic aids, as well as other information about the evolution of palliative care in the United States since *Crossing Over* first appeared.

hospice programs appear to apply inconsistent criteria in judging whether a patient is "appropriate." In the Authors' Comments for Shamira Cook's narrative we suggested that race- and class-based biases may play an important, though usually unacknowledged role in this process. If we again compare Mr. Gray's case to that of Ms. Cook, and to those of Frances Legendre and Jenny Doyle, another intriguing hypothesis arises. All three of the latter cases raised recurring questions in the minds of the palliative care team as to the appropriateness of the patient's involvement with the program. Mr. Gray's case raised noticeably fewer questions, even though he remained in hospice significantly longer, and his symptoms were by no means any more acute. In fact, Frances Legendre, Jenny Doyle, and Shamira Cook all experienced much more severe pain and other physical and emotional symptoms than Mr. Gray, and they all died after much less time in palliative care. Why, then, did they provoke so much questioning when Mr. Gray did not?

The answer may be that each of the women actively resisted her disease and sought treatments for it while Mr. Gray did not. In other words, from the hospice team's point of view, the mere length of time a patient has to live, or the severity of their symptoms, might be a less significant criterion for retention in the program *than the patient's attitude toward the disease*. In other words, hospice professionals might be more comfortable with patients who accept death—and are willing to extend those patients' hospice stays as long as they maintain that attitude—than they are with patients who actively resist death, even when those patients suffer more and die sooner. Our sample is small. We would need more data and more case studies like these to test this hypothesis adequately.

A final comment concerns Mr. Gray's fervent religiosity. We noted in the General Introduction that, despite increasingly prevalent assertions in the palliative care literature of the importance of the spiritual dimensions of patients' end-of-life experiences,[5-7] palliative care workers often struggle when patients express their beliefs very strongly. In the narratives of Martin Roy and Jasmine Claude, the staff wondered if the serenity with which these patients were approaching their deaths was a façade, calling for careful probing behind their statements of faith to make sure that unexpressed fears or anxieties were allowed to come to the fore. In other cases, such as Stanley Gray's and Katie Melnick's, hospice staff simply felt worn out by nonstop immersion in their patients' religious worldview. In Mr. Gray's case, the hospice chaplains even felt called upon to try to "loosen" their patient's religious attitudes in the belief that he would benefit from a less narrow and rigid connection with the divine. Perceiving Mr. Gray's religiosity as rooted in guilt and judgment, they tried to offer him a different, less punitive, pathway to a connection with God. Here we can appreciate the chaplains' attempt to occupy a middle ground between radical acceptance of a patient's religious belief and the concern that such belief may place undue burden, to the point of fear of eternal damnation, on a terminally ill person. At the same time, we can also see how thin the line can be between spiritual interventions that intend to help people reach inner peace in preparation for letting go and ones that promote, in a way similar to views of the "good death," the religious worldviews that hospice staff themselves embrace or consider "preferable" for their patients.

References

1. Percival T. *Medical Ethics: Or a Code of Institutes and Precepts Adapted to the Professional Conduct of Physicians and Surgeons*. Manchester, England: J Johnson; 1803.
2. Christakis, NA. *Death Foretold: Prophecy and Prognosis in Medical Care*. Chicago: University of Chicago Press; 2000.
3. ePrognosis. University of California at San Francisco. https://eprognosis.ucsf.edu/index.php. Accessed November 12, 2021.
4. Seattle Heart Failure Model. University of Washington. https://depts.washington.edu/shfm/index.php?width=1280&height=720. Accessed November 12, 2021.
5. Steinhauser KE, Fitchett G, Handzo GF, Johnson KS, Koenig HG, Pargament KI, Puchalski CM, Sinclair S, Taylor EJ, Balboni TA. State of the science of spirituality and palliative care research Part I: Definitions, measurement, and outcomes. J Pain Symptom Manage. 2017;54(3):428–440.
6. Steinhauser KE, Balboni TA. State of the science of spirituality and palliative care research: Research landscape and future directions. J Pain Symptom Manage. 2017;54(3):426–427.
7. Gijsberts MHE, Liefbroer AI, Otten R, Olsman E. Spiritual care in palliative care: A systematic review of the recent European literature. Med Sci. 2019;7(2):25.

14

Martin Roy

"Why Be Dead Before You're Dead?"

Narrated by Anna Towers

Martin Roy was only 37 years old when he learned that his cancer was far advanced. By his own account he had already had a full and fulfilling life, and he spent his final months preparing his family for his death. Although controlling Martin's symptoms was not easy for the palliative care team, with a combination of inpatient and home care they succeeded in finding a style of care that kept him comfortable and suited the family. Something other than symptom control proved challenging to the staff, however: Martin seemed almost too accepting of his situations. What accounted for his exceptional ability to adapt to dying at an early age? Was he simply a "good coper" or was he "euphoric" and "in denial"? What was really going on with him?

A Life of Travel and Social Justice

Martin Roy was a well-traveled French-Canadian who loved life. The center of attention at any social gathering, he loved parties and dancing. He made and kept friends for a lifetime. He was gracious, soft-spoken, with a charming smile, and looked straight into one's eyes when he spoke. He was a slight man, and when I met him he was very thin as a result of his illness, but he had been a well-built athlete before cancer began to ravage him. After receiving a master's degree in sociology, Martin had worked for the Peace Corps, then managed a travel agency and a solar energy firm and had been a scuba-diving instructor in the South Pacific. Martin and his wife Alexandra had lived in

Nepal for eight years. Their two children, Justin, 8, and Caroline, 6, were born there.

The eldest of five children, Martin now lived in Montreal, as did his brothers and sisters. His wife and his sister Diane provided his main emotional support, being the only people with whom he felt totally comfortable. Martin also had many friends from various walks of life, including some whom he had known since his childhood.

I met Martin about three years after he had been diagnosed with stomach cancer. Martin related the onset of his illness to a boating accident in Nepal. He was alone, sailing a small craft in a busy harbor, when he was hit by a larger boat. He explained:

> When I had my accident, I saw the first moments of death as Dr. Raymond Moody describes in *Life After Life*. It's true what they say. I saw the image of my son Justin appear, when I stopped a 23-foot-long boat with my head and my shoulder, at 55 km/hr. A ton! That's when everything started, I think. Something blew inside. I was in a state of burnout for about six months, and the cancer appeared after that, and I think it was because of that trauma. All that centrifugal force that I had to summon up to stop [the boat] just made something burn out inside me.

Although his travel agency was doing well, Martin and his family moved back to Montreal, mainly so the children could go to school there. Returning to Canada was a big change. He explained to me,

> It wasn't easy to come back, I have to be honest. [In Nepal] we lived without money, no kidding. At our house it was always a great food party. Some people stopped at our house; they thought it was a restaurant. Other people thought it was a bar. So we said, "Come in, have a drink."
>
> Traveling, when you change country, money, food, history, clothes, expression—everything changes. So I've never been afraid of change. I spent 10 years of my life in Nepal, Bhutan, Indochina. I've lived in many countries, and I've been through a lot. I've experienced discomfort, places where they had had drought for three years, illnesses, epidemics, the heat. But we lived 24-hour days, intensely. We lived off love. We loved what we did, we did it with people who loved. You see that the people are poor, but they're beautiful, they're gentle. They were kind and they never, never let me down.

So then I come back here and there's violence, murder, pollution. So I would go traveling again. I would do different things, go to the Pacific, go swimming with dolphins. I lived with iguanas, herons, turtles. . . . Scuba-diving in the Pacific Islands, I saw things under the sea. . . . You know, there are beautiful things on this planet!

Elaborating on his philosophy of life, Martin continued,

I'll take the best from all these places and I'll make something new, something good. For me it's Martin Luther King, Gandhi, or it could be Jesus Christ, or Mother Teresa. Or it could be a little boy that I meet in a poor village. If we want to lessen pain, suffering, evil, then we have to realize that we have the means and put ourselves to work. I read everything that Gandhi and Martin Luther King wrote. I got inspiration from them because in the Catholic religion I didn't feel very much at home.

But now his illness had interrupted everything. On his return to Montreal, Martin had received the definitive diagnosis of stomach cancer, and underwent an esophagogastrectomy. As Martin explained to me during our first long conversation,

It was working, except this wrench came into the works . . . a large wrench. . . . I'll tell you honestly, a large wrench. It's hard for me to talk about it. When I talk about it for the first time with someone . . . [sobbing] excuse me . . . I was saying, a large wrench, but not necessarily. Because death is a subject I've read about over the last 20 years. And with life, I think, there's quantity and there's quality. . . . In the sum of a life, be it 30 years, 40 years, or 100 years, there's an equilibrium. It's normal that I'm used up at age 37. I've done what some do in 100 years. It's like an automobile, the motor is finished, I've gone over 300,000 km. "Sorry, Mom, Dad. I've run for too long. I need a new motor, and they can't install one."

Martin and Alexandra had been together for seventeen years. She was the same age as Martin, a small, rotund woman with a calm demeanor. Barbara, the home care nurse from the hospital-based Palliative Care Service, described her as a "saint" because of her patience and warmth. She always had a hint of a smile on her face; none of the staff ever saw her upset. It seemed as though she could cope with anything. Alexandra described her husband as a joyful and charismatic person, a comic and a clown, who always spoke the truth.

After Surgery . . . More Surgery

Following his surgery, Martin had a long convalescence. He felt "cut up, amputated . . . a whole train had passed over me." Because Alexandra worked full-time as a dental assistant and could not look after him, Martin went to live with his parents for five months in their modest, one-story dwelling about ten miles away. Alexandra and the children visited every two or three days. Martin's mother helped nurse him, in addition to looking after her handicapped brother Robert, who had suffered from severe neurological dysfunction since contracting meningitis as a child. Mrs. Roy had been looking after her brother for eight years, since their mother died. Robert was bedbound, tube fed, and had a tracheostomy that needed frequent care. He lived in a hospital bed that Mr. and Mrs. Roy had set up in what was once their dining room. When Martin and his brothers and sisters were growing up, their uncle Robert was a key person in their lives. They called him "Bo-Bo," and would play together, considering him like a brother.

A year after his surgery, Martin developed headaches and was found to have a brain metastasis. He had a craniotomy with excision of the tumor, followed by radiotherapy and chemotherapy. Since he seemed not to have any tumor elsewhere, the oncologists offered to treat him as aggressively as possible, even though they did not expect a cure. Following the brain surgery Martin was left with double vision. He had to give up reading, one of his greatest passions. During this second convalescence he had plenty of time to think and reflect. He described some experiences that he had at this time that made him aware that he could use mental techniques to control pain.

> After my brain surgery it took me four, five days to come back. And I remember that I was very happy. I wasn't tired, I was totally comfortable. And I noticed my surroundings differently, because I wasn't in my conscious mind; I was in my subconscious. I was feeling so good that I didn't want to sleep, and I didn't sleep for five days. Then I realized that my subconscious doesn't know what fatigue is. It doesn't know what pain is. My subconscious

is total comfort. It's when we're in our physical body that we can suffer, but when we're in our subconscious, it's universal, it's grand, it's peace, it's infinity. It's eternal life. It's in that state that we feel the most loving, collegial, relaxed, devoted.

I only speak about this with my wife and my sister, because I know that not everyone can understand this. It's incredible! I didn't want to come back into my conscious mind. I was feeling so good in my subconscious! I was in paradise. I had no pain. And I wasn't taking any medication, not even Tylenol.

The day after my stomach surgery, when I started to feel pain for the first time, morphine didn't help at all. And the pain was so strong that I couldn't breathe or move. So I got a hold of myself, and the pain disappeared within five minutes. Forever. They had opened my ribs and I had this sword-like pain that came in front of my chest here and came out my back. So I got a hold of myself and reminded myself that I have certain powers, which I had discovered in my travels, like when I was in that boating accident. I learned that I had a physical and mental power whereby I could, by necessity or instinct, summon all the energy I needed in a thousandth of a second. There could be consequences afterwards . . . but I found that I had great powers.

The subconscious doesn't go to bed and doesn't sleep. It's there all the time. If I have pain, I know that I can seek refuge there.

Six months later, in January 1996, Martin was found to have multiple lung and liver metastases. He wanted no further chemotherapy and was referred to the Palliative Care Service. Barbara, the home care nurse, visited weekly. She was an experienced, efficient, no-nonsense nurse who had a good sense of humor. She monitored Martin's symptoms and reported back to Dr. Peter Lawrence, who became his regular palliative care physician. Barbara was the first to comment on Martin's demeanor in the face of his devastating disease.

In January, I found he was too euphoric, inappropriate, too good to be true . . . When you're that young . . . I wondered if he had a problem from his brain metastasis. I think that he might have been denying things. He was a non-stop talker. I think that when he was stressed, he became very intense. It was very draining for me because of the energy he had. It made me think of Rasputin—he had that intense look in his eyes.

Reflecting on Death

I met Martin in early April 1996, when he came to the hospital to see his palliative care physician. He looked tired after his one-hour journey. He wanted to tell me about his two children, and how he had explained to them that their father was very sick. He told them that "I would become an angel soon. You won't be able to see me, but I will be able to see you." He felt that the children were not coping too badly with this.

Because Martin's current regimen of acetaminophen and codeine was not controlling his lumbar and epigastric pain, Dr. Lawrence suggested switching to morphine. Martin was reluctant to do so, thinking he would try harder to control the pain with other means. Barbara continued to visit him weekly and to monitor his symptoms.

In mid-April, I interviewed Martin in his home, a two-bedroom apartment in a working-class neighborhood. As he opened the door to welcome me, he looked thin and tired but had a big smile for me. Their dwelling reminded me of a student's apartment; the sparse furniture looked second-hand. There were framed photographs of mountains, scenes from India and Nepal with family, and friends. In family photographs from three years earlier, Martin appeared fit and muscular, very different from the frail man in the reclining chair next to me now.

Martin spoke with me for three hours on this occasion. He was eager to discuss his travels and his illness. Words flowed out of him.

It's not serious being sick. I have been meditating on death since I was 15 years old. And I saw a lot of death, in the revolutions, the social upheavals. All my life has been a series of adventures into the unknown. I never retreated; I went forward because I wanted to get to know the unknown. There is nothing worse than dying ignorant! Not to know that there are beautiful things at our doorstep, and not touching them, examining them, observing them, or at least tasting them! But I led a good life. Maybe I abused my body because I lived too intensely. But I saw that we were about to contaminate our planet, and I wanted to see things before they got polluted. I had the chance to see that. So I can't complain.

I don't have 100% proof that there is a life after this one, but I've had several experiences, like that in the hospital with my pain, and after the brain surgery, where I spent five days in my subconscious. That was the ultimate! But I can't discuss this with people because it's not something that is valued in our society. And it's a shame, because that's where we find the joy in living, the realization of one's self. And it's hard to grasp. As we approach it, it moves away a bit. But we get a taste and that makes us accept death. And I've accepted death for a long time, because otherwise I wouldn't have gone to those countries where I saw all sorts of things and risked my life.

We have to teach and learn about death in our society, not from a negative point of view, but constructively, because to see death negatively is to strip it of all its value. There are countries where death is nothing serious. When we watch a funeral in Bhutan, or we see the infant mortality in some parts of India—they see death every day. They're not afraid of it. But here, as soon as we talk about death, well, no, death doesn't exist. "Come on! Is my car still in the parking lot? Good. OK." *That's* important. But death, that's *not* important. And what makes me feel sorry for [people here] is that they allow death to take them by surprise. If they were ready to face death, they would assume the task of dying without destroying the life of others. Because there are those who destroy others in their dying, with their agony, their perceptions, their views and by what they say.

Because death is beautiful also. I had a taste of it at the time of the boating accident. . . . I'm not afraid of death. I don't run after it, but I am blooming, flowering, I have realized myself. And I know one thing: you also have to trust in death. I know it's going to come. What's difficult, though, is when we suffer, before. Dying, apart from the emotional problem of leaving others and seeing them suffer, is nothing. It's the suffering of others that concerns me more than my own—my wife, children, brother, sister. I worry about my children's future and what kind of world they will live in.

Coping with Physical Symptoms

Two weeks later I saw Martin again at his home. He seemed peaceful, accepting, as before. Alexandra was at work. She had a lot to deal with: she had to work full-time, wanted to find an apartment in a more convenient location, and had all the usual family concerns in addition to Martin's illness. When I arrived, Martin was making arrangements with her over the phone about putting supper on.

He spoke more about his physical symptoms and how he coped with his illness on a daily basis. We discussed his pain, which had become more severe over the past two weeks. He had tried every means he could to control it, but the pain in his chest and flank was getting worse. He had finally agreed to take long-acting morphine and was now on 45 mg taken twice daily. He said it helped a lot and explained how he had been in pain for two years since his surgery. In the past week, since he had started to take morphine, he was pain-free for the first time.

Since his stomach surgery, Martin tolerated snacks better than meals. He had a significant problem with reflux. In spite of his improved appetite, he only felt like having milk, milkshakes, and cookies. He had to take frequent naps, even though he was sleeping twelve hours per night. He tried to make himself useful with the little energy that he had. After he got the children off to school he would watch TV, listen to music, or meditate. He was unable to read more than a page at a time because of the double vision. Otherwise, he seemed to adapt well to his vision impairment, and he didn't complain about it.

Martin spoke with friends on the telephone, but he was becoming more selective about his company: "I find that I can't tolerate foolishness, if someone says something stupid, illogical. . . . If I meet someone who's really zero, zero, zero across the board—well then, I'd rather not be there! I used to have a lot of time for that, but now I don't." Martin wanted to spend time either alone, with his family, or with people "of substance," which to him meant people who shared his humanistic concerns.

Preparing the Family

Martin focused a lot of his mental energy on preparing his family for his death. As he put it to me,

> Inside, I'm at peace. Alexandra is also doing well with this. We have informed everyone. So that's a lot that's already done. It feels like a hurricane has just gone by. Because to make the whole family aware and not to hurt them, and to comfort them in all this—it takes time. No one has died in my immediate family. So, for them, it's something new. We have to consider that. I've tried to help them, with all the precious advice I've been given [by palliative care], and all the information I've been able to pick up, here and there, to try to make them see the positive side of things.

Only Alexandra, and perhaps Diane, knew how the illness was affecting him: his pain, his lack of appetite, his lack of energy, his sadness. Alexandra told me,

> We have been in another phase since January. Before that we thought there was some hope. I tried always to show my hopeful side, to hide my tears from Martin. But after January it became clear that he was in the terminal phase. We decided to share our feelings, to cry together. So after that, I didn't hold back the tears.

In May, Martin started to spend weekends at his parents' house. His mother, who was in her early seventies and fit for her age, wanted to look after Martin's needs, but she felt physically and emotionally overwhelmed. She was upset with how fast Martin's illness was progressing. She was also concerned about her husband's reactions and how her other children would deal with the situation. Martin was concerned about her.

> [Being here] gives me a chance to prepare my mother. She is having trouble. She has to realize that this is reality and that we have to accept what destiny presents. My mother is a good person but she's not very spiritual. She doesn't accept human limitations. She is trying to fight this. My mother has already lost her parents, brothers, and sister. Nevertheless, she is suffering with this. Perhaps it's more difficult because I'm her son. She has had six children, so you'd think it would make it easier, but perhaps it doesn't.

Coming into the Palliative Care Unit

By early June, Martin was feeling so weak that he stayed in bed all day. He started to have more vomiting and abdominal pain. Alexandra could not look after him anymore because she still needed to work. Martin therefore moved into his parents' house full-time, but after a few days his parents realized that they could not cope with the situation either. Therefore, despite Martin's desire to die at home, he came into the Palliative Care Unit.

Alexandra came to the hospital every evening after work while Martin's brother and sister-in-law looked after the children. Justin and Caroline came to see their father every other day. Diane visited several times per week and would stay for several hours. She would take her brother out into the hospital gardens to enjoy the summer sun, where they would sit, chatting together, for long periods of time.

Alexandra shared Martin's view that one had to enjoy the present. "How does it help to be sad?" she would say. "Why be dead before you're dead? We want to live in the present, to make the present pleasant. We're not sad now. In January perhaps, we went through a phase where we would cry together. But we don't cry now. Martin and I have seen the world together. It has been a spiritual experience for us. We share the same spiritual views. That has helped us deal with this. Even when he is very ill I tell him, 'I find you beautiful.'"

Martin's mother, on the other hand, found it difficult to accept that her son had entered the final stage of his illness. "The first time I went to the hospital to see him," Mrs. Roy told me, "he said, 'Now I'm all organized.' He had his funeral organized. He wanted his brother Simon to sign his advance directives. He was very clear about what he wanted for the funeral, all the details. We didn't expect this—we had to leave the room—we couldn't take it."

"That Man Is Euphoric"

Within a few days Martin's pain and vomiting were controlled by moderately increasing the dose of oral morphine and antiemetics. He continued to show good spirits. The head nurse, who observed Martin when he was admitted to the unit and the first interactions he had with the staff, said to me, "There's something not right about that man. He's too light. That man is euphoric." Dr. Lawrence's reaction was, "That's okay. I think it's better to be a bit euphoric."

The possibility that Martin may have been euphoric was not something that had crossed my mind in the many meetings that I had had with him over the previous three months. I had formed the impression that he was a man who felt things deeply. The ward staff's label of "euphoria" took me aback. Had I missed something? Was I too close to the situation to see that Martin's reactions were unusual, and perhaps abnormal? My doubts grew when I read some of the other staff's notations in the chart. The occupational therapist, for example, wrote: "The patient is euphoric, extremely positive (over-positive). Seems to push himself too much and does not respect his limits." Nurses' notes read: "Lots of hopes and wishes. . . . Smiling and engaging everyone in conversation. . . . Very nice man. Smiling, joking and socializing with staff. Spirit very good and +++ high."

I observed myself as researcher slipping into the institutional mode and taking the opinions of fellow caregivers more seriously than the data that Martin was presenting to me. I subsequently alternated between the two points of view—seeing Martin as a remarkable man or looking for pathology in him—and was never able to integrate the two viewpoints in my mind.

I was not alone in alternating between admiration and doubt. Dr. Lawrence recalled that the main question Alexandra had for him was, "Should the children come after the death to see the body?" Peter continued,

> It's amazing. You meet them together or alone, and there is that serenity, that feeling of completion. And at first I had trouble assessing whether this was a pathological reaction. But now I've come to the conclusion that, although I don't understand it totally and we're not used to that, I see both of them coping the same way—very nicely, very peacefully. . . . It's a spiritual process, not religious, but a spiritual process. It's almost a rebirth. . . . It's a question of surrendering. She has that sense of completion as well, in her life with him. Not that she's tired of it, but when I asked her, she said, "He was given to me and now he's needed elsewhere."

Alexandra explained her sense of completion to me by saying that she and Martin had asked a lot of questions at the time of the diagnosis. "But now we don't need to know anything, so we're not asking many questions. Martin and I are talking to each other." Alexandra found Peter's advice (about having the children view the body) very helpful. "Dr. Lawrence said that we shouldn't leave a doubt in their minds about the reality of the death. I found this logical and sensible."

The staff and I (in my researcher role) were deeply impressed by this couple's attitudes. And yet, Peter spoke for all of us when he commented,

> I'm careful, because you know, you don't have so much light without shadow. With Mr. Roy there is not much shadow presently. Then, you're always saying, well maybe if it's totally repressed, what will happen when he stops being able to repress? Because at one point, and that is my experience, there's a period when the filter between your unconscious and conscious becomes more and more porous. And then the shadow becomes more evident and then sometimes it can be quite ugly. So I feel much better when I see both sides.

A Video for the Children

The unit provided video equipment for patients to use. In mid-June, Martin made a video for his children, to leave for them after his death. When I went to see him one afternoon, we watched it together. He had set up the camera in his hospital room, enabling him to address the children privately. In the video, he is lying in his bed, speaking directly into the camera, addressing his children unscripted. Here is some of what he said:

> The body is the prison of the soul. What will happen is that Daddy will become an angel. But stay strong. I hope that you will accept my departure with a bit of wisdom. Look after each other, and your mother, too. You know that Alexandra, your mother, is eternal love. She loves you as Daddy does.
>
> Daddy is proud of the two of you [crying]. I could say that you saved my life. Eight years ago, there wasn't much in Daddy's life, and then big Justin came along. I remember your first steps, and Caroline, who jumped in the swimming pool.
>
> You will create your happiness by doing the things that impassion you. The important thing is to have pleasure in the realization of your being. What you do, do it well, for the good. In the final count, one must love continuously. In life, it's important to be able to get close to others. The friendships that we create, outside of blood ties, are important. We need to love and help our friends unconditionally. We shouldn't attach ourselves to material things; suffering comes from possession.
>
> Don't be afraid to take risks, calculated risks. We are in a difficult era in the world, socially, economically. You'll need to read a lot, find out, equip yourselves. Carry a book with you and read whenever you can. Don't waste your time in life. Protect life on the planet.
>
> Death isn't something frightening, in itself. I have taken many risks in my life, I had many adventures, some of which made me afraid. I've had close brushes with death. God is generous and gives us a lot of chances. I should have been dead a long time ago, but God let me live a bit longer so that I could prepare you. Eternal life exists. Daddy still exists in the message of love on this video.
>
> I will wait for you in God's kingdom, and I imagine that it will be restful, peaceful. I'm sure that it will be beautiful in paradise. Not that it's not beautiful on earth—the blue sky, the clouds that we see when we fly—they enrich our soul and bring us closer to God, and eliminate our fear. Justin,

Caroline, your dad will surely be sad to leave you [cries] but while we were together, you gave me pleasure and happiness. You are like two jewels. You have creative beings within you. Let your imaginations loose and create, no matter how small or large. I am confident that you will succeed in life.

"You Have to Do Something"

Toward the end of June, Martin began to have more epigastric pain and gastric reflux, and he developed a cough. His pills left a bad taste in his mouth because of the reflux, which he found unbearable. Feeling that he was at the end of his rope, he told the nurses that he was uncomfortable and he wished it were all over.

"You have to do something," he said.

In an attempt to achieve better symptom control, Dr. Lawrence stopped the oral medication and ordered subcutaneous medication through a special pump (syringe driver). Martin received morphine 70 mg and metoclopramide 30 mg subcutaneously over 24 hours. The chest X-ray showed increasing metastatic lung disease, but no pneumonia. He was put on an oral antibiotic for bronchitis and on famotidine to reduce stomach acid secretion and help his epigastric pain.

While his symptoms improved over the next couple of days, the staff noted that he appeared increasingly tired, thinner, and sadder. He expressed the need for more privacy. He rested with eyes closed most of the time. He expressed some anxiety over his wife and children moving to a different apartment on July 1. He said he hoped that they would be able to manage on their own.

After their move, Martin began to go home for four days every week, maintaining his medication schedule with the syringe driver. He wanted to be with his children as much as possible, and Justin and Caroline seemed more settled now that they saw more of their father. At the end of every visit he would hold the children and cry.

Back on the ward, he looked happier. He expressed no concerns to the nurses and continued to be pleasant and agreeable. Alexandra continued to visit every evening during the week, and his children visited every other day, even though the hospital was one hour away from their home. Martin insisted on Alexandra's company every day, which was not easy for her. She commented to me,

It's almost selfish of him. I have to keep the family together and work and look after the children, to keep everything together and he just thinks of his own needs. When I arrive at the hospital through the traffic I have to take a big breath to calm myself before I can talk to him. He lives in a different relaxed space and he doesn't need to think of my troubles. I have to make the transition, in order to see him and relate to him, from my busy practical world to his world. But once I move into his world it's like being in a sanctuary. I forget everything, all the stresses.

When Is Death Going to Come?

By the end of July, Martin looked weaker, but he was still cheerful, calm, uncomplaining, and outgoing. He would joke about his illness, "I'm not fat, am I?" and seemed to want to enjoy every moment. "Until you die, you must appreciate life. You can't just think about death," he would say. The syringe driver had improved his symptoms considerably. He had no pain or nausea. Whenever he could, he would slowly wheel himself out to the hospital gardens where he enjoyed the trees, flowers, and birds. Often, his sister Diane would be there with him. They had a deep connection with each other that they could share in the silence. His other brothers and sisters felt less comfortable visiting. They would ask Diane, "What do the two of you find to talk about?" They couldn't understand it.

Dying was taking a long time. Martin had thought he would die within a few weeks of coming to the Palliative Care Unit. He was fed up with waiting, and felt guilty because he was taking up a bed that someone else might need. "Let it come," he would say. "Let's get it over with."

By early August, he showed signs of increasing anxiety. He started to take up smoking again, which he had quit following his stomach surgery two years previously. Over the next few weeks this turned into chain smoking. He sometimes smoked while alone in his room, which was against the rules. Occasionally, Dr. Lawrence smelled cannabis in Martin's room and on his breath.

"My time is approaching," Martin said around this time. He had suffered with his stomach for over two years, and he saw death as a liberation. He felt he had no unfinished business. He was ready to die.

On September 16, he developed a cough. The chest X-ray was suggestive of mild bilateral pneumonia. In his discussion with Dr. Lawrence, Martin expressed the wish for death to come and requested comfort care only. He didn't want to get weaker and become a burden to anyone. They agreed not to start antibiotics unless Peter felt that it would help control his symptoms by decreasing lung secretions. When I saw Martin the next day, he looked extremely weak and spoke very slowly. I wrote in my notes: "He looks like his battery is winding down."

Death Comes

When Martin went home as usual for his weekend pass two days later, his brother had to carry him up the three flights of stairs to the apartment. Martin was out of breath, his cough was getting worse, and he was getting weaker. Alexandra felt that she would not be able to cope with him for the whole weekend, but she knew that he was dying and wanted to remain as calm as possible, for his sake. Neither of them slept. They talked all through the night. Martin needed reassurance that his family would be there when he died, that he would not be abandoned. Alexandra said to him, "Even if you can't do anything physically, we can still talk, we can still relate. You can express your needs. It means a lot to me, to be able to relate." Martin replied, "Me too."

The next morning, Peter gave Alexandra instructions over the phone to give Martin some extra morphine, but after 30 minutes he was still very short of breath. Alexandra and Diane realized that they could not keep him comfortable at home. They convinced Martin that they should call an ambulance and take him back to hospital. Once he made that decision, he seemed at peace with it. Before the ambulance arrived, he asked to see the children. He squeezed their hands and opened his eyes to say good-bye to them. Diane knew that this would be the last time the children would see their father alive. Judging from the look on Martin's face as he looked at his children, he knew it, too.

"I am going to die," Martin announced to me when he arrived on the ward on a stretcher, with Alexandra in tow. He was in great respiratory distress. He was rushed into his room where he improved slightly with oxygen. Alexandra said to him, "Stay calm. We prepared for this. Stay calm and think of yourself, don't think about us."

Peter and the nurse adjusted the oxygen to make Martin as comfortable as possible. Alexandra stood at the bedside, holding Martin's hand and trying to comfort him. I also stood beside him. The whole scene was so peaceful.

I had practiced obstetrics for many years, and it felt to me as if Martin and Alexandra had rehearsed for this moment as one rehearses for a birthing. Martin reached out to grasp my fingers and looked at me with acknowledgment and gently shook my fingers in gratitude and farewell. It was such a peaceful look, even though he was cyanosed, congested, and breathing rapidly at a rate of 60 breaths per minute. When Peter finished adjusting the oxygen, he told Martin that they would give him an injection to make him more comfortable. He then put his hand on Martin's shoulder and held it there for a few moments.

Martin's parents and brother arrived, and they took turns being in the room with Martin while the palliative care team worked. Dr. Lawrence ordered a small dose of midazolam to try to reduce Martin's awareness of respiratory distress. Alexandra stepped briefly out of the room. She looked tired and dazed. She said, "We were expecting this to happen, but when it does happen, it's still a shock."

Martin died with Alexandra, his parents, his brother, and his nurse John present. He had remained as calm as a person could under the circumstances. Given that normally this can be a most distressing way to die, his was the most peaceful respiratory death out of dozens that I have witnessed. The family contacted Diane, and she arrived a half hour later with the children. Justin and Caroline, guided by Alexandra, spent some moments saying goodbye to their father. The team then organized a brief ritual at Martin's bedside, where everyone congregated and recited a Universal Prayer.

The First Year: Carrying on with Living

At the funeral service, Justin was very protective of his father's body. He said, in an aggressive tone, "No one will bury my father. I will bury him. He's my father. I will take the shovel and bury him." He wanted to help carry their father's coffin after the service and was allowed to do so. Justin was upset with his mother because he would have liked to have been there when his father died. Alexandra said afterward, "I think it might have traumatized him, and it would have been difficult for Martin if Justin had been there. I think it was okay the way it happened." Justin couldn't quite understand what had happened to his father's body after it was cremated. Alexandra decided to keep the ashes in a wardrobe at home until the children were older. Then they could decide what they wanted to do with them.

Two weeks after Martin's death, it was Alexandra's and Justin's birthdays. They knew that Martin would have wanted them to celebrate, so they did. In the months that followed, the family did their best to resume a normal life, for Martin's sake. Two months after the death, Alexandra commented,

> The fact that the family was there when he died—his mother, father, and brother—that helped a lot. That helped his mother accept. Martin would have been happy with how things went. There was no significant loss of autonomy. Bowel or bladder incontinence would have been unacceptable to him.
>
> During the illness I did not have much time to think. Now I revisit the memories. I'm trying to let go. But I'm functioning okay. Martin and I talked a lot, so we were somewhat prepared. He said, "Be ready. Be ready." But now there's a void. We communicated so well, sometimes without words.

Justin showed some aggressive behavior at school during the first three weeks, but this subsided. His teacher expressed surprise at his maturity. Both children did well in their school work. They spoke about their father often, saying how they missed him. They also felt his presence. Alexandra said, "Last week I was crying and Caroline came up to me and said, 'Mom, why are you crying? Daddy is among us!'" Justin often identified with his father. "I want to be a comic, like my father," he would say. And he tried to make people laugh.

Three months after Martin's death, Alexandra and the children took a trip to Nepal "to try to make closure," revisiting their old house and meeting old friends. Alexandra said, "It was a big shock for me, because we had spent most of our married life there. All the memories came back. The children used the time to fill in holes in their memory."

Alexandra considered the first six months to be the worst. She cried often. Then she noticed a shift. Things started to improve as the warm weather came. She went out as often as possible with the children; they would enjoy the outdoors, for Martin's sake. Alexandra also began to feel Martin's presence more. She continued to have this sense of Martin's presence well into her second year of bereavement. She told me,

> First there was a void. A part of me was gone. We were together 17 years— that's half of my life. I felt like something was torn inside me. Then I started to sense Martin talking to me. Now we have conversations. Whatever I am

doing, I hear him making comments. We knew each other so well. I know what he would say. It's as if he's with me all the time now, and I feel less sad. I hear him talking. Maybe it's my imagination, but does it matter? The void is gone.

She smiled. "And I feel him alive within me. Whenever I see something beautiful—the sky, the clouds—I think of him. Because we experienced a lot of beauty together."

It was not until one year after the death that Alexandra could bring herself to view the video that Martin had left for the children. She decided to wait until the children were older before showing it to them, so they would understand better what their father was saying to them.

Six months after Martin's death, I visited his parents in their home. They had plenty of time for me and spoke very freely about their son, so that I had trouble getting away even after two and a half hours. They told me how Martin's death had brought his brothers and sisters closer. Mrs. Roy's brother Robert had also died in the meantime, three months after Martin's death. Mr. and Mrs. Roy experienced Robert's death as a release, whereas the loss of Martin was exquisitely painful.

Mr. Roy said, "It was worse when we found out the diagnosis. The end was not too bad—he was well looked after."

Mrs. Roy said, "It made it easier that he didn't suffer."

Nevertheless, their pain was now profound. Of all the family members, Mrs. Roy seemed to be the most affected by Martin's death. She explained,

When you lose a child, you feel like you're missing something, a part of your body. I hope that time make it better. But it's getting better. At first, when he was dying, I was thinking of him the whole time. Now in my mind, I often see the image of him being ill. I dreamed about him for the first time last week. He was ill and then he died. I was so glad to have that dream. I cried.

She began to cry.

Mr. Roy said softly, "My wife cries a lot."

"Martin wouldn't have liked that," Mrs. Roy said, drying her tears.

Mr. Roy agreed. "He hid his emotions. You know that."

"But he cried when he spoke of his children," Mrs. Roy remembered.

"It's not easy to lose a child," Mr. Roy said with tears in his eyes. "I hadn't planned this—that he would leave before me."

Authors' Comments

Mr. Roy was a well-travelled man who had lived in several non-Western cultures. Some of these cultures have a different and—some would say—more natural and accepting view of death and dying. Is this what we are seeing in Mr. Roy? In palliative care, our assessment antennae are always working! We are trained to label, categorize, and make interpretations—for example, was Martin Roy euphoric or not? The assessment training is embedded in palliative care providers and is almost a reflex. By necessity the process involves objectification, which has implications for the way we view the person. We cannot objectify and empathize in the same moment. We have a duty to go through this process, for example, to screen for depression or to detect masks that may be covering up a lot of emotional pain. Yet psychological assessments are often difficult to make. A case like Martin Roy's shows us how complex these issues are—perhaps more complex than what our literature and concepts can explain. Who knows what Mr. Roy's inner life was really like?

Is the palliative care viewpoint as expressed in this chapter too Westernized? It certainly displays what might be called "the hermeneutics of suspicion"; that is, a perspective that assumes the difference between surface and depth, overt and covert, manifest and hidden—and that the second term in each binary is somehow closer to the "truth." Psychoanalysis is a prime example of such a stance. We will encounter this attitude among palliative care staff taking care of Jasmine Claude in a later narrative, where the staff's concerns were centered around their personal unfamiliarity or discomfort with the patient's expressions of strong religious faith.

Mr. Roy and his wife Alexandra prepared their children for his death, and it is moving to see how Alexandra involved the children after their father died. Part of palliative care practice involves guiding parents, counseling them on how to communicate with their children about death and dying according to the child's level of maturity.[1,2] Mr. Roy's parents seemed particularly affected by the death of their 37-year-old son. The death of one's child often leads to complicated grief, even when that child is an adult.

A further ambiguity in this narrative occurs when, "feeling that he was at the end of his rope, [Mr. Roy] told the nurses that he was uncomfortable, and he wished it were all over.

"You have to do something," he said.

What did Mr. Roy mean by this? Was he asking for better control of his symptoms, or for euthanasia? The latter would not have been legal at the time, but today it would be.

References

1. Christ GH, Christ AE. Current approaches to helping children cope with a parent's terminal illness. CA Cancer J Clin. 2006;56:197–212.
2. Fearnley R, Boland JW. Communication and support from health-care professionals to families with dependent children, following the diagnosis of parental life-limiting illness: A systematic review. Palliat Med. 2017;31(3):212–222.

15

Richard Johnson

"Do Not Go Gentle into That Good Night"

Narrated by Anna Towers

Many people, especially those who are relatively young, opt to fight their illness to the end. Richard Johnson refused chemotherapy at first, but when his disease became far advanced, he asked for aggressive treatments. Although he understood that his chemotherapy was a purely experimental treatment, he nonetheless hoped that his life would be prolonged. It made him feel safe to be on a medical ward where he thought that he might get aggressive biomedical interventions for as long as possible. Both Mr. Johnson and his wife Linda wanted to be totally involved with the decision-making concerning his illness, down to the last detail. Yet Mr. Johnson did not involve his wife in some of the crucial choices he made. Mrs. Johnson disagreed with his aggressive approach at the end, when she saw him get sicker and realized that he was dying. Mr. Johnson died a conflicted death, and the course of his wife's and son's bereavement reflected this.

"A Good Little Family"

Mr. Johnson was a 51-year-old engineer who had advanced carcinoma of the prostate when we met him as part of our project. Even when ill, he was a handsome man who looked younger than he was. He was a gracious man who communicated in an intense way, making good eye contact, articulating his words carefully. He seemed wise, spiritual, able to surrender to life events and learn from them. He could be warm and relate cordially with others. "I feel supported and loved by the people around me," he said to me soon after I met him. "I'm very lucky. That's what's important. Family and friends. I have a good little family. I see people who are collecting toys [instead of focusing on true values]. I have a brother-in-law like that. He's a doctor in the States. He wants a Porsche. I used to be like that. But now, even though I don't have my health, I feel that I have everything I need. I'm a rich man."

However, there appeared to be another side to Mr. Johnson. I also observed an intense determination to control and fight, a need for things to be perfect. He did not like to take medication, especially tranquilizers and analgesics, because he was afraid they would make him lose control. Dr. Allan, his palliative care physician, described to me how both Mr. Johnson and his wife Linda kept note pads on which they wrote down everything he said—every observation, every prediction, and every dose of medication that Mr. Johnson received.

Mrs. Johnson described her husband as a nervous man. His tendency toward depression and generalized anxiety were documented regularly in the hospital chart, which dated back 15 years. He had a history of manic-depressive illness and had required lithium and a tricyclic antidepressant for many years. When he was 31, his mother died of cancer on the palliative care ward of the same hospital in which he was now a cancer patient.

Mr. Johnson had never really found a direction in his professional life. He didn't care much about his engineering work, which he found very stressful, nor did he enjoy working for others. He had tried to change careers and started a full-time business of his own that did not work out. Nevertheless, Mrs. Johnson seemed proud of her husband's achievements. One advantage of the five-year period when he worked from home was that he became very close to their son Simon, who was now 12 years old.

Mr. Johnson was raised a Roman Catholic and went to church every Sunday with Simon. Although his wife was Anglican, she went to church with them occasionally. Mr. Johnson had a deeply spiritual view of the world and said that his faith helped him throughout his illness.

Linda Johnson, a bright, beautiful 38-year-old woman of English origin who worked as an assistant manager in a bank, was a capable individual who liked to be well informed. She had been married to Mr. Johnson for 16 years. Simon, a well-spoken, handsome boy, went to a private high school and was a good student. He was quiet, a loner, and according to his mother had always been that way.

Refusing Chemotherapy, At First

Mr. Johnson was diagnosed with adenocarcinoma of the prostate in the summer of 1994. He had consulted his doctors, complaining of genital pain, and was diagnosed within a month. Two weeks later, scared and angry, he was recovering from a radical prostatectomy. After the surgery. Mr. Johnson's father, who lived in the same city, came to see him. They had not been close and they could not talk now. The distance between them increased as Mr. Johnson's illness progressed. Mr. Johnson was not close to his three brothers or sister, either. His wife was the only family member who was there to support him during his illness.

At the time of the surgery the tumor had spread to the lymphatic system. Although the urologist suggested chemotherapy, Mr. Johnson chose to undergo hormonal treatment. He made this decision himself, without involving Mrs. Johnson. His wife thought the tumor had been removed completely at the time of surgery and that her husband was cured. This discrepancy exemplified an issue that persisted throughout Mr. Johnson's illness: his wife felt left out. In his mind, Mr. Johnson was trying to protect her. As a result, however, when he was unsure of what he should do, he didn't know how to ask his wife for help.

In January 1996, Mr. Johnson developed pneumonia and was readmitted to the hospital. He was found to have liver metastases and recurrent tumor in the pelvis. The oncologist offered him experimental chemotherapy. Again Mr. Johnson refused.

Once again, neither Mr. Johnson nor his physicians involved Mrs. Johnson in the decision, so she tried to get information on her own. She would be on the Internet for hours looking at cancer research, searching for alternative treatments. "But by January," she told me, "it was too late." She resented the fact that she had been kept out of the decision-making process. The doctor had asked her to leave her husband's bedside when they had discussions with him. "Sometimes doctors seem to treat people like they're stupid," she commented. "But doctors have to realize that people have access to treatment information. They read up about it. And doctors should talk to family members because patients will only hear what they want to hear and sometimes the messages don't get through."

The oncologist, Dr. Ron Logan, was a sensitive and mild-mannered man who was ordinarily regarded as having excellent communication with his patients. But he found Mr. Johnson to be a challenge. Mr. Johnson had strong feelings about how he should be treated, and sometimes these feelings seemed to prevent him from hearing information. Two days after Dr. Logan had presented the option of experimental chemotherapy, he had gone back to see Mr. Johnson in his hospital room. Mrs. Johnson was not present. What Dr. Logan had intended to be an exchange of information and a therapeutic encounter turned into a tirade by Mr. Johnson about how oncologists were "just out to poison people." After this meeting Dr. Logan put a note in the chart that expressed (for him) unusual frustration.

> I have spent more than 30 minutes with Mr. Johnson. He swore at me and accused me of entertaining an "infantile approach" with him. Mr. Johnson is very upset because he thinks that I plan to use chemo. My reply to him was that this was a misunderstanding. There will be no chemo. He can read my consult [to this effect] in his file ad libitum.

Mr. Johnson opted to receive more hormonal treatments. In the meantime, his tumors were growing rapidly. He started to experience abdominal and leg pains due to sciatic nerve involvement from a new tumor mass in the pelvic wall. He was given carbamazepine, which helped relieve the pain, though the nurse noted that Mr. Johnson often refused analgesia even if he was in pain. He was afraid to take morphine, especially if it was given by injection.

Toward the end of January, Mr. Johnson went home with a weekend pass. He spoke to Simon about his cancer—for the first time. On his return to hospital, he asked for psychological support for himself and his family. The nurse gave him the name of the cancer support volunteer agency, which he phoned to obtain a referral for therapy that involved visualization techniques. A psychologist taught him this method, which Mr. Johnson subsequently used to try to control his pain.

About Turn

In May 1996, Mr. Johnson was found to have widespread bone metastases and his liver tumors were growing. He complained of fatigue, increasing pain in his right upper abdomen, and right shoulder. All of this was because of his huge liver, most of which was now involved with tumor.

Mrs. Johnson pleaded with him to get another opinion regarding possible treatments. Mr. Johnson was not keen to have treatment, but he did go along with her to see a specialist in another province. The specialist told him about some experimental treatments that were available. Mr. Johnson decided that he was not ready to die. He had been against "poisons" of all sorts and had preferred vitamins and meditation. He had thought for sure that the hormonal treatment would work. Now he saw that he was in trouble. He asked for the experimental chemotherapy. He wondered whether he should have had chemotherapy before this. Linda wondered if she should have pushed her husband sooner.

Back in Montreal, the Johnsons found another oncologist, Dr. Alexander Peters, who agreed to give him the experimental treatments. Mr. Johnson still had many concerns. "Don't take a good day of my life and turn it into a bad day with your treatment," he admonished Dr. Peters. "If I would live 1 month and your drug makes me live two months, but the second month is poor quality, then don't do it."

"No, the odds are better than that," Dr. Peters replied.

Mr. Johnson was admitted to the oncology ward to receive the experimental chemotherapy. His pain was not well controlled. He preferred to put up with pain rather than take an opioid dose that would produce mental clouding and make him feel he was losing control. For pain from his enlarged liver and neuropathic-type pain in his right leg, he was receiving 4 mg hydromorphone orally every 6 hours, 400 mg carbamazepine orally three times daily, and 25 mg amitriptyline at bedtime.

When Dr. Patrick Allan from the Palliative Care service was consulted, he noted that Mr. Johnson was very drowsy from the hydromorphone. He switched him to morphine elixir to "facilitate fine-tuning." Mr. Johnson was also receiving steroids, 30 mg prednisone by mouth daily, which was not only part of the chemotherapy protocol but was also to alleviate his liver pain.

Mrs. Johnson took a leave of absence from her work and spent a large part of every day at her husband's side. She dutifully recorded the medication orders, and every dose that he received, in her notebook, which came to serve as a diary of her husband's condition. Some of Mr. Johnson's physicians had difficulty with this. "At first," Mrs. Johnson recalled to me, "the doctors asked me to leave the room while they did their rounds. And then they realized that I have a few brains, so they started to give me information and asked me what I thought. The junior doctor especially didn't understand why I had so many questions about the blood tests and everything that was happening to my Richard."

After two weeks, Mr. Johnson was discharged home. By the end of June, he began to feel worse. He took to his bed and could not eat solid food. He became more somnolent and had tremors and mild confusion. The physicians felt that this was due to his deteriorating liver function. He was started on 30 ml lactulose by mouth three times daily. Within 2 days he seemed more alert, and the oncologist resumed the experimental chemotherapy.

By July 4, however, Mr. Johnson had not eaten anything in three days because of nausea and vomiting and was readmitted to the medical ward. He had lost 14 pounds in one month, was confused, and showed signs of hepatic encephalopathy. He complained of increasing back pain, abdominal distension, and pain in his swollen right leg. The physicians thought that he might have an infection, so they started intravenous antibiotics. Dr. Peters, the oncologist, noted in the record,

> He is obviously very ill and he knows it. He feels that all his systems are shutting down. I agree that he should be a "no code." However, if he was to improve a bit, I would like to restart his experimental drug, perhaps by the weekend. This admission, and the deterioration, are due to his cancer, not the [experimental] drug. I would ask Palliative Care to see him with a goal of putting him on as little medication as possible.

The medical goal at this time was to try to improve Mr. Johnson's functional state by readjusting any medication that might be making him somnolent, with a view to continuing the experimental treatment. Dr. Peters also wanted Palliative Care to get to know him and the family, to facilitate transfer to the Palliative Care Unit (PCU) when the time was appropriate.

Do-not-resuscitate (DNR) orders were written. These were discussed with Mr. Johnson but not with his wife. When Mrs. Johnson saw the "no code" in the chart, she asked her husband about it. He replied, "Yes, I told them, and don't you change it because I'll never forgive you." He admonished her like this several times.

"How Long Do We Carry on with This?"

Dr. Peters resumed the experimental treatment on July 6. Now, however, Mrs. Johnson wanted it to be stopped. She would follow Patrick Allan, the Palliative Care consultant, into the corridor after many of his visits to her husband. Wiping away tears, she would ask, "How long do we carry on with this?" She looked exhausted. Patrick appreciated how hard it was for her to watch her husband, whom he knew was dying. Still, he would usually answer her by saying something like, "We have to meet him where he is. As long as he wants drugs, I'm not going to tell him to quit. Not because I believe that drugs are going to help, but because I believe that's what he wants."

Mr. Johnson's physical condition seemed to fluctuate dramatically from one day to the next. Over the next few days, Mr. Johnson felt better—his appetite improved, and he became more alert. He began to organize his affairs, preparing his will and discussing plans and finances with his wife. But then his appetite got worse again. When Dr. Allan went to see him this time, he was lying in his bed, his head in the pillow, crying silently. Patrick sat with him.

"I feel so discouraged," Mr. Johnson said, "and so useless. My appetite is gone. When I tell my wife about it, she's upset that I'm not eating more. What am I supposed to do?" Then after a while he said, "What if the pain in my leg gets worse?"

Patrick tried to reassure him. "You know I will continue to do my very best to make sure that you get the right medications that will keep you comfortable."

"I'm sorry," Mr. Johnson said, holding back his tears, "I think I just haven't had enough sleep."

Patrick continued to sit quietly at the bedside. "How's Simon doing?" he asked.

"Oh, he's okay"—the reply that Patrick always heard when he asked after Simon.

Simon was waiting for the day when Mr. Johnson would return home. Although aware of his father's illness, he did not seem to realize its extent or seriousness. Simon found the change in his routine to be difficult. Mrs. Johnson's parents looked after him, but Simon missed his own parents. The social worker arranged a counseling session with Simon and continued to see Mr. and Mrs. Johnson regularly. Other members of the family visited Mr. Johnson infrequently, and his brothers and sisters didn't visit him at all. Mrs. Johnson said that they were afraid of hospitals after what had happened to their mother.

When Patrick saw Mrs. Johnson later that day, she pleaded with him again: "Do you think that we should stop the chemotherapy treatment? Richard is dying." The staff often saw Mrs. Johnson in the family lounge, by herself, crying. But she tried to control herself in the presence of her husband and her son.

By this time, I was visiting Mr. Johnson as part of our project. I saw him in his room on the medical ward. He lay in his bed, dressed in the standard blue hospital gown, too weak to sit up. He was friendly and alert, but his cheeks were sunken. He seemed to be relating well to the other patients in the room; as I walked in, he was trying to support and encourage the man in the bed opposite him.

He spoke with me openly and at length about his life and his values. Even though this was only our second encounter, he spoke about very intimate things.

> Maybe the chemotherapy is working because I feel better this week. I have a great oncologist. He and Dr. Allan—they are doing everything possible. Last week I thought I was dying. But I'm ready to die. I have a lot of faith. I keep saying, "God, if you want to take me, I'm ready." I didn't used to be this way. Five years ago, I was ready to leave my wife. You know, you get married, you go through the honeymoon that could last a few weeks to a couple of years, then children come, and it gets hard. It's not so much fun anymore. I wanted things to be perfect and they weren't perfect, so I wanted to leave. Not that there was another woman. But then something happened to me. I decided to stay. I committed myself, and I began to see things in a different light. I matured. It was a gradual thing, but I realized that my priorities had changed. I know men who get involved in serial marriages, and they don't have solid relationships. There's nothing solid there.

Mr. Johnson spoke about the effect of the treatment on his sexuality. "This room is quite noisy, so I wouldn't mind moving into a single room," he said. "The men around me are very ill, but you know they dream at night, and they have very hot dreams. I know because I can hear them talking in their sleep. You know, I had a chemical castration in March and since then I haven't had such feelings."

"That must have been difficult for you," I said.

"You know, I don't miss it," he replied. "It's good not to be a slave of those feelings."

More Physical Problems

By mid-July, Mr. Johnson had developed clinical signs of ascites and increased leg swelling, which was thought to be related to his low albumin.

He also continued to have abdominal pain. Although there were days when he felt a bit better, the residents felt that this might be the time to ask for a transfer to the PCU. Mr. Johnson was now so weak that he spent all his time in bed, mostly sleeping. Nonetheless, he continued to ask that the chemotherapy be continued.

I went to see him and found him asleep. Linda was seated at his bedside, reading. We went to find a quiet room, and she was tearful as she spoke to me. "I'm all right as long as I don't talk about it," she said. "It's hard for our son. He and his father have been so close. For a large part of when he was growing up his dad was working from home, so they saw a lot of each other. Yesterday Simon said, 'Is Daddy coming home soon?' I couldn't let him know how sick he is. He is used to his dad being in and out of hospital, so I don't think that he realizes that his father is near the end."

She paused and then continued, "Richard wants to have this experimental treatment. That's how he is. He wants to keep on pushing. And I don't know what to say to him. I don't know if Richard wants me around as much as I am. Yesterday I left the hospital early so he would have a break from me."

"He told me that he really appreciates your being here," I said to her. Instead of relief at this remark, however, Linda looked distressed, anxious, and confused.

Over the next few days, Mr. Johnson appeared to be doing better again, his abdominal pain now well controlled. He got out of bed, moving about his room with his walker. He asked that the morphine dosing time be adjusted to decrease sleepiness during mealtimes—perhaps he would then feel like eating more. He became anxious about developing bedsores, wanting everything done to prevent that. According to the nurse, there had never been any signs of bedsores.

A few days later, Mr. Johnson developed shortness of breath, a symptom that is particularly frightening for patients. The resident told Mr. Johnson that his shortness of breath could be from his lung metastases or he could have "water on the lung." The scan for pulmonary emboli was negative, so the resident offered to treat him with diuretics. That evening Mr. Johnson was anxious and frightened that a tumor could be starting to compress his lungs. But the shortness of breath responded to diuresis, so the physicians concluded that he had developed pulmonary edema. Throughout these episodes Linda continued to ask the doctors many questions. Why was the albumin in his blood low? Why had he developed pulmonary edema? As she explained to me, "This keeps my sanity and makes me feel like I have some control. It's just to keep it together. It's my way of coping."

Dr. Peters monitored the prostate-specific antigen (PSA) every week to see if the chemotherapy was working, and every week, Mr. Johnson and his wife would wait anxiously for the result. So far, the PSA had been stable, but the oncologist suspected that it was now rising. Mr. Johnson agreed that he would transfer to the PCU if this were the case. Dr. Peters also offered him another option. If he was responding to the chemotherapy, Mr. Johnson could still go to the PCU and continue to receive the oral chemotherapeutic agent there. Perhaps he would be more comfortable with the specialized nursing care on the PCU, and Dr. Allan could supervise his care more closely.

When I went in to see Mr. Johnson that evening, he was pondering his options. His wife had left for the night. He looked very weak and ill, out of breath despite the oxygen mask. He said, "I would like to go to PCU, no matter what. The only thing is my mother died there 20 years ago. I remember it was a nice sunny place, but she died there, and I still have feeling about that." He paused. "One of the things that bothers me about palliative care is that there is no life there. The nurses are there when you need them, but they come in less often because they are single rooms. Here there are four in a room so there is more action, more life." He talked about how sad he was to leave his son. "I know I could die tonight," he said, "or I could die three months from now."

Mr. Johnson was feeling particularly ill the next evening, so Mrs. Johnson decided she would spend the night with him. Because of general bed shortages in the Canadian hospital system, there is often a wait for beds on the PCU, and this was the case now. The nurses brought Linda a cot so she could sleep beside her husband. This was the first night that she had spent with him since he was admitted to hospital. She was glad that she stayed, for she could note when he had pain and note his reactions to the morphine. She didn't get much sleep, but she didn't care.

The next day Mr. Johnson's pain seemed better, and Mrs. Johnson went home to sleep. Simon was not very happy to see her. He wouldn't talk to her or let his mother kiss him.

"What's wrong? she asked him.

"You didn't come home last night."

Mrs. Johnson explained to him that his father was sicker. She did not tell him that he was dying. Simon did not say anything more that night. The next morning at breakfast, he seemed his old self again. "I understand that Daddy needs you now more than I need you," he said.

The Life Review

Something now changed with Mr. Johnson. He had come to trust Dr. Allan and began to speak to him about his life. He spoke for about 40 minutes, longer than he had ever talked before. He talked about everything. "I've done my work," he said at one point. "I never liked engineering. My father pushed me into it and I did it anyway." He talked about guns, planes, and pain. It seemed to Dr. Allan that he just needed to say who he was. Mrs. Johnson had to leave the room because she was crying so much.

He spoke of the things he had liked, armaments and planes, saying at one point, "When you come to think about it, I would get depressed that all these wonderful inventions do one thing, kill human beings." He was philosophical, asking, "Who am I? Who are we as individuals? We're all nobodies. Nobody's big. If you die, you die, and the world goes on." And then, Dr. Allan recalled, Mr. Johnson related to him that when his mother was dying, somebody called him on the phone and told him he should come right away if he wanted to see his mother alive. "I just could not bring myself to her side," Mr. Johnson recalled. "I went over, but I waited outside and drank coffee or whatever, and then she died. I've sort of felt guilty about that all my life." But then he dropped the subject and started to talk about something else.

Later that day Mr. Johnson said to his wife, "If I go to PCU, it means I'm going to die sooner." It was as if a door opened for the first time. In the meantime, Dr. Allan suggested to them that Mrs. Johnson might want to visit the PCU to get an idea of what it was like.

"It Seemed Gloomy"

Simon saw that arrangements were being made. His aunt had now come to stay with them, and his mother was spending more and more time at the hospital. Mrs. Johnson told me that Simon had come into her bedroom that evening and was more open with her than ever before. He said, "I know that Daddy is dying. He's going to be with his mother, and he'll be able to look down on us. He'll see everything that we do." Mrs. Johnson hugged him, and they cried together. She said to me, "He is 12 years old and he's telling me all this. I hadn't mentioned anything about his father dying."

On the morning of July 27, Mr. Johnson was asleep when I went by the ward. His wife was there, and she followed me out of the room. She said, "He's sleepy because of the morphine. He was having more pain, so they had to increase the morphine from 3 to 4 mg every four hours, by injection. Dr. Allan mentioned something [methylphenidate] that might wake him up a bit. I will ask him about it."

Mr. Johnson was very sensitive to morphine and required very small doses. He also developed side effects very readily. Patrick was trying to fine-tune the medication in a very delicate situation, in the interest of keeping Mr. Johnson as awake and aware as possible, which is what Mr. Johnson wanted. Patrick was considering starting a syringe driver which might better control Mr. Johnson's pain while minimizing somnolence.

Mrs. Johnson said to me, "I went to have a look at the Palliative Care Unit yesterday afternoon. I didn't like it. It was dark. It seemed gloomy. I didn't say that to my husband. I said that it was quiet, there were carpets, so you didn't hear the nurses walking down the hallways, but I didn't like it." However, she did like the idea of her husband being in a single room.

The next morning, Mrs. Johnson left a message for me at the PCU. She knew I was on call and covering for Patrick. She said that her husband had had a bad night. Could I go and check on him? I said I would. For the next two days I added to my researcher role the role of Mr. Johnson's treating physician.

There were no PCU beds available, so Mr. Johnson was still on the medical ward. I checked his medication record and noted that he had required morphine injections every two hours. Mr. Johnson was now on 40 mg of morphine per day subcutaneously, a relatively small amount, but he was receiving it by frequent injections. The syringe driver was not started until later that day. Mr. Johnson had also been more short of breath during the night. The resident had assessed him and had ordered heparin in case he had pulmonary emboli. She ordered a chest X-ray to ensure that Mr. Johnson had not developed a pleural effusion, which could have been drained to relive his breathlessness.

Mr. Johnson was asleep when I went into his room. He had had his 4 mg morphine just one hour before; he was so sensitive to these injections that he became sleepy even with small doses. He wore an oxygen mask, and he looked ill and frail. Mrs. Johnson looked anxious and perturbed, her face pale and puffy. I spoke with her outside the room. She had spent the past two nights with her husband. There was never anyone with her to help her take shifts.

"You look very tired," I began.

"He had a bad night with the pain."

"He might be more comfortable on PCU where the nurses are more used to managing pain medication," I suggested. I could see the hesitation on her face.

"I think he's dying," I whispered to her.

"I know he's dying," she said, somewhat impatiently. "I know that. Dr. Allan said it would be a couple of days. I know that that's just a probability. It could be three weeks. Last night he said, 'I want to go home. I want to go home.'"

"He was confused?" I suggested.

"No, he wasn't confused. I don't know if he meant that he wanted it to be over. But he wasn't confused."

The Palliative Care Unit

Mr. and Mrs. Johnson agreed to transfer to the PCU when a bed became available. Mrs. Johnson hoped that the symptom control would be better there. She asked again about the medical management policies there and was reassured to hear that, apart from the fact that we did not usually use continuous IV drips, the medical care would be no less aggressive. I told her that because her husband was so weak, we were at the point where no further diagnostic tests would be done, whether he stayed on the medical ward or came to the PCU.

Mr. Johnson was transferred on July 29, arriving on the unit with Linda and Simon. Simon stood calmly at his mother's side. I noticed that he looked big for being 12 years old. His blond hair was neatly combed, and he was tastefully dressed. He smiled shyly when I spoke with him. Simon was having difficulty adjusting to the reality of his father's illness and was getting some counseling through his school. The PCU pastoral worker noted, "Simon looks 'too well.' People expect him to behave older than his 12 years because he looks older."

As Mr. Johnson was being settled into his room, Simon said to his mother, "I'm glad Daddy's here. It means he'll get better."

"Daddy's very sick," his mother replied.

Later that day, he said it again: "Daddy's going to get better."

The PCU resident physician noted Mr. Johnson's strong desire to remain alert and to be advised about any proposed changes in medication. The Johnsons' need for meticulous control had been clear to the Palliative Care Service from the beginning. A few days before, Dr. Allan had been visiting on the medical ward when Mr. Johnson needed to use the bedpan. "The angle of the bed had to be just so," Patrick told me. "He asked his wife to adjust the angle, and a few degrees seemed to make a big difference to him."

When I saw Mr. Johnson that afternoon, he was alone in his large single room. There was a comfortable chair beside the bed and plenty of room for a cot if anyone wanted to stay overnight. The room had a pleasant view over the city but was otherwise bleak as Linda had not had the opportunity to bring anything from home. Mr. Johnson did not seem to be in pain but was somnolent and confused, and he looked very ill.

He said to me, "I feel the whole thing is out of control. I don't know what's going on."

I replied, "Your wife is telling us what to do—the medication, everything. It's in her control now. Is that okay?"

"Not one hundred percent," he said.

He said he was thirsty, so I gave him something to drink, even though it was hard for him to manage to drink now. Then he fell asleep. He was still sleepy despite the efforts to minimize the morphine dosage. Dr. Allan had increased his steroids (dexamethasone) in an attempt to keep the morphine dose as low as possible and still control the pain in Mr. Johnson's liver. The challenge was that there was such a narrow margin for error in Mr. Johnson's case. When Mr. Johnson was at home, he would get 6 mg of morphine by mouth and he would be fine. Raising the does to 8 mg would make him somnolent.

"Control is so important to him," Patrick said to me. "I think that he must feel terrible when he is confused. The big question is to decide with Mrs. Johnson when to stop attempting to give him a clear mind. She is always asking, 'Is he getting a little too much morphine?' He was willing to bear pain for the sake of mental clarity. He has been totally clear-minded until today. I discussed methylphenidate with her [an amphetamine to make him more awake], but she refused. Both he and she did not like the idea of any more pills."

"I Don't Know Now Whether I Did the Right Thing"

Mrs. Johnson was getting tired, and she was full of doubts. "I worry that I'm making the wrong decisions," she said to me outside her husband's room. "I want to know what's going on, but then I worry about having to decide. In March, we could not accept that he was dying. We went to see Dr. Peters and asked if he had any treatment at all. I don't know now whether I did the right thing to have encouraged him to do that. Maybe he would have lived longer if he had not followed the treatment?"

She burst into tears. "It's hard seeing someone so young die. And I'm afraid that I won't know what to do after he dies. I've been so involved in looking after him."

She had some questions about how aggressive we were going to be on the PCU. "Would you give him [furosemide] if he developed water on the lung again?" she asked.

"We would do whatever was necessary to keep him breathing as comfortably as possible," I explained. "Sometimes this does involve giving a diuretic."

"How do I know when it's time to restart the morphine again?" she asked doubtfully.

The syringe driver had been temporarily turned off since her husband was so somnolent. Dr. Allan had hoped that he would wake up a bit, but 8 hours later, he had still not awakened. This signaled to me that Mr. Johnson was dying.

"You decide, when you think he's getting uncomfortable again," I suggested, knowing that until now she had wanted to maintain control of the dosage interval.

"I decide? I think a doctor should decide," she replied anxiously—the first time I had seen her wanting to give up control.

On August 1, the nurse reported that Mr. Johnson was confused and restless and sometimes would lash out. At one point the nurse said to him, "I'm your nurse," and Mr. Johnson responded, "Nurses don't—nurses don't deal with cemeteries." He began calling out, "Mommy, help me! Help me!"

The resident physician was notified of Mr. Johnson's distress, and he ordered an immediate subcutaneous does of 2.5 mg midazolam. He also added 5 mg midazolam to the syringe driver, which contained 35 mg morphine and 1 mg haloperidol, to be administered over 24 hours.

The next day, Mr. Johnson was restless when he was turned, but was otherwise unresponsive. He could barely be coaxed to drink small quantities of juice or to suck water from a mouth sponge. Mrs. Johnson was alone with him when I went to visit. Simon had come earlier, with his aunt, but had left. Mrs. Johnson seemed sad, but relatively calm and accepting. She said to me, "He was agitated before and they gave him the tranquilizer and he's more peaceful now. He's bad, isn't he? But I'm talking to him. I'm sure that he can hear me. I think I'll stay with him tonight."

I replied that it might be a good idea. Her father and Mr. Johnson's father also came. Mr. Johnson died at 7:00 that evening, with the three of them present.

"I'm Too Young to Go Through This"

The next week at the PCU rounds, the team signaled Simon as a bereavement risk, noting that even up to the day that his father died, Simon had been hopeful that he would get better. Simon was keeping to himself. Counseling was available through his school, but he refused it. "I don't want anyone to mess with my head," he said.

One month after her husband's death, Linda felt a lump in her breast and underwent a biopsy. Her mother had just been diagnosed with breast cancer. Linda looked extremely anxious and overwhelmed when I saw her. Her biopsy result revealed carcinoma in situ. She was relieved that all she needed was careful follow-up.

Linda went back to work three months after her husband's death. She had regular counseling sessions with a social worker, but, five months into her bereavement she seemed to have more problems than average. She suffered with poor concentration and insomnia. "We tried to get a routine," she told me when I spoke with her at this time. "It was a shock to go back to work. I notice that my memory is not as good as it used to be. I used to have a great memory for details. I can't handle the same volume that I used to, especially when it comes to multitasking. I guess that's normal. I'm taking something to help me sleep that [my family doctor] gave me in October. That's the last time I saw him. Even then I'm usually up at 5:00 A.M."

She continued, "Sometimes I can't understand why Richard's cancer couldn't be controlled. Prostate cancer is supposed to be one of the easiest cancers to control. The surgery went well, but then I don't know what happened. I have a copy of the whole medical file but I can't bear to look at it." She became tearful. "I think about it a lot—everything that happened.

I'm not at peace with everything yet. I think about whether he could have had different care, a different kind of treatment, whether he should have had more aggressive treatment earlier on. Sometimes I think that it's something that I have to live with. I can't let it kill me inside. Sometimes I feel that I'm to blame."

Mrs. Johnson spoke with the social worker at the hospital four or five times, but then the social worker went on maternity leave. Mrs. Johnson didn't want to go for group bereavement counseling, even though this was an option. The social worker said that she would look for one-on-one alternatives for her. The volunteer counselor from the Palliative Care Service also contacted Mrs. Johnson, and they spoke on the telephone a few times. But this did not help. "I still think that bereavement is for older people," Linda said. "I'm too young to go through this."

Mrs. Johnson told me that Simon had some problems paying attention in school, although he managed to get good grades. He would sometimes disrupt class, which his mother believed was an attempt to get attention. He was more socially withdrawn than usual and had given up his sports activities. He didn't talk to anyone except his one good friend. "He doesn't talk about his father much," Linda said. "He keeps it inside. I bring it up but he never brings it up. I give him the opportunity as often as I can. I talk about his father. He was very close to his father. I'm sure that he thinks about his father every day."

At six months, Mrs. Johnson cancelled an interview that I had arranged with her. She sounded tense, like she was trying to keep the lid on things. "I've been up and down and I'm up right now," she explained. "I'm afraid that if I talk to you, it will bring things up and I'll be down again."

She decided to see the Palliative Care Service psychologist and received counseling for three months. Then they somehow lost touch, and Mrs. Johnson decided she would try to handle things on her own. She started to take a benzodiazepine daily, commenting to me, "I don't think it's a good thing to take in the long term, but it's a security for me."

One year after her husband's death, Mrs. Johnson was still having difficulties. Even with the tranquilizer, she slept only two or three hours every night. The volunteer bereavement counselor continued to telephone her, asking her if she wanted more intensive counseling. Mrs. Johnson was considering this. Simon, meanwhile, was back to his old self—the quiet loner.

Authors' Comments

This narrative is disturbing for several reasons. First, Mr. Johnson was a relatively young man, dying of prostate cancer—a disease that usually affects older men. Second, he was very sensitive to opioids, easily developing side effects such as somnolence. He had neuropathic and bony pain that proved difficult to control. This is another case where present protocols might include the early use of methadone. Third, a child was involved: Simon was twelve years old when his father developed advanced cancer. This case shows the reaction of a child, and it demonstrates how school and community services can work alongside palliative care services to assess and provide support to children who are facing the death of a parent.

Mr. Johnson had some comorbidities and had experienced life events that likely contributed to the difficulties that he experienced at the end of his life. He had a history of bipolar disorder. His mother had died on the same palliative care ward when Mr. Johnson was 31 years old. He suffered from generalized anxiety, made worse if he felt that he was not in control of a situation. He seemed to be a socially isolated man.

Mr. Johnson was afraid to die but found it difficult to discuss his feelings with the healthcare team. He was even afraid to share feelings of fear or sadness with his wife, though she was constantly at his side. He pushed hard to get aggressive cancer treatments even when there was a low chance that these would prolong his life.

Mr. Johnson's fear of losing control was with him to the very end. He was unable to trust his wife to make decisions on his behalf. He trusted no one. He stated that he was a religious, church-going Catholic. Yet his faith seemed to bring him no comfort. Compounding the situation was that his wife seemed to have similar difficulties. She wanted some control, but then experienced doubt and guilt. These feelings continued throughout the bereavement follow-up period, leading to what palliative care practitioners refer to as *complicated grief* or *mourning*. Many programs offer bereavement services to families to try to address these problems.

Complex medical and psychosocial scenarios such as this are common in palliative care. Sometimes, even with our best efforts, we fail to make the situation "all better."

16

Jenny Doyle

"It Is So Nice to Know that You Have Not Been Given Up on"

Narrated by Yanna Lambrinidou

Jenny Doyle, a 47-year-old White American woman with inflammatory breast cancer, received end-of-life care for eight-and-a-half months, much longer than is typical for a US hospice program. Her time with hospice was tumultuous, marked by periods of anger and resentment amid others of gratitude and affection. She fought her disease bitterly to the very end. Her struggle led her to a series of doctors and created serious tensions for the hospice team. Throughout this journey, the legacy of early years of strife with her children created additional stresses and strains, which persisted in the bereavement period. "At least let the moment of her death be peaceful," her family prayed. But even that was not to be.

A Rebel with a Cause

Jenny Doyle was a stout, White American woman with wavy brown hair, a pronounced chin, rosy cheeks, and a smile that emphasized her bright eyes. Her high-pitched voice, fast speech, and excited tone revealed an intensity about her that many of her loved ones cherished. Since 1983, she had worked as an administrative assistant for a manufacturing company. Her office was on the first floor of a dilapidated building with leaky pipes, excessive damp-ness, and a steady wave of insects. The mold on the walls and monthly spray of insecticides that lodged into the carpet brought out allergies in many employees. Some filed complaints with the company's management, even though they lacked proof connecting their declining health to their workplace. When two of Mrs. Doyle's co-workers announced they had cancer, Mrs. Doyle was convinced that her office building was contaminated. In May 1995, after a series of doctors' appointments, medical tests, and missed workdays, she was diagnosed with occupational asthma. Her physician gave her a letter stating that her work environment was detrimental to her health. She was immediately transferred to a branch office. For the days that she had to skip work, she filed a workers' compensation lawsuit against her employer.

Two months into the trial, Mrs. Doyle was diagnosed with inflammatory breast cancer, an aggressive form of the disease that often makes its first appearance as a dermatological irritation. She was 47 years old with two adult children. She had been remarried only nine months earlier. Her dreams for a new life with a man she loved were shattered. Her initial desire for worker's compensation suddenly turned into a desire for revenge. Although her lawsuit addressed her asthma, not her cancer, she was determined to win it.

In September, Mrs. Doyle started four courses of chemotherapy. The treatment was hard on her, but she continued to work. Her co-workers recognized her for being the only employee to take a stand against the company. Affectionately, they named her "the rebel with a cause." Mrs. Doyle was flattered. "If the cause is my life, you bet I'm going to be a rebel!" she laughed. She made a T-shirt saying, "I am not calling in sick. I am calling in dead." She was going to give it to her supervisor when she won the lawsuit.

In November, after disputing the company's claim that the air at work did not pose a health risk and refusing to return to the main office, she lost her job. She was now forced to rely on her husband's limited income as well as donations from co-workers, relatives, and friends.

Then a fourth co-worker was diagnosed with cancer.

To educate herself about her disease, Mrs. Doyle joined a support group. She liked these meetings because they gave her the opportunity to learn and help at the same time. She exchanged information and advice. She cried and laughed. The third time she went, a woman announced that her cancer had metastasized to her liver. Six weeks later, she died. Mrs. Doyle was shocked. For the first time, she had come face-to-face with the deadliness of her disease. She wanted access to new treatments.

Mrs. Doyle's oncologist, John Silverman, invited her into an experimental study for early-stage inflammatory breast cancer. The research was looking at the effect of bone marrow transplant on the disease. Mrs. Doyle agreed. Since her tumors had not spread beyond her breast and local lymph nodes, she was admitted to the hospital for three weeks. There, she underwent a preventive double mastectomy as well, and she consented to a five-week course of radiation to her chest wall and lymph nodes. She returned home with renewed hope. She had finally entered the frontline of the battle against inflammatory breast cancer. By September 1996, 13 months after her initial diagnosis, she had done everything she could to contain her disease. That thought in itself reassured her. Now, every day, she waited anxiously for mailings with updates on the bone marrow study.

In January of the following year, after a bout of intense pain between her shoulder blades, she learned that her cancer had metastasized to her spine. Dr. Silverman said that she had one year to live. To control her pain, he prescribed slow-release morphine. He also suggested radiation, chemotherapy, or radioactive strontium. Mrs. Doyle chose the first. Radiologist Larry Stein explained that this round of radiation, in contrast to the first, would be strictly palliative. "A lot of what we try to do [at this stage]," Larry told me, "is keep people as functional as possible during their care. Jenny makes it easy because she is very positive, and she always gets better. One of these times she won't, and that will be sad, but [up until now] all of our interactions with Jenny have been good because she gets better, so that makes it a lot easier on everybody—myself, the therapist who gives her the treatment, and Jenny."

Mrs. Doyle remained optimistic. But she noticed that the mailings about the bone marrow study had stopped. To her dismay, she learned that she had been dropped from the research because her cancer had spread. When I saw her, she exclaimed,

> You are no longer part of the study, so they don't share any information with you then. You lose your information rights, so to speak. You think, "What? Is it only for women who they think have been cured by the bone marrow transplant?" You get the feeling that you are detrimental to their program or their funding. Like if they cannot show a certain amount of success rate they would lose their funding. And I think that's what it's all about.

Calling Hospice

Mrs. Doyle envisioned herself dying as quickly as the woman in her support group. "Since the girl ahead of me with this disease died so very quickly," she said, "I thought it was probably to my advantage to have hospice. It took her about six weeks to pass away. She went very quickly." She was admitted to the home care program of the Hospice of Lancaster County on February 6, 1997. The next day, she met Lucy Stephens, her hospice nurse, and Sandra Dunn, her social worker. Sandra spent her first visit asking Mrs. Doyle about her life.

Mrs. Doyle was born and raised in Lancaster County, where both of her parents still lived. She married in 1966 and had a daughter, Kim, who was 28, and a son, Peter, who was 25. That marriage dissolved. Kim maintained a cordial but distant relationship with her mother, and Peter was not in speaking terms with her. In 1992, Mrs. Doyle met Andrew Doyle. They wed two years later. But there was something inauspicious about her second union. Nine months in, Jenny was diagnosed with inflammatory breast cancer, and a year later her husband had a heart attack. Mr. and Mrs. Doyle's short life together had already been burdened by chemotherapy, a bone marrow transplant, a double mastectomy, radiation, and bypass surgery.

Sandra noticed that the upbeat, positive, and energetic tone of Mrs. Doyle's delivery didn't match the gravity of her words. Mrs. Doyle spoke fast. She came across as self-assured, fearless, and good-humored. She expressed concern about the coping abilities of her family but said little about herself. She worried for Kim and Mr. Doyle, who had lost many members of his family to cancer. Her husband had no support system of his own and seemed to cope with his wife's illness by pretending it didn't affect him. Mrs. Doyle wanted him to get help.

Mrs. Doyle assured Sandra that she was all right. She was working with a wonderful counselor, who offered her services for free. She had a strong faith in God and a supportive spiritual community. The only help she wanted was asking the landlord for permission to break their lease. She was already having difficulty climbing the stairs to the second floor. She and Andrew had found a first-floor apartment they liked, but could not possibly afford two rents. Sandra called the landlord immediately. On March 1, the Doyles moved into their new apartment. That day, Mrs. Doyle noticed that when she tried to lift light items, she felt a dull pain in her shoulder.

In the new apartment, Mrs. Doyle found herself spending her days watching television and visiting with friends. On the weekends, the Doyles took day trips to the seashore or went to dance clubs. Traveling and dancing were Mrs. Doyle's favorite activities. Although she was still ambulatory, she followed Dr. Silverman's recommendation to get a wheelchair. Prompted by Lucy and Sandra, she also named the people who would be able to help her when she needed more intensive care. Andrew was one. Her father and daughter would also be available. So would her mother, even though Jenny did not feel comfortable around her. She was too negative, critical, and unsympathetic. Her son, Peter, lived in New York and would not be able to stay with her for long periods of time.

In early April, a second woman in the support group died. Mrs. Doyle was devastated. Five days after the funeral, she awoke with excruciating pain in her left shoulder. It took her a double dose of oxycodone to get back to sleep. But she continued to feel low-grade discomfort. Tests showed further metastasis. She now had two small tumors in her shoulder socket and one on her collar bone. She started a third course of radiation. After the first treatment, she told Lucy that her arms felt sore, she coughed frequently, had lost her appetite, and was tired. "Otherwise, I am well," she asserted, moving on to a happier subject. Kim had gotten engaged. She and her fiancé had just announced that they were getting married in Europe in October. On the first weekend of November, they were going to hold a wedding reception in Lancaster County. Mrs. Doyle was delighted. November seemed far away, but she felt confident she would be well enough to make an appearance at her daughter's reception.

Lucy was relatively new at hospice and had never met a dying patient with the feistiness of Mrs. Doyle. She told me,

> She is so upbeat and accepting of everything, much more so than me. I am just wondering if it's all show for everybody, and if underneath she is really scared to death, or if this is really just Jenny. But everyone says this is how she had been with everything all along. I actually admire her for being able to handle it like that, because I know I could not. I am an upbeat person for the most part, but if it came to something like that, I know I could not be as upbeat as she is. I know when her time comes it is going to be difficult for me. I am feeling somewhat attached to her. I try not to be, but you cannot help but be sometimes with her. It is just that she pulls you in. I actually miss the weeks when I don't get to go out and see her.

Sandra, the social worker, had a different reaction. "I find it almost a difficult thing about Jenny," she observed, "that you talk about hard things, and she always uses this very bright tone of voice. The affect and the content just don't go together. Maybe she is dealing with things internally or with her counselor. I don't know. Sometimes you are not sure exactly where she's at." Mrs. Doyle's independence, self-sufficiency, and close relationship with her counselor made Sandra feel like "a fifth wheel" in her care. Still, she found it important to build a good relationship with her patient. She wanted to be prepared for the day when Mrs. Doyle would be unable to visit her counselor and would turn to hospice for emotional support.

"I Know I Have Done Things Wrong"

At the end of April, Mrs. Doyle invited Kim and Peter to one of her counseling sessions. She had something to tell them and needed her counselor's support. In the counselor's office, she admitted that she had not been a perfect mother. "I know I have done things wrong," she said. She didn't delve into details, but her implied repentance made Kim and Peter cry. Both promised to stay by their mother's side until the very end. The rift between Mrs. Doyle and her children went back 15 years, when Kim and Peter's father abused Kim. Mrs. Doyle sent her daughter away temporarily with the promise that she was going to make things safe before letting her back. But that promise was never realized, and, after some time, she invited Kim to return. Kim refused. She moved in with her grandparents and kept minimal contact with her parents. From her perspective, they had not only betrayed her, but they were now pouring all their love into her little brother.

When Peter was in college, Kim remembered telling her mother, "Mom, it looks like you screwed up so bad with your first kid that you just brushed that one under the rug, and you did everything you could to make the second one work out okay. I mean, you didn't send him to live with someone else, you sent him to college, you supported him, you were at his high school graduation. You didn't do any of those things for me, and I didn't just vanish. I am still here, and I am still hurt, and I am still wondering why." As if in reply, Mrs. Doyle stopped paying for Peter's education and asked him to move out of the house. In 1994, Peter relocated to New York. He developed a drinking problem. "I felt responsible for that," Kim said to me. Since then, Kim recalled that she and her parents vacillated between periods of closeness and distance. Peter hadn't made any effort to stay in touch with his mother. When he learned about her terminal diagnosis he said, "Well, it's not like I know what it is like to have a mom right now anyway."

"They Tell You in the Video: 'This Is Not a Cure'"

In the first week of May, Mrs. Doyle began using the wheelchair. The palliative radiation to her spine had caused her blood count to drop, which made her weak. She had lost her appetite and experienced increased constipation and shoulder pain. Her hips ached. Her radiologist suggested radioactive strontium. Just one shot of this substance, Dr. Stein told her, had the capacity to bring her long-term comfort. Mrs. Doyle's understanding was that the strontium could alleviate her pain for three to six months, free her of her need for narcotic analgesics, give her flexibility, and possibly prevent further metastases. She consented to it after watching a promotional video and confirming that her health insurance would cover the medication's high cost. Although she spoke excitedly about it, she always added, "They tell you in the video: 'This is not a cure.'"

Because of its radioactive properties, strontium needed to be handled with care. For one week after receiving it, Mrs. Doyle was instructed to ensure that no one was exposed to her bodily fluids. And, if she were to die within six months, her body would be considered hazardous and, therefore, ineligible for cremation. Lucy was apprehensive. "Jenny is really almost hoping for a miracle," she said. "Not as far as a cure, but as far as being able to go off almost all her medications and increasing her level of functioning. But my understanding is that strontium either works—and when it works it is fantastic—or it doesn't work. There is no in-between."

Mrs. Doyle had the injection on May 23. I saw her five days later. When I arrived at her apartment, she opened the door, greeted me with a big smile, and walked back to the couch with ease. She was wearing sweatpants and a white T-shirt. She looked comfortable. She told me that the reason she agreed to participate in our study was because she wanted to educate others about inflammatory breast cancer and remind the medical establishment that this disease deserved further investigation. She was almost pain-free and had gained flexibility. She had been able to cut her nightly dose of oxycodone in half and hoped that soon she could eliminate it. She had also been able to dance. If these improvements were to last six months, she calculated, she would be eligible for a second shot and would live well for a whole year. "I am a little radioactive," she giggled, explaining that she had to wash her clothes separately from her husband's, flush the toilet twice, bring her own utensils to restaurants, and wash her dishes with special care. "We circled on the calendar when I do not have to do this anymore," she said.

Mrs. Doyle told me she had noticed that Kim was looking at her curiously. She suspected that her daughter was surprised by her restored limberness and afraid of her radioactivity. At the same time, Kim's newfound optimism about her condition bothered her. Mrs. Doyle was aware that she had not been cured and that her prognosis had not been extended. When Kim asked her to buy herself a dress for the wedding reception in November, Mrs. Doyle told her that she preferred to wait until she was sure she would be able to attend. "That's a defeatist attitude!" Kim exclaimed.

Strontium's magic didn't last. Within three weeks, Mrs. Doyle returned to her original medication doses. Her blood count remained low. She felt extremely weak, and pain returned to her right hip and left shoulder. Dr. Stein said that it was normal for her condition to worsen before it got better. This gave her hope. For the July 4th holiday, she and her husband booked a four-day vacation to Las Vegas. They had always wanted to visit Las Vegas. "I will put $10 in the slot machine, and then that will be it," Jenny laughed. The Doyles could not wait to attend variety shows, go dancing, enjoy the sun, and relax together. Until then, they intended to spend a quiet month at home.

"We Kind of Feel as If We Have to Be the Voice of Reality"

In the middle of June, the pain spasms in Mrs. Doyle's right hip worsened. Her discomfort persisted even after a doubled dose of oxycodone. In a matter of days, she lost nine pounds. An X-ray revealed cancer metastasis to both her hips and pelvis. John Silverman, the oncologist, instructed her to replace the oxycodone with 100 mg of slow-release morphine twice a day. He also advised her to take the Las Vegas vacation immediately. The way her cancer was spreading, he said, made it difficult for him to imagine how she would have the strength for a long trip in July. Mrs. Doyle found her doctor alarmist.

Hospice staff were startled to hear that Mrs. Doyle questioned Dr. Silverman's judgment. In their estimation, her disease was progressing much faster than she realized. Her life expectancy had probably dropped to weeks. A supervising nurse asserted that it was time for her to start preparing for her death. She instructed Lucy and Sandra to pay their patient an informational visit in order to explain to her the gravity of her condition. Nervously, Lucy called Mrs. Doyle and made an appointment for the following day. "I dreaded that visit," Lucy told me later. "It is like when you have an exam, and even though you studied, you just have this sinking feeling in the pit of your stomach you don't want to take it, even though you know the answers. I just had that sinking feeling in the pit of my stomach all day long, because I felt like I was dropping a bomb." Sensing the nervousness in Lucy's voice, Mrs. Doyle asked her husband to join the meeting. She also called her attorney, told him she was dying, and urged him to put pressure on the judge to make a decision about her case—two years had already passed since the filing of the lawsuit. And she called her travel agent to cancel their vacation.

The next day, in the Doyles' living room, Lucy looked Mrs. Doyle in the eyes and explained that hospice was concerned about her. The strontium had failed both in alleviating her pain and preventing a new metastasis. Radiation was not a solution, either. It worked only temporarily. Plus, many of the spots on her body had already received the maximum amount. Her disease was progressing rapidly. Her prognosis was now in the range of weeks rather than months. If she still wanted to go to Las Vegas, she had better leave soon. And if she wanted to make her will or tie up loose ends with loved ones, this was the time to do it.

Everyone cried. Mr. Doyle hugged his wife and assured her that he would take family medical leave to stay at her side. Mrs. Doyle told Lucy and Sandra that the trip to Las Vegas was off. She talked about the anger she harbored for her supervisor at work. She felt it was time to send him the T-shirt, but her attorney advised her against that. Mrs. Doyle gave Sandra permission to contact her parents and children, as she would need their support. At the end of the meeting, a tearful Mr. Doyle escorted Lucy and Sandra to their cars. Softly, he asked if cremation was going to be an option. Lucy explained that it was not. The crematorium would not accept Mrs. Doyle's body before November.

Mrs. Doyle bought baby gifts for the grandchildren she expected would arrive but that she would never get to see. She also got into the habit of checking her mailbox daily for the judge's decision. And she returned to Dr. Stein for radiation to ease the pain in her sacrum and ilium. To her surprise, Dr. Stein gave her a different picture of her condition. Having seen not only her X-ray but also her most recent blood tests, he concluded that her death was not imminent at all. Yes, her cancer had spread to her hips and pelvis, which meant that the strontium had probably not worked, but there was no reason to believe that her prognosis had changed. Her major organs—lungs, liver, and kidneys—still seemed healthy.

Mrs. Doyle suddenly saw the meeting with Lucy and Sandra in a different light. She was furious that, on the basis of a single X-ray, her hospice team had felt it was their duty to convince her that she was dying. "How could they do this?" she asked angrily as she told me about the news from Dr. Stein. "Lucy had the need to show me that her way was right—almost maybe to scare me into seeing what she thought was the truth, and that caused a lot of pain, a lot of pain. I guess it kind of opened my eyes. This is one of the complaints that I understand there is with hospice. They sometimes tell the patient the way they perceive things, and that is not always correct."

When Lucy heard Dr. Stein's assessment, she said to me, "I don't think [Jenny] is going to go downhill as quickly as I was thinking before our meeting. My nursing supervisor really thought that she would not be here come the 4th of July. I don't know. Jenny is a fighter. Now here we are, June 18, and I cannot see her not being here in three weeks." Sandra was also disturbed by the fact that she had sounded what now seemed like a false alarm. At the same time, she saw a positive side to the meeting: it at least prompted Mrs. Doyle to think seriously about her death. She elaborated:

> Because of what we do, we maybe tend to lean more on the negative— forecasting the worst—and then sometimes it does not happen that way. I guess I feel like it is still better to err that way and have things turn out better than to be looking on the bright side and not be prepared. We may tend to lean more on the negative, because we know that out there in the world people don't know about death, don't understand about death, don't expect death, and therefore are working hard to believe that it is not coming. We kind of feel as if we have to be the voice of reality.
>
> I don't think that talking to somebody about dying really hurts that much. For us to do that with Jenny did not make it happen any sooner, it did not really do anything to hurt, it probably was good. The vision of Jenny going out to Las Vegas and dying there was pretty upsetting, and that was enough to make you get in there and really say something.

Sandra was confident that Mrs. Doyle understood hospice's perspective. In her last conversation with her, she had sensed no anger or tension. But she did wonder if Mrs. Doyle was always transparent. Did she feel resentment toward hospice after that meeting? Did she hold a grudge against her and Lucy? Had she lost her trust in them, but was unable to say so?

Mrs. Doyle considered complaining about Lucy and requesting a new nurse. Yet she liked Lucy. Lucy had shared many aspects of her life with her. Among other things, she had told her that she was a single mother. She had also shown her photographs of her youngest child who was chronically ill. Mrs. Doyle did not want Lucy to lose her job. At the same time, she saw herself as stronger and healthier than the patients hospice seemed designed to serve. "Maybe I shouldn't be in this program yet," she said to me. She was clearly not ready to die. To the contrary, she planned to start driving again as soon as her hips allowed.

The day I saw her, she was pale and cold. I could hear a catch in her breathing. Sitting under an electric blanket and a heating pad, she attributed her chills to the radiation. She had just finished her 52nd treatment. She was thankful for all the therapies she had received. Even the strontium had been worth it to her. She wanted to get it again as soon as she could. It had eased her shoulder pain and, in her opinion, couldn't have possibly prevented her metastasis. The pain in her hip had appeared before the administration of the shot. To her, this suggested that the metastasis had occurred before her treatment. She was disappointed that Dr. Stein had a different opinion about the strontium's success. And she was hurt by the fact that he didn't kiss her on the last day of her treatment. Larry always kissed her goodbye. She worried that this shift signaled his discouragement.

A Sister in the Struggle

By July, the occasional catch in Mrs. Doyle's breathing had become more regular. Her slow release morphine was increased from 100 mg to 130 mg twice a day. The rest of her medications included the hormonal treatments anastrozole and megestrol, a diuretic, an antiemetic, and prednisone. To Mrs. Doyle, every day that passed without a new intervention that could prolong her life seemed like a waste. She was eager to meet Dr. Valerie Richards, a friend's oncologist. Valerie told her that she wasn't hospice-appropriate. Mrs. Doyle's voice filled with fervor when she recounted the doctor's words: "When I see someone functioning as well as you are—walking, talking, breathing, telling me that they are caring for their apartment, telling me that they are looking to get back to driving and things like this—this does not spell 'hospice patient' to me," she asserted.

Dr. Richards conducted experimental research trials. She told Mrs. Doyle that if her major organs were cancer-free she would be eligible for new treatments. Mrs. Doyle was filled with hope. When she informed Dr. Silverman about this development, he sounded disapproving. He doubted that enrolling in another experiment would benefit her. His pessimism disturbed her. But it didn't stop her from traveling a long distance to see Dr. Richards. Mrs. Doyle described her new physician as an extraordinary person who was determined to fight breast cancer with all her might. Valerie had lost her own mother to breast cancer and was a breast cancer survivor herself. "It is a relief to know that we have a sister in the struggle," Mrs. Doyle declared. She then told Lucy that if her cancer had not affected her major organs, she would leave hospice. "It is so nice to know that you have not been given up on," she told me.

More than anything, Mrs. Doyle wanted to attend Kim's wedding reception in November. If she could, she also hoped to see her first grandchild. The next time she spoke with Lucy, she announced that she was switching physicians. Lucy was happy for her. "Be it beneficial or not physically," she said to me, "this is something Jenny needs to do, and if she needs to do that, I have to stand behind her. I think emotionally it is helping her a lot." Lucy felt reassured that her patient didn't see Dr. Richards's interventions as a cure. She also called Dr. Richards to confirm that her work with Mrs. Doyle was strictly palliative. Valerie assured her that her goal was to give Mrs. Doyle comfort and, in the best of circumstances, buy her more time. "That pretty much falls right in line with hospice's philosophy," said Lucy after hanging up the phone.

On July 10, Mrs. Doyle received an infusion of the bone resorption inhibitor, pamidronate. Valerie thought this was an appropriate treatment, for it had the potential to strengthen Mrs. Doyle's bones without compromising her blood count. Already, Mrs. Doyle's platelets were so low that she was covered with bruises. Her appetite and overall energy quickly improved. Her spirits soared. Now that she had gained some strength, she started dreaming of a weekend trip to the Atlantic coast.

"Stay Tuned for Jenny. She's Always a Surprise!"

The Doyles returned from the coast rejuvenated. Mrs. Doyle's blood count had started to rise, and her bruises had faded. On July 23, Dr. Richards announced that, according to Mrs. Doyle's test results, her major organs were healthy. Once her platelets reached a normal level, she would be able to receive chemotherapy. Mrs. Doyle was ecstatic. "We made it over that hurdle!" she exclaimed with relief. But six days later, she woke up with excruciating pain. She assumed she had broken a rib. Soon after her husband left for work, she started to vomit. Somehow, she managed to hit the speed dial button on the phone to speak to Lucy. Lucy rushed over. From the Doyles' apartment, she called hospice to arrange for 24-hour in-home nursing care. She also contacted Dr. Richards, who asked to see Mrs. Doyle as soon as possible.

Dr. Richards determined that Mrs. Doyle had not fractured a rib. The problem was that her blood count had dropped even further. In response, she administered a second infusion of pamidronate. A few days later, Lucy told me that I would not believe the changes in Mrs. Doyle. She had regained her energy. Although her appetite remained poor, she felt no pain. Once again, she was able to walk by herself to the mailbox at the bottom of the driveway. Another hospice nurse was standing nearby listening to Lucy's report. "Stay tuned for Jenny," she interjected laughingly. "She's always a surprise!"

"Before I Opened the Letter, I Said a Little Prayer"

On August 22, when Lucy arrived at the Doyles' for a scheduled visit, she found a note on the front door. Mrs. Doyle had won the lawsuit. She had been awarded worker's compensation from the day her company ordered her to return to the main office until the last day of her life. I saw her a few days later. She beamed with happiness. "Everybody is really happy for me over this!" she said. And she continued,

> Before I opened the letter, I said a little prayer. I said, "Please, God, please!" At first, I just read the back part for myself that I had won. I was so happy that day. I just feel vindicated. I feel that justice did prevail, and it makes you believe in the system again.

Our conversation turned quickly to Kim's wedding reception. Two hundred people were invited to a sit-down dinner and ballroom dance. Mrs. Doyle not only planned to attend, she also took it upon herself to organize a bachelorette party in September. She giggled. Kim had requested a male stripper, and it was Mrs. Doyle's job to find one. Things looked good. The Doyles decided to use some of the worker's compensation payments to rebook their vacation to Las Vegas. This time it would be a 10-day trip, and it would include not only Nevada but also New Mexico and Arizona. It was tentatively planned for the beginning of September. When I asked Lucy what she thought about it, she said,

> Thrilled for her and baffled for me. She is like a Timex. She takes a licking and keeps on ticking. No matter what setbacks she has, she seems to come out of them with flying colors, so you are not quite certain if the next setback is going to be the final one, or if she is going to bounce back again. I am really stunned that she's doing so well, but have a feeling when she really, truly does start to go back, it is going to be a quickie, because she had so much metastasis in there. I know she wants to make it to her daughter's wedding, which is in November I guess, and boy, at the rate she's going, there is a chance she might.

Mr. Doyle saw this vacation as an opportunity to "regroup" with his wife and experience intimacy in an environment that wasn't dominated by her illness. Mrs. Doyle's cancer had become greater than a mere disease, he told me. It was a way of life. The undivided attention it demanded had led them to neglect other parts of their lives. "We have lost a lot of the physical contact," Mr. Doyle said. "Not that I want the moon, the sun, and the world, but it's time to get away and try to get back to a little bit of normalcy, along with relaxing and doing things couples do."

When the Doyles returned from the Southwest, Mrs. Doyle felt hopeful and strong, despite the fact that she was tired, puffy from her corticosteroid, and low on platelets. She was dismayed, however, to learn that, while she was away, Lucy had left hospice. Mrs. Doyle had grown close to Lucy and trusted her as a nurse. Dr. Richards, too, was sorry to hear the news. She worked well with Lucy. And she liked the fact that Lucy had shown a real interest in keeping Mrs. Doyle out of pain. Valerie appreciated the "free rein" given to her by hospice. She was confident that the pamidronate infusions helped Mrs. Doyle with her pain and spared her from further radiation. But she saw a fine and unclear line between mere symptom management and aggressive treatment. On the one hand, she asserted that what she was giving Mrs. Doyle was palliative. On the other hand, she explained that the category "palliative" was contestable. "I think everything I do is palliative," she said, "but there is 'palliative' and 'palliative.' I mean, there is palliative like giving morphine, and there is palliative like giving intravenous hydration, blood products, the pamidronate. That is kind of pushing it."

Mrs. Doyle's case was transferred to another nurse, Roberta Smalley.

"My Mom Is a Very Big Part of My Life"

The male stripper brought laughs and blushes to Kim's bachelorette party guests. The wedding was now around the corner. Kim was scheduled to leave for Europe on October 11. She would be gone for three weeks. The possibility that Mrs. Doyle wouldn't be alive when she returned frightened her. She instructed Peter to keep her abreast of every emergency. She explained to her fiancé that if her mother were to decline, she would return home.

Mrs. Doyle seemed well. For the first time, she even talked about the dress she planned to wear at Kim's reception. She expected to be alive for at least a few more months. She even hoped that her platelets would allow her to start chemotherapy. Kim was less optimistic. She had learned not to take anything for granted. Tearful, she said,

> I think things are good, and that is when I get scared. Am I missing something? I was with Mom last night, and I was paying attention to her, and I did not see anything. She looks great, she is acting fine, she is energetic to the point that she can really talk about her trip. My mom is a very big part of my life. She is this vital person, this source of energy and enthusiasm, and she is a friend. She is someone I want to embrace and hold on to. I am going to lose so much. My criticisms of her are just kind of part of the background now. I can see her, appreciate her, and love her just because she is who she is.

For the first time in her life, Kim said, she felt proud of being Jenny Doyle's daughter.

Mrs. Doyle saw Kim and her fiancé off to Europe. She gave them her blessing and insisted that they stop worrying about her. "I wished they could take me with them," she told me. Upon her return home, she found her first worker's compensation check in the mailbox. Three days later, she started to vomit uncontrollably. She experienced severe pain and shortness of breath. Mr. Doyle took her to the nearest hospital. Her platelets had dropped so low that she was instructed to stay for inpatient treatment. She had multiple bruises on her arm, abdomen, and back. Her face, neck, and arms were puffy. She received a blood transfusion immediately.

Sandra, the hospice social worker, was shocked to hear about this development. When she visited Mrs. Doyle at the hospital, Mrs. Doyle spoke non-stop, leaving no room for conversation. To Sandra, this was a façade. Behind Mrs. Doyle's confident appearance, she saw fear. On her way out, she looked at Mrs. Doyle's chart. In it, she saw a letter from Dr. Richards, written a few months earlier. It said that Mrs. Doyle was too active to be hospice-appropriate. "Well, you know," Sandra said to me, "if Dr. Richards communicated that to Jenny, that certainly puts a distance between Jenny and us."

"I Think I'm Dying"

I visited Mrs. Doyle on October 17. She was lying in bed with an oxygen mask. Her nose was bleeding, her head and extremities looked hard and swollen, and her eyes were yellow. She struggled to stay alert. She kept her words to a minimum, but she managed to tell me that she was "hanging in there." Mr. Doyle was sitting by her side. The rhythmic sound of machines filled the heavy silence.

Suddenly the phone rang. It was a friend of Mrs. Doyle's. Mrs. Doyle started to cry. "I think I'm dying," she said with a frightened tone, as tears rolled down her cheeks. Her friend told her she would be there right away. Mrs. Doyle turned to us and said she was confused. She had a look of horror on her face. She sobbed. She wanted to know what was happening to her. Mr. Doyle leaned over the bed railing and looked his wife in the eyes. "Your platelets are low," he said softly. He started to cry. His voice shook. "Probably they won't be able to raise them, Jenny," he said. Had any doctor said she was . . .? She couldn't say the word. Mr. Doyle shook his head. The tension on Mrs. Doyle's face eased. If she were dying, she said, she wanted the opportunity to speak to her parents, her cousins, and Peter. Mr. Doyle reminded her that her parents had visited her that morning and lived close enough to come again. Her cousins were available, too, and Peter was on his way from New York.

Mr. Doyle invited me to join him in the lounge. He looked distraught. He had not slept in days. He cried. He told me that he didn't know what to do. He knew his wife was dying, but he didn't know how to tell her that, or when. Peter was scheduled to arrive the next day. Kim had just gotten married in Europe, but because Mrs. Doyle did not want to ruin her trip, Mr. Doyle wasn't going to notify her about her mother's condition. Lucy was the only person he would have felt comfortable calling for help. When I mentioned Sandra, he had difficulty remembering who she was. He cried some more, then he laughed, then he cried. He was tired, he said. Somehow, he needed to take care of himself as well.

Before I left, a nurse walked into Mrs. Doyle's room. As she was giving her a blood transfusion, Mrs. Doyle pointed upward to show us a bird flying in the room. We all looked up, but saw nothing.

"Jenny Is Gone in Spirit, but Her Body Is Still Here"

Two days later, Mrs. Doyle was informed that her cancer had metastasized to her liver. She asked to be kept comfortable and spared from further blood transfusions. She was no longer able to get out of bed. She required a urinary catheter. Her respirations were shallow and labored. She was given an anti-anxiety medication for a panic attack. She requested a pill that would help her die. Peter was by her side. He left a message on his sister's answering machine, asking her to call the hospital. Mr. Doyle declined Sandra's offer to transfer his wife to the hospice inpatient unit. He felt that Mrs. Doyle was comfortable enough and would not want to be subjected to an unnecessary move. He requested, however, a visit from Lucy.

When Mrs. Doyle opened her eyes, she asked to see her husband, her parents, two of her cousins, and Peter all at once. She seemed alert. Once everyone gathered around her, she told them she was dying. Looking at each one, she spoke about the things she appreciated about them. She said she loved them. She instructed her parents to give the baby gifts she had bought for Kim's and Peter's unborn children. And she led a prayer. When she finished, she closed her eyes. Mr. Doyle encouraged her to let go. Mrs. Doyle moaned with every breath. Bruises were visible under the surface of her yellow skin. On her right arm she had a large, fluid-filled blister. Mr. Doyle applied water to her lips to keep them moist. He spoke to her affectionately without knowing if she could hear him. He assured her that he loved her. Suddenly, Mrs. Doyle opened her eyes, gave him a kiss, and said, "I love you, too." Her gesture made him laugh and cry. A friend called. "Jenny is gone in spirit, but her body is still here," he said softly. He had already inquired about funeral arrangements. To his relief, he was assured that Mrs. Doyle was now eligible for cremation.

Kim and her husband took the first flight home. Softly, Mr. Doyle told his wife that her daughter was expected soon. Mrs. Doyle's breathing started slowing down. At times it stopped completely. Every three or four breaths, someone would shake her and she would start up again. Her body was very hot. With a friend's help, Mr. Doyle wrapped ice cubes in rags and placed them on pulse points to cool her down. Mrs. Doyle's mother, anxious and distraught, took sedatives to calm herself. Then Kim walked in. She hugged her mother, crying and crying.

The next day, at the recommendation of a hospice nurse, Mrs. Doyle's intravenous hydration was stopped. The following morning, the family gathered in the room and watched. Mr. Doyle brushed his wife's hair and sprayed perfume on her body. Mrs. Doyle was swollen and covered with black, blue, and yellow patches. All her family hoped for was that she would leave this world in peace. But to everyone's horror, her last gasp came with vomit. "She threw up all this brown, pus-looking, oatmeal stuff," Mr. Doyle recalled. "It must have been bile backing up from her liver. We had to carry her mother out of the room."

Half an hour later, a hospice nurse arrived. When she asked how she could help, Mr. Doyle said, "Could you give me another 30 years with my wife?"

"That will be in Heaven," Kim responded.

"For Me, Jenny's Death Was Sort of a Mess"

Two hundred and fifty people paid their final respects at the viewing. The next day, Mrs. Doyle was cremated.

Mr. Doyle was having trouble sleeping. His wife's death had fallen upon him quickly and unexpectedly. Kim was depressed. She couldn't understand how her mother could have declined so rapidly. She cancelled her wedding reception, which was scheduled to take place in six days. Dr. Richards was disappointed that her interventions had failed to raise Mrs. Doyle's platelets. "We had tried to get her on an experimental drug," she said, "and the red tape was a real stumbling block. But I am not so sure, even if we had been able to actually get it into her system, it would have made a difference. But I guess Jenny took the approach that she wanted for a period of time. She did not beat the cancer, but she gave it a run for a while." Sandra was disturbed. "For me, Jenny's death was sort of a mess and not the way I would have liked to see it go for her," she said. "She was treating herself as if she was not a hospice patient, when really, underneath, all this stuff was going bad and then just caused her to totally crash. I could not escape the feeling that she was not dying comfortably." Sandra suspected that if Mrs. Doyle had not sought aggressive treatment all the way to the end, she and her family would have been better prepared for her death. She didn't think they denied reality. She thought they ignored it. At the same time, she acknowledged that her own preference for a more gradual ending in the inpatient unit of hospice might not have been Mrs. Doyle's priority.

Not everyone at hospice shared Sandra's feelings. Roberta Smalley, the nurse who replaced Lucy, said to me,

> Jenny was a very powerful person. I wrote in the chart that we need more people like Jenny Doyle in this world. Just her strength, her vision, her drive to stay alive, looking out for her family even though she knew she was dying, not talking about dying. If I were her, I would be the same way. I wouldn't want to give up at her age. Hospice people think you need to talk about your dying. No. These people are so sick, they know. Deep inside, they know. Why do I have to badger her with that? She knew she was dying. She was just visionary. Just a perfect hospice kind of patient.

Five weeks after Mrs. Doyle's death, Mr. Doyle had melted their wedding bands into a cross that he placed over her urn. He felt guilty about his wife's final moments. Why did she vomit? Could he have prevented that? The hospice support groups he attended brought him in touch with other widowers, but they consisted of people much older than him, which he found depressing. "It is a transition period. And I don't particularly care for it," he said. "I still choke up five or six times a day. Like, last week I hated love songs. But I moved stuff around a little bit, and I know after a while I will have to put a picture away or something along those lines, but there is no rush right now." One thing he didn't want to repeat was spraying his wife's perfume in the house. The memories that brought him were overwhelming.

"I Am Angry at Her, and I'm Hurt"

When I saw Kim two months after her mother's death, she told me she was reluctant to participate in another interview. She felt uncomfortable talking because her feelings toward her mother were not all positive. At the same time, she didn't want to squelch them. On the one hand, she explained, she missed Mrs. Doyle, but on the other, she resented her. "I am angry at her, and I'm hurt," she said. Her mother, she told me, had left her and Peter only a minor fraction of her assets. The rest of her estate had gone to Mr. Doyle. Kim emphasized that her hurt had nothing to do with dollars. That was a point she wanted to make sure I understood. The problem was that, once again, Mrs. Doyle had left her children to fend for themselves. "I remember my mom saying to me she was going to make sure I was taken care of with her death benefit," she said. "That was how she was going to make it up to me."

"Now I'm wondering if all the healing that went on in our relationship was just strictly for her benefit," Kim continued. She felt like a fool for having forgiven her mother. At the same time, she questioned if holding a grudge against someone who was gone would help. "I can either let this hurt me for the rest of my life or accept it," she said. "I think it will just take some time." The memory she thought would ease her anger was that of her mother regaining consciousness when she came back from Europe. She had heard that Mrs. Doyle was unresponsive. She said, "Once I got to the room she started breathing really strong, and her heart was good for almost two days. She could not talk any more, but she gave me a kiss. So she stuck it out. I really appreciate that she stuck it out." Kim didn't want to go through her mother's clothing. She didn't want her jewelry. All she would have liked was photographs from her childhood, but she knew that her mother had thrown those out.

Kim was unable to make use of hospice's bereavement services. She told me that hospice, as an agency, reminded her too much of her mother. Then she said, "There were many years that I did not have contact with my mom, and in a sense, it just feels like that period again. I am 15 again and don't know if I will ever see my mom again. So I tell myself, my mom is dead. I remind myself, 'It is not that your mom is not coming, your mom is dead. Your mom is dead. *Gone*. She is not living anymore.' I don't miss her. That I don't like. But I don't think it is the result of anything I have done."

Mr. Doyle told his hospice support group that he was in the "second half" of his grieving period. To the support group leader, he gave the impression that he was moving on with his life. In fact, he was contemplating moving out of Lancaster County altogether. He was lonely, and he felt rejected by Mrs. Doyle's family. They had accused him of being greedy, selfish, and too eager to get rid of his wife's belongings. "The second six months is more difficult, because I have to find out who I am as an independent person and what I want to do, because at my age in life that gets a little worrisome," he said. "I have to build up a whole different network that I don't have. It still gets lonely and quiet around here at night, but I am sleeping a little bit better. You can't run through this period. You just have to walk through it. I think I would just like to find ways to walk through it quicker."

Authors' Comments

At a pivotal point in her illness, Jenny Doyle found herself torn between conflicting interpretations of her medical condition. She enjoyed three weeks of
improved health and buoyant spirits after receiving a strontium injection on
the recommendation of her radiologist, Larry Stein. Together with her husband Andrew, she made plans for a Las Vegas vacation a few weeks hence.
Although her condition then seemed to worsen, Dr. Stein remained cau-
tiously optimistic, which gave her hope. But when an X-ray showed that her
cancer had spread, her oncologist, John Silverman, painted a grimmer picture, even advising Jenny to leave for Las Vegas right away.

Mrs. Doyle was in a difficult spot—one that we will also see in the narrative of Costas Metrakis. When patients receive authoritative but seemingly
contradictory messages from different medical experts, deciding whom to
believe and what to do can be agonizing. In a situation like this, hospice's
role is clear. As patient advocates who are committed to helping people live
their remaining time according to their own values, hospice workers are
well-situated to bring together patients, families, and healthcare providers
to facilitate clarifying conversations about matters that can be complex and
inherently uncertain. They can invite medical experts to lay out their interpretations, along with the reasons for their views. They can support patients
to ask questions, process answers, and weigh options. And they can serve as
catalysts for consensus-building on a treatment plan that combines as much
as possible differing expert perspectives with patient and family values,
preferences, and goals.

In Jenny Doyle's case, this did not happen. What did happen, at the insti-
gation of a supervising hospice nurse who may have never met Jenny, was an
intervention with the Doyles that might best be described as bullying with
benevolent intent. Rather than attempting to shed light on the conflicting
views of Dr. Stein and Dr. Silverman, the hospice staff arrived at Jenny and
Andrew's home as fervent and relentless partisans of the oncologist's more
pessimistic position, without an explanation for their rationale. In a later reflection, the hospice social worker Sandra Dunn justified the visit with the
breathtaking claim that hospice must be "the voice of reality."

We might well ask what criteria were used to assess "reality" and whose
"reality" was ultimately served? The "reality" within which it would have
been upsetting were Jenny to die during her Las Vegas vacation? The "reality" within which it is better to accept one's impending death rather than

seek "desperate" and ultimately "futile" life-prolonging treatments, as we also heard in the case of Shamira Cook? Although it is certainly true that Jenny died the following October, within Dr. Silverman's one-year prognosis, conflating the accuracy of his prediction with "reality" is to ignore what, for Jenny Doyle, the "rebel with a cause," was the more important question: How shall I *live* while dying? Jenny herself gave us the answer when she reflected on her meeting with her second oncologist Valerie Richards: "It's so nice to know that you have not been given up on." Like Shamira Cook's "reality," Mrs. Doyle's "reality" seemed to be that a life lived fully meant standing up for oneself and never giving up the fight. Hospice, except for nurse Roberta Smalley and, belatedly, nurse Lucy Stephens, seemed to miss this. Or, if they saw it, they reinterpreted it as Jenny's self-destructive avoidance of the "truth," again, echoing hospice's claims of patient "denial" in the case of Ms. Cook.

By the end, and especially after reading Valerie Richards's note about Jenny not yet needing hospice—itself a questionable judgment in our view, though common among oncologists—the hospice team appeared to better appreciate the context of the multiple medical opinions that Mrs. Doyle was trying to navigate. After the fateful intervention in mid-June, when a doctrinaire embrace of a top-down ideology of the "good death" seemed to divert Jenny's team from its patient-centered focus, hospice staff seemed to reorient themselves to the institution's mission. Even Dr. Richards expressed her appreciation for their subsequent willingness to accommodate her proposed treatment. Still, Jenny's death was a difficult one. As long as hospice—defined and constrained by its rules and eligibility requirements—is the patient's gateway to any palliative care, patients like Jenny will face intolerable dilemmas. At the time we wrote this narrative, that was essentially the situation in the United States. Today's environment at present-day Hospice and Community Care and other hospices participating in Medicare's experiment with more permissive rules would no doubt ease some of these treatment decisions.

As we look at the narrative as a whole, for both Jenny's husband Andrew and her daughter Kim, the first year of bereavement was filled with ambivalence and hard feelings. Andrew, besides coping with his own heart attack, was often overwhelmed by his memories of Jenny. One aspect of his suffering that receives scant attention in accounts of life-threatening illness was the impact of Jenny's disease on the couple's sexual relationship, to which he alluded in discussing the trip they were planning to the Southwest: "Not that I want the moon, the sun, and the world, but it's time to get away and try to get back to a little bit of normalcy, along with relaxing and doing things couples do." In the previous narrative, Richard Johnson spoke ambivalently about the impact of his cancer treatments on his sexuality, commenting that "it's good not to be a slave of those feelings." Some have advocated the establishment of specialized clinics to help couples address sexual issues that arise during cancer treatment.[1] Kim struggled with the legacy of long-standing resentments and hurts that had marked her relationship with her mother. Such burdens are rarely within a hospice team's ability to address. The course of one's grief will often depend as much on a family's history as on the interventions of even the most skilled counselors or bereavement volunteers.

Reference

1. Walker LM, Wiebe E, Turner J, Driga A, Andrews-Lepine E, Ayume A, Stephen J, Glaze S, Booker R, Doll C, Phan T, Brennan K, Robinson JW. The oncology and sexuality, intimacy, and survivorship program model: An integrated, multidisciplinary model of sexual health care within oncology. J Cancer Educ. 2021;36(2):377–385.

17

Jasmine Claude

A Study in Faith

Narrated by Anna Towers

When Jasmine Claude's lymphoma was first treated with chemotherapy, the cancer was put into remission; however this was short-lived. She was only 37 years old when the tumors started to grow again, and her oncologist tried three different regimes to get her into remission. In her fourth year of treatment she began to develop abdominal pain. The oncologist consulted the Palliative Care Service to help control her symptoms, and the service followed her as an outpatient. She continued to receive palliative chemotherapy for many months after this. When the oncologist told her that the abdominal tumor was growing despite the chemotherapy and that he would have to stop the treatment, Mrs. Claude began to receive palliative home care. She was feeling tired and less able to go out but was otherwise not feeling too bad. She carried on with her daily routine as much as she could and seemed surprisingly cheerful and serene. It was unusual for the palliative care staff to witness such serenity, which derived from an unshakable faith in God that Mrs. Claude had developed over the years. Their reactions ranged from curiosity, fascination, and inspiration to skepticism. This narrative describes not only an experience of palliative care, but also an exploration of the experience of faith, as seen within a palliative care context.

The Birth of Faith Through Adversity

Jasmine Claude had not had an easy life in her native Haiti. In her early twenties she experienced terror at the hands of the Tonton Macoutes military police that destroyed her young family. Her husband died while a political prisoner, leaving her to raise their son, then only three years old. Twelve years later, Mrs. Claude developed lymphoma. She was working as a secretary at the time and had managed to save some money. She moved to Montreal, where there is a large French-speaking Haitian community, to have further medical investigations and receive treatment. Mrs. Claude knew some friends with whom she could stay until she was settled. She had been a devout Jehovah's Witness in Haiti and was able to fit into a new "family" in Montreal. She also kept in touch with old friends in Haiti and others who were spread out across North America. She continued to be concerned about the unstable political situation at home. The democratically elected leader Aristide had been ousted by the Haitian military and an economic embargo was in force. Mrs. Claude, like most Haitians, had invested great hope in Aristide, and she corresponded with friends who were hoping for restoration of democratic rule.

I first met Mrs. Claude in December 1995, one month after her oncologist had stopped her chemotherapy, as her abdominal tumor continued to grow. She lived near a densely built working-class section of Montreal. Mrs. Claude's modest two-bedroom apartment was in a 10-unit building near a major highway. She shared it with her 20-year-old son Paul, who was a full-time student.

When Mrs. Claude answered the door, I was struck by her gracious, aristocratic bearing and warm, engaging eyes. A tall and slim woman, she looked much older than her 41 years. As we settled around her kitchen table, I noticed her markedly protuberant abdomen. Only by frequently shifting her position did she manage to remain seated throughout the interview. The apartment was spotless, and I surmised that she must be spending all of her physical energy cleaning. She said that Paul helped with the household chores.

She looked very sad as she spoke of her husband's death in prison, but she brightened as she spoke about her faith. "I was very depressed after my husband died," she said, "even suicidal at times. Then something happened to me about six years ago. Things changed. I started to have faith. I felt strong again. So now, no matter what happens, I know that God is there for me. I often wonder why this had to happen to me, of all people. I don't know what it all means. But I can look death squarely in the eye. Don't get me wrong: I do feel angry and frustrated about all this, but I won't allow it to get me down."

She spoke about her hopes for Paul. "He's in college and he's doing great," she told me. "I brought him up alone, but I did my best to bring him up well. I want him to grow up in a way that would have made his father proud. And he's a good boy. He gets on well with people and he adapts well to change. I don't think he'll go back to Haiti after I die, because of the political situation there. But with his skills he could go anywhere in North America. So that's what's important for me—to make sure that my son will be okay and settled."

Mrs. Claude's abdomen was so bulky that she felt like she was nine months pregnant, and she found it difficult to breathe. Still, she kept busy with chores in the apartment as much as she was able to, counseled needy members of her church community on the telephone, and wrote letters to her friends.

"One thing I do enjoy is writing letters to my friends," she said. "I write to them about all sorts of things. I try to encourage them. So many of them ask me for advice about their problems."

"Do you write to them about your illness?" I asked.

She answered without hesitation. "No, I never do. I never write about my illness."

"Whom *do* you talk to about your illness?"

"Oh, my son is good. Whenever I get upset or depressed, he has a way of sitting me down at the kitchen table and having a chat with me. We talk, and he doesn't give up until I feel better."

Mrs. Claude still had close ties with her family in Haiti. She was trying to arrange for her mother to come to Canada to help look after her during the terminal phase of her illness. That was her wish, to stay at home under her mother's care. She also had two brothers in Haiti and a sister who was a nurse in Switzerland, with whom she spoke regularly on the phone. She had several close and supportive friends in her church community who helped her both practically and emotionally. Her friends regularly took her shopping for her groceries, so she didn't have to go by bus. She organized the schedule herself.

By the time I met Mrs. Claude, Susan, the palliative home care nurse, had been visiting Mrs. Claude weekly for quite some time. Cheerful, outgoing, and able to see the humor in situations, Susan cared deeply for her patients and went out of her way to help them. Around the same time as my visit, she made the following observations in the journal she kept as part of our project:

> There's been a remarkable change in this lady in the past year. She is much more optimistic; very, very peaceful. She has made all her arrangements. She is going to have her last will and testament done on Monday. She's quite a remarkable lady, I think. Every day I've gone, for about the last month or six weeks, she's had a radiance on her face, even though she'd been very uncomfortable with ascites and edema in both legs. She knows she's very sick, she knows she has a short time to live but she takes every day as it comes and tries to live it the best she can. There's just something very wonderful after being with her. It's a feeling of being wrapped in soft, soft cotton, a feeling of peace that I have when I leave her. She knows there are hard times ahead, and yet I come away feeling that I've been touched by something blessed. She's not looking for consolation or comfort or anything—that seems to be within her. And I take this serenity with me when I leave her.

"A Calm Heart Is the Life of This Body of Flesh"

Around Christmas, Mrs. Claude began to have more physical symptoms, and Susan noted that she was becoming more subdued. Her abdomen was getting bigger and more cumbersome, so she could hardly walk. She was losing her appetite, getting weaker, and was now bedbound. Her sister visited from Switzerland, and one of her brothers came up from Haiti. Mrs. Claude expressed to Susan the feeling that there was a lot of power inside herself to change the course of the illness, possibly leading to miraculous improvement. At the same time, she was exhausted from too much company over the holidays. There was a sign on the inside door of her apartment, requesting that visitors not stay for more than 30 minutes.

By early January, Mrs. Claude's sister and brother had left, and Mrs. Claude insisted that she wanted to be alone. She refused additional help at home through the community health services, saying that she was capable of looking after herself with some help from Paul. She just wanted her family around her, her religious magazines, and her Bible. She wanted to be alone to reflect and meditate, without having to be sociable. An inspirational quotation was mounted on the wall above her bed: "A calm heart is the life of this body of flesh."

When the oncologist had stopped the chemotherapy two months earlier, he had told Mrs. Claude that she might live another year. Mrs. Claude's health had markedly deteriorated since then, but no one else had discussed her prognosis with her, and she seemed unaware that her disease was progressing faster than her oncologist had estimated. Mrs. Claude was still waiting for her mother's visa to come through and was looking forward to her mother coming in about three months—again seemingly unaware that her prognosis was likely shorter than that.

Bursts of Anger as Energies Dwindle

Once, in late January, Susan's weekly home visit with Mrs. Claude had to be delayed because of another, more urgent, visit. She telephoned Mrs. Claude to let her know, offering to come one hour later than her scheduled appointment of 2:30 P.M. She added that she would be accompanied by a physician who had been visiting the Palliative Care Service. Mrs. Claude replied in a curt tone that Susan had not heard from her before, "You will either come before 3:00 or not at all."

"But, Mrs. Claude, that's not possible," Susan replied., "And I really want the doctor to see you because he'll be leaving us this week and it's the last chance for him to see you."

"A doctor isn't necessary because I have the Lord who will look after me," Mrs. Claude replied. She sounded angry now.

"But you really need to be seen," Susan persisted, "and we can't come sooner because we have another patient whom we urgently have to see right now."

"Well, I'm sorry, but I need my rest."

Susan paused for a few moments. "Well, I guess I'll have to come next week then."

"I think that would be better. Because if you come later today it will interrupt my rest."

Susan was upset by this encounter. Mrs. Claude's manner was a real surprise, and Susan's other patient really did have an emergency: he was dying and, in fact, died shortly after Susan got off the phone. A week later, when Susan arrived, she was greeted by an angry Mrs. Claude. Susan started cheerfully. "So, Mrs. Claude, how has it been having your brother and sister here? You had lots of other visitors, too. That was a lot of company."

"It's really tired me out," Mrs. Claude said, irritably. "It was good to see my family, but some other visitors are really inconsiderate when they come to see you, and they have all kinds of advice to give that you don't need."

"I'm sorry I couldn't make it last week at the time we'd agreed," Susan said. "I had a patient who was in a crisis situation."

"Some people will say anything to get attention, and they'll call any little thing a crisis," Mrs. Claude responded bitterly.

"No, Mrs. Claude. My other patient was really sick. The crisis was that my other patient was dying."

Mrs. Claude sighed and softened her tone. "I'm sorry," she said. She then resumed in an angry tone. "But I'm having problems here. My mother can't get a visa from the Canadian consulate in Haiti. She ought to be here now to help me, but we need the papers."

"You asked the doctor to give you a letter last week," Susan said. "And she faxed the letter to Haiti. Didn't that help?"

"The visa is still delayed. I'll need a stronger letter." Mrs. Claude puffed up her face and clenched her teeth in anger. "They treat people from poor black countries like we are all criminals!" she said.

Once more, Susan felt hurt and unfairly treated. I had had a similar encounter with Mrs. Claude around this time, though I had reacted differently from Susan—possibly because as a researcher rather than as Mrs. Claude's physician, I was not actually responsible for her care. Mrs. Claude's expression of anger actually made me respect her more, for I now knew that she could express her needs directly and that she could be angry when she felt she had to be. Rather than putting distance between us, it strengthened the bond that I had with her. To me, the fact that she could get angry made her serenity all the more authentic.

On February 14, Mrs. Claude called Susan to say that she was experiencing abdominal pain and it was hard for her to breathe. Susan discussed this with Denise Morin, the palliative care physician, and they suggested to Mrs. Claude that she come to the hospital for a paracentesis to remove fluid from the abdomen. She could then go back home. However, an ultrasound test revealed a solid tumor. There was no ascites fluid to be extracted. It was the tumor that was making her abdomen protrude to the size of a massive twin term pregnancy. Susan felt that she should be admitted to the Palliative Care Unit (PCU), and Mrs. Claude reluctantly agreed. She assumed that her stay would be short. Paul was taking exams at this time and Mrs. Claude did not want him to quit his studies to look after her. But she expected her mother to obtain her visa any day, so that she could go home under her mother's care.

"Now I Want a Rest"

On the PCU, Dr. Morin started Mrs. Claude on diuretics and steroids. The music therapist found classical music that helped relieve her abdominal pain. Paul came to see his mother every evening, and Mrs. Claude's church friends busily organized medical aides and worked to prepare for her eventual return home. Two friends, Jacques and Brother Demers, a church leader, visited almost every day.

When I went to see Mrs. Claude in her room, she was still too uncomfortable to lie down and so was propped up on several pillows in a reclining chair. She had some difficulty breathing because of the pressure from her abdomen and had to stop in mid-sentence to take a breath. But she was generous in cheerfully taking the time to chat with me. We got talking about her relationships. "I was always the organizer in the family," she explained. "When I'm not there, the people around me don't know what to do—they stand there with their arms by their sides. So, I'm trying to organize my mother to come. But it's not easy because I have to get Paul to phone, and he's young and not so able to organize things."

"Why don't you get a phone in your room?" I suggested.

"If I get a telephone then too many friends call me, and they want to talk for a long time and get advice about their problems."

"They want *you* to help *them* even though you're sick?"

Mrs. Claude replied calmly, "I'm always the one who has helped other people with their problems and now I want a rest. I don't want to see any visitors except my son and two men friends from my church." She had a hint of a smile as she paused. "I prefer male visitors—they don't talk as much as the women."

"That's true, isn't it?" I replied. We both laughed.

Along with Mrs. Claude's sense of humor, the staff appreciated and found fascinating her ability to get her needs met without making them feel manipulated. Instead, they felt worthwhile and successful. I discussed this with Rosemary, her ward nurse, who had worked on the unit for many years. She had formed a close bond with Mrs. Claude.

"Rosemary," I began, "what I find interesting is that she has absolute control over her world, but it's something positive as far as the staff are concerned. I mean, there are patients who take charge—"

Rosemary finished my sentence, "And they abuse. On thinking about it, it's that she doesn't control me. She controls her affairs but without controlling those around her. She uses me, but it's okay for her to use me; it's part of my role. But I know that she isn't going to abuse my services or abuse my goodwill. I can be myself. I'm not risking my skin in helping her. She is realistic in her demands. She expresses real needs."

On February 16, within two days of her admission, Mrs. Claude's breathing and leg swelling started to improve, presumably in response to the diuretics and steroids. She still got short of breath when she talked, but she was now able to walk down the hallway. She liked to stay up at night writing letters, and she seemed to have a voluminous correspondence. Since she didn't nap during the day either, I wondered whether her insomnia might be a sign of fear or anxiety, but Paul told me later that his mother had never slept much.

Mrs. Claude was trying to process the fact that nothing could be done to markedly reduce her abdomen, that there was no fluid to remove. She expressed the desire for space and time to think, limiting her visitors even further to those whom she truly wanted to see. During the second week of her admission, she developed new symptoms: nausea and increasing abdominal cramps. The pain was quickly relieved by oxycodone, a strong opioid, but Mrs. Claude was reluctant to take the medication regularly. She was under the common but mistaken impression that if she took regular analgesics now, the medication wouldn't work if and when the pain got worse. Even after we explained to her that this was not the case, she continued to be stoical about her pain.

When I visited her on February 24, she was lying on her side, her face slightly contorted. She was holding her abdomen.

"Mrs. Claude, do you want me to tell the nurse to bring you a painkiller?'

"No, I think I'll wait. A little rest might ease the pain. Anyway, my spirits are good. I have a spirit of steel. It's been four years that I have lived with this, and my spirits have always been good. They say that if one can keep one's spirits up, it's 90% of the battle. But I am eating less, and I'm feeling weaker." She paused. "I'm not afraid of dying. I consider it a deep sleep. I think my son is also more prepared now, about my going."

When I asked Dr. Morin later about her relationship with Mrs. Claude, and the issue of Mrs. Claude's faith, she said,

> At first, I was a little skeptical. But after two or three discussions with her, I realized it's clearly all right for her to be like that. The deeper you go into her history, the more you realize that she needs her religion. I don't make it a habit to confront people because religion is something personal. I said to myself, "This woman—if we push her, if we challenge her too much about her personal beliefs—it would be to her detriment." So it wasn't something that I tried to challenge, but it's something that I tried to listen to. One day I asked her, "What about your son? Is he a believer?" Her answer was very interesting. She said, "He can't really understand this. He is too young." So, for her it was clearly a long spiritual journey that she had undertaken.

Denise herself did not have such a powerful, unquestioning faith. But alongside her skepticism was a real fascination with Mrs. Claude's faith, and she often found herself drawn back to the subject when she interacted with her. "I often brought it up," she told me. "It was clear that one couldn't play around too much in there, to question too much. I didn't try to do that, but I certainly used the patient, in the sense that I made her talk about how she got to believe what she believed. People with these strong fixed beliefs have always intrigued me. What's going on in their heads? How can they believe something so totally? It penetrates to their very marrow."

I also interviewed a ward volunteer who had looked after Mrs. Claude and who had been with the Palliative Care Service for 21 years. She described Mrs. Claude's faith as "radiant."

"You have a tremendous faith," the volunteer had said to her.

"Yes," Mrs. Claude had answered, "with so many evil forces around the world. The wild dogs are out there. I don't know what my son will do. I despair about my country. I worry about the political situation, about Aristide. It never gets better. My country is torn to pieces, and there are so many negative forces in the world. But we have to keep our faith in the Lord."

The volunteer was very moved. "I couldn't get over it," she said to me as she recounted her time with Mrs. Claude. "She had been through so much in life, and still she could look so calm and radiant. She was not in despair for herself, she was not afraid of anything, I haven't seen a patient like her in all these years. When I sat with her, she communicated so much. Her eyes, her body language just spoke 'peace' so clearly!"

The Last Days

Meanwhile, Mrs. Claude's increasing abdominal cramps heralded trouble. On February 20, she vomited and had other symptoms and signs of small bowel obstruction. Because of the extent of the tumor, she was not a candidate for surgical treatment to relieve the obstruction. Dr. Morin explained all this to Mrs. Claude, who remained fully alert and continued to ask for as much control as possible over her medical and nursing care. She did begin to accept regular doses of opioid medication for pain relief.

She looked weak and dehydrated when I went in to see her that day. "I'm having more pain," she told me, "but my breathing is better." She smiled and said, "I had a great whirlpool bath yesterday! So pleasant. I even told my sister in Geneva when I spoke with her on the phone yesterday. I said, 'You have money in Switzerland, but here we have whirlpool baths!'"

Mrs. Claude told me she was thinking that she would go home again. She said that she was looking forward to seeing her brother, who was planning to come from Haiti in two months' time. Again she didn't seem to be aware that her prognosis was shorter that 2 months, and the staff decided to leave it at that for the time being.

The next day it was clear that Mrs. Claude was seriously obstructed. Even if she took nothing at all by mouth, she vomited bile. Medication controlled the nausea and reduced the vomiting, but she could not eat or drink. I spoke with her again, with Rosemary present at the foot of the bed.

"Mrs. Claude, you know your bowels are blocked," I said gravely.

"Yes. I was so afraid this would happen." She looked calm and dignified.

"There's a 50% chance that this will get better either by itself or with the help of medication. But that would be only a temporary improvement, I'm afraid."

"Well, I've told my brother to come sooner. I've also organized everything: my funeral, money for my son. I even wrote my own obituary notice to be printed in the newspaper in Haiti after I die."

"Your own obituary notice! Amazing!" I cried. "You're a great organizer. I think I'll hire you!"

Mrs. Claude smiled. "To work with you in the next life?"

"Yes," I said softly. "In the next life."

I reached out and held Mrs. Claude's hand and she started to cry. This was the first time I had seen her cry. I continued to hold her hand for a minute or two, and then she spoke again.

"I can't cry in front of my son. I must be strong for him."

"So who is there that you can speak with?"

"There is my friend from the church."

I sat silently with her for a couple of minutes more. When she was more composed, I left, and Rosemary continued to chat with her. I remember feeling at the time that this exchange had deepened the bond I had with her. It was the type of meaningful encounter that happens occasionally in palliative care, and so often at unexpected moments.

The next day, February 28, the home care nurse Susan returned from a vacation and went immediately to see Mrs. Claude. When she got to the room a volunteer was sitting next to the bed, gently rubbing Mrs. Claude's stomach. Susan had heard about the bowel obstruction, and, for a few moments, they discussed the serious implications. But Mrs. Claude soon changed the subject. "She asked about my vacation," Susan recounted to me, "and wanted to know if I had any photographs. I promised I would bring them. She then said, 'You look good!' and flashed that amazing smile of hers. I was so touched. I found myself crying as I walked down the hall."

That evening, Mrs. Claude called her two church friends, Brother Demers and Jacques, and said, "I'm not feeling well. Come see me." When they arrived, she discussed her life with them, the funeral arrangements, and she was able to cry with them. Brother Demers was too emotional to speak with her and had to leave, but she and Jacques spoke at great length. "We will see each other in another world," she reassured him. She reviewed her life, every phase of her illness. It was the only time that Brother Demers and Jacques had seen her cry. She cried with Paul that night, too, the only time that she cried in front of her son. She told him, "I'm satisfied with my life. I am going in peace."

Paul phoned his mother early the next morning, as he did every morning. For the first time, he found that his mother was confused. He was concerned and came immediately to check on her. He looked worried when I met him on the ward. I told him that his mother's condition had changed. He visited her briefly and looked even more worried as he came out of the room. But he had to go to school to write some exams. He was already late, he said, and quickly disappeared into the elevator.

Around 2:00 P.M., Rosemary left Mrs. Claude's bedside to attend to another patient. She returned to find that Mrs. Claude had suddenly died. No one had expected her to die suddenly that day. Usually, patients who develop bowel obstruction live on for days, sometimes weeks. Denise Morin guessed that Mrs. Claude had probably had an internal hemorrhage. Although Rosemary is an experienced palliative care nurse, she was shocked and distressed and could not carry on working. She went to sit in the nurses' lounge for the remaining hour of her shift.

I went into Mrs. Claude's room, to spend time there alone. Her body was still warm. I touched her and thought of how much I respected this woman. The death had been so sudden. We all knew that she was dying, but it wasn't supposed to be today! She didn't fade away. She went, just like that. It was a shock for me as well.

In the meantime, Denise and several other staff were milling around the nursing station. Denise had tried to reach Paul at school to tell him of his mother's death; however, the exam was over, and Paul had already left. Repeated phone calls to his home failed to reach him. Everyone was afraid that Paul would arrive without having been forewarned.

Paul arrived around 4:00 P.M. The nurses were in their change-of-shift meeting, and the only staff around was a volunteer who had just started her shift. She was not yet aware herself that Mrs. Claude had died. Paul went to his mother's room, which she had shared with another patient and found that his mother's bed was no longer there. (If a patient dies in a two-bed room, the practice on the ward is to give the grieving family more privacy by moving the body into another, quieter room at the end of the corridor.) The volunteer saw Paul come back out to the hallway looking worried and puzzled and immediately realized the situation. She took him to the meditation room where his mother's body had been taken. He looked completely bewildered. It was dark outside, but he did not want the light on. He just wanted to sit in the dark room with his mother. When Rosemary heard that Paul had arrived, she went immediately to the meditation room to see him and put her arms around him. She had stayed well beyond her shift to wait for him.

When Paul got his bearings, he said he had to make some phone calls. The volunteer offered to help him get through to his aunt in Switzerland. When he had finished his business, he ate some food the volunteer had found for him and then sat in the darkened nurses' lounge for half an hour. He went back to be with his mother's body and then returned to the lounge. After another half hour, he went to pick up his mother's belongings. The volunteer watched him collect everything in sight, even the half-dead flowers.

The psychologist who was there that evening spoke briefly with Paul and with Brother Demers, who had also arrived. She reassured herself that Paul had some good support immediately available. Over the next few days, it was Brother Demers who helped Paul look after all the affairs. Mrs. Claude's mother did not get her visa papers until after her daughter's funeral. She arrived from Haiti three weeks after Mrs. Claude died.

Rosemary

The next day, I spoke with Rosemary. She described her reaction to Mrs. Claude's sudden death:

> She went fast. I left her room to give anther patient some medication. It took five or ten minutes. I came back and she had died during this time. I was so surprised because—you know, we expect people to die here—but it was so sudden, she was already gone! Everyone expected that there would have been time for the family to come from Haiti. So I cried. It's bizarre, isn't it? I've been working here for 12 years, and thought that I had built a shell around me, but it had been a while since I had cared continuously for a patient many days in a row. She always told me she was happy when I was there. That same morning, the day she died, she told me, "You're a marvelous nurse."

Rosemary interrupted herself to look at me and say, "She was kind, wasn't she?" Then she continued,

> It's me, and it's a very personal reaction. When I'm with a mother and a child—when it's the mother that dies, but not when it's the child—there's a kind of unconscious identification, that I can't control. I couldn't control myself when she died yesterday. And I couldn't leave without having made the bridge between the mother and the son. He arrived, and I was there. I was waiting for him to come. I was waiting for something. I don't know what. I had to make the connection. I was there when she died and I had to make the bridge between her and her son. And I felt responsible! I've noticed that on several occasions, it happens when it's a sudden death. It's

like an abandonment. She left, without giving us a chance to prepare, not like the others.

Rosemary paused. "Mind you," she continued, "I was adopted at the age of 20 months, so I have these crises of abandonment."

Paul

When I spoke with Paul afterward, he, too, commented on what it had been like for his mother to die so unexpectedly that day. "I spoke with Rosemary and Dr. Morin," he said, "and they told me it was okay for me to go to my exam. I looked at the chart and Rosemary had written that my mother was confused, that she was speaking Creole. Rosemary couldn't understand what she was saying, but I could have, had I been there." Paul wondered aloud to me, "Did she have a final message for me in Creole before she died? I feel that I should have stayed with her."

Dr. Morin thought that Paul was at high risk for bereavement complications. He was relatively young and was now orphaned. He might still have unresolved feelings about having lost his father. He was a recent immigrant and seemed socially isolated. Denise thought he was at risk for developing prolonged grief reactions or a depression that would interfere with his daily functioning. She planned to speak with the bereavement co-ordinator to try to get extra help for Paul over and above the usual follow-up offered to families.

As it turned out, the members of Mrs. Claude's church community looked after Paul, even though he was not a member of the church. The church friends came by, telephoned, and generally treated him like a member of the family. Though Paul failed the exams that he was writing at the time of his mother's death, he rewrote them the next month and passed them all.

Two months after his mother's death, Paul told me that things were getting better. He had spoken with many of his friends and found it easier to talk about his mother. Now, whenever I spoke with him, he seemed calm, confident, well-organized, and in control. He was also more open and talkative with me, very different from the way he had been when I saw him with his mother, when he seemed shy and more of a little boy.

By four months, Paul had gotten himself a temporary job, and he hoped to study electronics at the university the next year. When I spoke with him around the time of the first anniversary of his mother's death, things were continuing well, although he described some common signs of grief. "Every day is a battle," he said. "I'm anxious. Every time the phone rings, I'm afraid that someone is phoning to give me bad news, that someone has died. I'm also more sensitive to the grief of others. I talk more. I'm more open. There have been many changes in me over the past year."

He continued to sound confident. He was coping with his job, had retained his hope for the future, and was planning to further his studies. There seemed to be no cause for concern about the course of his bereavement.

Authors' Comments

After Mrs. Claude's death I continued to explore the theme of faith, which had emerged as such a major thread in this narrative. Palliative care units offer pastoral services. However, Mrs. Claude was (in her own words and according to staff observations) well supported by two church friends who visited almost daily, one of whom was also a church leader. Therefore, PCU pastoral services were not involved in this case.

Paul shared the palliative care team's admiration for his mother's spirituality. When we spoke several months after her death he said,

> Everyone who met her said what a remarkable person she was. Looking back on it, I see that religious people believe, but this was different—the way her faith played a role in every decision that she made, everything she faced. I am not sure that I could have done it. She witnessed in a special way. In the funeral speech the theme was the faith that she had, even in the end. It prevented her from being afraid. She didn't worry. She knew that it wouldn't be the end, that there was a future.

The physicians expressed intellectual and scientific curiosity, but also skepticism, regarding Mrs. Claude's spirituality and were ambivalent about the issue of faith. On the one hand, they assumed, tacitly, that religion isn't adequate. They took a psychodynamic view that was often taught in medical school at that time and saw faith as a maladaptation, even as pathological. At the same time, however, they could not deny, and even admired, the enormous power of what they had witnessed, a power that called into question the narrowness of their skeptical psychological interpretations. Indeed, medical education itself has evolved to incorporate significantly more nuanced, less pathologizing appraisals of religious faith today.

The comments of a resident physician were typical of the attitudes I encountered in the aftermath of Mrs. Claude's time on the PCU.

> Unquestioning faith has always been difficult for me because that is not my approach. It is not my experience. I have always admired people who can just be that convinced. And yet I wonder what else could be going on. And I think that maybe I am not getting at the underlying fear, or the underlying questions, because I don't know how many people are really fearless. Maybe I was being presumptuous or parental or something, but I just would get the feeling with her that things were much more fragile than she made them out to be, and I wanted to help and yet didn't, or couldn't.

The physicians did not openly negate or disaffirm Mrs. Claude's faith. It was hers, and they respected it. But they were torn between admiration and suspicion. Dr. Morin expressed the ambivalence of several of her colleagues when she said to me, "It always creates a difficulty for me, a faith like that, because I have a hard time adhering to something that dictates everything in advance for me. But it was clear to me that it helped her to get through everything she had to face."

In addition to being the narrator of this case, I am also a palliative care physician. I could easily relate to the team's fascination with Mrs. Claude's faith. We are all struggling with our own questions of spirituality and transcendence. We learn on different levels, and we plateau at different levels, as caregivers and as persons. In palliative care we are actively relating to the mystery of living and dying as a vital entity. We learn to relate to the mystery through the care of our patients.

18

Katie Melnick

Living and Dying with God

Narrated by Yanna Lambrinidou

God was omnipresent in Katie Melnick's life. She saw signs of him everywhere she went. Even during the last stages of her lung cancer, after the disease had spread to her brain, Mrs. Melnick felt a deep sense of peace. Her hospice caregivers marveled at the depth and resoluteness of her faith. Mrs. Melnick's dying took four months longer than her doctors prepared her to expect. In contrast to her own serenity, family secrets caused pain, confusion, and guilt, especially for Mrs. Melnick's adult daughter. As the Melnicks relived old hurts, they also found unexpected opportunities for love and reconciliation.

"I Am with You"

"I am very busy for a dying woman!" Katie Melnick exclaimed the first time I spoke with her on the phone. Mrs. Melnick was a 52-year-old, third-generation Polish mother with a 14-month history of lung cancer. Following her diagnosis in August 1995, she underwent a lobectomy of her left lung. But the cancer metastasized to her brain, and doctors' appointments were filling up her calendar. First, she was to see her radiation oncologist in Lancaster for a 14-course radiation treatment and then she was to travel to New York City for a second opinion from a brain tumor expert. Her lungs were too weak to survive brain surgery, she was told, but perhaps something more could be done about her increasing seizures, forgetfulness, difficulty seeing, and tingling in her right arm. She had been offered stereotactic radiosurgery, an alternative to conventional brain surgery that treats tumors with highly focused radiation beams.

Mrs. Melnick felt ambivalent about this intervention. The last thing she wanted was to compromise the quality of her remaining life. She knew she was dying and had already contacted Hospice of Lancaster County herself. Yet her three children—Paul, 31, Carl, 29, and Lena, 22—insisted that she get a second opinion before turning down a potentially beneficial treatment. She and I agreed to meet after her return from New York.

I met Mrs. Melnick in her second-floor apartment on November 21, 1996. She was a tall, thin woman. She had a soft voice and elegant features—youthful skin, high cheekbones, a delicate nose, and light brown eyes. Her hair had only recently fallen out from the radiation. Mrs. Melnick prided herself on both her physical and emotional strength. "I am like the matriarch of the family," she asserted. She was sitting in an overstuffed chair at the corner of an unadorned living room, alone. Her husband John and daughter Lena were at work at the family dry-cleaning store. By her side was a coffee table with her essentials: medications, cigarettes, ashtray, and her beloved Bible. She smoked nervously, joked and laughed, and asked me questions about our study. She expressed eagerness to start with the interviews. At her suggestion, we moved to her bedroom to avoid the squawks of Anabel, the family's African gray parrot. "Anabel bird!" "Melnick bird!" Anabel shouted in between a polyphony of undecipherable sounds.

Mrs. Melnick began with a story about the neatly folded, hand-knit wool blanket at the foot of her bed. It was an ivory-colored throw with a pink cross in the center. "After my lung surgery," she recounted,

> I still was not feeling that good, but I had still worked six days a week at our dry-cleaner's. I was pretty depressed. This lady came in one time to drop off some clothes. We had no conversation. She did not know me. She does not know whether I am Jewish, Christian, anything. She had no idea that I had the lung cancer. When she left, God put it on her heart to pray for me, and she makes these prayer blankets; at each stitch she prays for the person that she is making it for. She gets home and God kept telling her, "Pray for that lady," and she was, like, arguing with God, "I don't know her!" "Make a blanket for her!" So, she says, she was in the process of making one for somebody else, but God kept putting it on her heart. It took three weeks. She argued with God and said that even when she would go to bed, he would say, "Pray for that lady." Really! A total stranger! Anyway, she did.

So, in she comes with this blanket. She put it on my counter, and I figured she wanted to have it cleaned. I said, "Oh, isn't that pretty," and she goes, "It's for you." Well, I'm telling you, from a total stranger! That is why I have such a strong faith in God, that he could send a total stranger. It is just unbelievable! See the cross at the center? A total stranger! So to me that is confirmation of God telling me, "I am with you."

Mrs. Melnick was a practicing Catholic until 1988. She then switched to Protestantism and now attended a Pentecostal church. The Scriptures gave her inspiration and courage. Since starting to have difficulty reading for long periods of time, she limited her study to favorite verses—those that exhorted contentment with one's fate and confirmed God's love for all his people. "I know I should be experiencing anger, denial, and all these different things, but I am not," she told me. "I just pray. I say a little prayer to God, and I'm fine. I am just at peace. I am probably going to be like this right up until the end because He is with me—unless I tear my eyes away from Him and stop praying." Mrs. Melnick was not fatalistic. She considered every form of palliative treatment available. She attended healing services—Catholic, Protestant, and Pentecostal—in the hope of getting cured. She believed in the power of both medicine and God.

Her appointment in New York buoyed her. She learned that she was a good candidate for stereotactic radiosurgery if her cancer hadn't metastasized to new organs and if her brain tumor hadn't grown. The procedure would give her six months to a year of life. Without it, the physician estimated that she had two months left at most. But the mass in her brain, her radiation oncologist back home told her, had doubled. The 14-course radiation treatment she had started only weeks before had not helped at all. The oncologist seemed detached—his voice, cold. Ms. Melnick was startled to see a human being lose all emotion as he handed her what amounted to a death sentence. She felt sorrier for him than she did for herself. She recalled, "I hugged him, and I said, 'I'm fine. I feel so bad that you have to tell people this.' My heart went out to him, and he just, like, got a tear in his eye and hugged me. So, doctors are compassionate, but I guess they have to say these things over and over to people, and it is not easy. I have been really praying for the doctors because it is a tough, tough thing."

Since stereotactic radiosurgery was no longer an option, Mrs. Melnick was offered brain surgery—the very procedure that weeks earlier she had been told she wouldn't survive. After a period of prayer and conversations with Lena, she turned the proposition down. "I don't want to spend my last days fighting cancer," she explained. "So now I feel that the growth of my tumor is a blessing because I don't want to linger and watch my family suffer. So, I believe God answered my prayers because my tumor is growing. I am going to live shorter now. It is going to be a quicker death, and I would rather [it be that way]." Although resolute in her decision, Mrs. Melnick was shocked to hear, on December 2, 1996, how short her prognosis actually was. Without surgery, the brain surgeon said, she would live no more than two weeks. That was, she remembered, "the first time I have prayed for my life. All I was thinking was, 'God, help me make it to Christmas. Let me be around for Christmas, so I don't ruin the holiday for everybody for the rest of their lives.'"

A Family Secret

John and Katie Melnick had been married for 36 years. They had spent almost all their life in a small town in Maryland. Mr. Melnick worked at a fabric store, while Mrs. Melnick raised their three children. Although they loved each other, Mrs. Melnick told me, she and her husband weren't close. She liked openness and affection whereas he kept mostly to himself. "My husband is not a very warm person," she said. And she continued,

> I think he has hugged me twice since I got sick. He was never a huggy person. You'd think living with me all these years he would have changed a little bit, but he didn't. He is just not a warm person. He is not like me and my kids. I love him. He is a good man. But he just is not warm at all. He is just very cold, very cold. He was always like that. Because I am dying now, I would like him to be a little more warm, but he is not. I would like him to be a little more comforting or just say, "We'll get through this together," but he doesn't. But he does not have the same peace in the Lord as I do, either.

Mrs. Melnick poured all her love into her children. Paul, Carl, and Lena were the essence of her life. Motherhood was the most important part of her existence, the only aspect of herself she cried about losing. "The happiest time of my life was raising my kids," she would say when reminiscing about her past. She described herself as a playful mother who took part in water games, snowball fights, camping trips, dancing, and many other activities that brought happiness to her children's lives. In contrast to other parents, she said, she relished summers because her youngsters were out of school.

In 1993, after 27 years of work, Mr. Melnick found himself unemployed because the fabric store closed down. When he and Mrs. Melnick heard that a profitable dry cleaner in Lancaster County was for sale, they bought it and moved north. Neither was happy to leave Maryland. Paul was already married, had a child of his own, and was in the middle of culinary school. Carl flew commuter planes and was engaged. Lena worked happily at a hair salon. Lancaster County was four entire hours away, but daily phone calls between mother and children kept their bonds intact.

Life in Lancaster County was markedly different. Mr. Melnick grew unhappy in his new job. The long, demanding hours exhausted him. The responsibility of running his own business overwhelmed him. And the fact that he was an introvert—quiet and uncomfortable with strangers—made his interactions with clients an unrelenting challenge. Mrs. Melnick, on the other hand, thrived. She loved to work. She took charge. She orchestrated the store's remodeling, bought new equipment, and paid the bills and taxes. She relished meeting new customers and made a point of nourishing a personal connection with the regulars. But, eight months in, she was diagnosed with cancer. She was devastated. Mr. Melnick blamed her for chain-smoking and needlessly bringing a tragedy down on the family. Assessing that without her help the business would destroy him emotionally and financially, he put the store up for sale. No one showed interest.

Mrs. Melnick stopped smoking. When she was able, she went back to work—to a life that looked like it had returned to normal. In October 1996, she noticed feeling weak and unable to control her right hand. Tests showed that her cancer had metastasized to her brain. She immediately called Lena. "It's a brain tumor," she said. "Can you come out right now? Can you quit your job and come out right now?" Four days later, Lena moved in with her parents and started working at the dry cleaner.

Lena's decision to support her mother was difficult. Her relationship with Mrs. Melnick was, as she put it, "not a very good one." "I know it sounds sick," she said, as she explained that her move to Pennsylvania was motivated more by her love for her father than for Mrs. Melnick. "I have a lot of respect for him," she said, "and I know what he has been living with for the past how many years, and I know how rough it is. He has become dependent on my mother, and I wanted to help him." Lena shut her bedroom door so that Mrs. Melnick, who was sitting in the living room, wouldn't hear her. She then told me how, during her teenage years, her mother abused alcohol. Physical fights, injuries, obscenities, and unpredictable outbursts of anger were common. "There have been a lot of things that have happened over the course of my relationship with my mom that I thought were just irreparable," she said. "It was awful, and my dad has no recollection of that whatsoever. He is in denial, although he would sit up with her for nights, many nights. I remember one time I came in and he was choking her and another time she was choking him, and—oh my God! It was awful."

All three of the children became suicidal. Paul developed a drinking problem of his own. But Lena said she suffered the most. For reasons she did not understand, she became the target of her mother's violent eruptions. She suspected that Mrs. Melnick was jealous of her. Lena had many friends, she did not suppress her feelings, and she enjoyed a close relationship with her father. To protect herself, she "disconnected" from her family. For a while she moved in with her grandmother. Later, she rented her own apartment and visited her parents only occasionally. Even then, she felt discomfort around her mother. At times she "could not stand to be in the same room" with her. Now, however, she had come to Lancaster County "with an open heart" and a renewed belief in God. She had forgiven Mrs. Melnick for the pain she had caused her, and she had forgiven herself for the ways in which she might have contributed to her mother's rages. Her hope was that she and her mother would finally bond.

"I'm Going to Heaven"

The Hospice of Lancaster County had been involved with Mrs. Melnick's care for a month and a half before she refused brain surgery. Because she was younger than 65, she did not qualify for Medicare's hospice benefit. When she discovered that the benefits from her private insurance were limited, she was shocked. Her coverage included only "skilled nursing visits." Medical equipment like an electric hospital bed, a wheelchair, and a walker had to be paid out of pocket. Her insurance would not pay for continuous hospice home care either. Neither she nor her husband had the money to cover the support she would need to live comfortably through the last weeks of her life. The local Cancer Society provided her with a walker and promised an electric hospital bed and wheelchair, if and when she were to need them— interventions that Mrs. Melnick interpreted as further evidence of God's providence. Lena was named Mrs. Melnick's "primary care provider." Mr. Melnick, who would have been the most likely candidate for this position, did not want to get too involved. He did not cope well with crises, and the responsibilities of the business were more than he could handle.

Sue Elwood, the hospice nurse, tried her best to address Mrs. Melnick's symptoms with acetaminophen and codeine (for headaches), lorazepam and temazepam (for anxiety and insomnia), amitriptyline (for neuropathic pain in her arm), and prochlorperazine (for nausea). Mrs. Melnick's seizures, the symptom that upset her the most, were controlled with phenytoin. When free of pain, Mrs. Melnick was relatively comfortable. But her unsteady gait and shaking hand prevented her from carrying out day-to-day activities. "A lot of times she will try to feed herself and the spoon will go to her chin instead of her mouth," Sue observed. To keep her safe, Sue recommended that Mrs. Melnick not be left alone. Lena hired an assistant for the dry cleaning store to replace her.

Nadia Lantz, a personal care nurse from hospice, saw Mrs. Melnick five days a week. Nadia's primary purpose was to assist Mrs. Melnick with her personal hygiene. Mrs. Melnick was exceedingly modest. She did not want anyone to see her naked—not even her husband. She told me that she belonged to a generation in which "women kept their private parts private." Despite Nadia's reassurances that she was a beautiful woman, she felt shame about her body because she had lost weight. She insisted on washing herself alone. She always shut the bathroom door and had Nadia wait outside in case of an accident. The only help she accepted was a medical chair for the shower and an elevated seat with handles for the toilet.

Mrs. Melnick expected to die about a week before Christmas. She was remarkably pragmatic. She gave Lena durable power of attorney. She also passed on to her the ownership of the dry cleaning store and the responsibility for managing the family's finances. She instructed Nadia to keep her comfortable on the last days of her life and to remember to moisten her mouth and straighten her sheets when she was no longer able to speak. She asked her family to gather around her bed and pray when she died. She pleaded with her children to stay together after her death and make sure to take care of their father. Convinced that Mr. Melnick was incapable of carrying out such a task, she made her own funeral arrangements.

Mrs. Melnick despised the cliché about cancer patients' "courageous battle" against their disease, for she didn't see herself as a fighter. "You don't have a battle, you are stuck!" she often said in exasperation. "I got this disease, and there is no 'courageous battle.' It is a battle with your God and your peace, but not with the cancer. There is nothing courageous about it." She told me that she dreaded everything that would come prior to her death. She didn't fear being dead; she feared getting there. How much longer would she live? How much longer would she be able to maintain even a bit of independence? How much longer would she be conscious enough to comprehend what was happening to her? Would she lose her mind so fully that she would start lashing out? Would she be forced to give up her modesty, just to stay physically clean? More than anything, she feared being bedridden. To her, the inability to stand up in the morning and sit upright for the rest of the day seemed the most violent assault of all.

Despite her family's discomfort with "morbid conversations," Mrs. Melnick had no difficulty talking about her death. "I talk about my death like I would talk about going to work," she remarked. Through her openness, she said, she ripped some of the mystique away from the subject and prepared her children better for her imminent demise. She showed everyone around her that she was neither distraught nor devastated. "I just have this inner peace," she said. "I feel God is with me. Dying is not scary to me at all. I could die tomorrow, and I will be at peace because I know where I'm going. I'm going to Heaven. I am going to be with Jesus, so I am not afraid of that. God promised me that, and I live on His promise. I just believe in His word."

Her main concern was Lena. In one of our meetings in her bedroom, still trying to isolate ourselves from Anabel the parrot, Mrs. Melnick admitted that her daughter and she had not been as close as she wanted. When Lena was a teenager, she said, she cut Mrs. Melnick out of her life. She avoided spending time with her and resented her motherly advice. "She is our only girl, so we spoiled her and, oh, those teenage years were horrible," she remarked. "Lena was stubborn, she was going to do what she wanted to do. She even left home for a while and stayed with my mother. We had a couple of shaky years, and it is possible she is feeling a little bit guilty about that." In Mrs. Melnick's view, Lena went through a normal, adolescent rebellious phase. Now, she suspected, she had returned to repair the damage she caused and free herself from the guilt that burdened her. I wondered if she was going to say anything about alcohol, fights, injuries, or rages. She did not.

"My Nadia," as Mrs. Melnick had started to refer to her personal care nurse from hospice, was a young and vibrant woman. She applied lotion daily to Mrs. Melnick's scalp to moisten the skin that had dried out from the radiation. Standing behind her, rubbing her head with slow and rhythmic movements, she gave Mrs. Melnick precious moments of human touch. Hesitantly, Mrs.

Melnick started to call her into the bathroom. One time she asked for help scrubbing her back, another time, getting out of the bathtub, a third, drying her legs. To respect her privacy, Nadia walked in, assisted with the task at hand, and left the bathroom as soon as she was finished.

It took time for Mrs. Melnick to get used to Nadia's help. But she came to like Nadia's professionalism, warmth, gentleness, intelligence, humor, sensitivity, and—most importantly—her Christian faith. It was very important to Mrs. Melnick to be surrounded by Christians. She was delighted to discover that the other hospice staff on her team attended Christian churches as well. "Christian people are caregivers. Like nurses in the hospital, hospice nurses could not do it if they weren't. They couldn't do it," she asserted. Nadia said "Praise the Lord" at the end of every sentence that expressed a good thought. Anabel learned to say it, too. "Praise the Lord!" she would shout during my visits. "Praise the Lord!"

Lena complained that Nadia was cutting into her time with her mother.

Old Hurts Boil Over

It was December 16. "I feel as though I am going to make it for Christmas," exclaimed Mrs. Melnick. "After that, every day is going to be a blessing—what God gives me, you know." The approach of the holidays excited her, but it also filled her with a "bittersweet" feeling. As she explained,

> The hardest part for me is the loss. That is something you feel because of little remarks people will say: "I am going to do this this summer," "I am going to do this a month from now or two months from now," and I know that I may not be here and that will go through my mind right away. The sweetness is that I'm going to be with my Lord, my God. I am not going to suffer. I am not going to be bedridden as long. That is a blessing to me.

She pulled the family Christmas tree out of storage and asked Lena to decorate it. It looked like mother and daughter would be able to plan an unforgettable holiday together. Paul was due in four days with his wife and son. But the newly hired assistant at the dry cleaner's got sick, and Lena was forced to resume her normal working hours at the store. Days went by, and Lena did not find the time to decorate the tree. Mr. Melnick returned home overworked, irritable, and unable to devote his attention to anything other than the television. Lena was equally exhausted. To decompress, she went out with her friends and stayed up late. The household was filling up with tension. When Paul and his family arrived, everyone cheered up. But the Christmas tree was still leaning against the wall, long and thin and bound up unadorned.

On Christmas Eve, Mrs. Melnick told herself, "This is my last Christmas, and I am not going to get aggravated over a tree!" She mustered all her energy to pick the tree up, drag it into Lena's bedroom, and drop it in the corner. "Lena," she said, "if you don't feel like putting the tree up, we won't have it then, but I don't want to see it sitting in the living room. It's making me nervous!" Shocked and enraged, Lena carried the tree back to the living room and set it up. "Everything has been falling on my shoulders," she told me exasperated and exhausted. "I have got to take care of the business, I have got to take care of both parents, everything is my fault, I have got to take care of everything. Paul could have gotten the Christmas decorations out easily, but they wanted *me* to do it for some reason." She hunted for the decorations but couldn't find them. Paul had been drinking and was upset at the commotion. When Lena finally found the ornaments, she threw them on the couch. On her way out, she swore and pushed her brother. He, in turn, hit Lena in the face. "I still have a scar right here on my head," she told me. "He was choking me, he was trying to kill me. I have never felt so betrayed and so upset in my life." Mrs. Melnick took Paul's side. "Lena," she said, "that is your brother, and you don't expect your brother to stand there and get manhandled."

"I don't have any respect for my mom after the Christmas tree incident," Lena asserted. She concluded that she would never get close to her mother. It's not that she didn't love Mrs. Melnick; she did, she grieved for her. She was convinced that her mother was unhappy and saw her almost complete con-finement to her chair as the most brutal form of torture against her strong-willed and active spirit. But, at the same time, she wondered if this person who was now at the brink of death had grown from her experiences, recog-nized her mistakes, and changed inside in any way that made her a better person. Lena doubted it. She was angry and confused. Was she a bad person to feel resentment toward a woman who would soon be dead?

The Victory Tree

"The patient had an enjoyable Christmas with her family," wrote Sue, the hospice nurse, in Mrs. Melnick's chart on January 2, 1997. In the new year, Lena returned to spending her days at home on a full-time basis. Anabel had mastered the phrase "Merry Christmas," which she repeated ceaselessly. The fact that Mrs. Melnick had lived to see the holidays meant a lot to her. "To me, it's a victory," she said. "A victory in Jesus." She saw her survival as proof of God's power and the Christmas tree as a symbol of his presence in her life. She named it her "victory tree" and vowed to leave it up until the day she died.

When the undertaker who stopped by to discuss Mrs. Melnick's funeral left, Mrs. Melnick felt relief. Lena felt shock. She did not know that her mother had taken it upon herself to arrange her own funeral. She couldn't believe how coldly and calmly Mrs. Melnick had discussed the technicalities of her own interment. In tears, she called her father to report what she had witnessed, and he, too, sounded surprised. When he returned, he looked at his wife and said, "Aren't you jumping the gun a little?" Mrs. Melnick didn't expect such a reaction. "I have been tying up loose ends by myself," she said to me, "but that is what I have always done. All my life. It has worked. It is working still. I would have liked my husband to have helped me, but I know he would have never [done it]."

When I saw Mrs. Melnick in the beginning of February, I couldn't help but notice her decline. For the first time she appeared small in her chair. Her world had shrunk to what seemed like a little circle—her walker, a newly acquired bedside commode, several feet of cable that brought the telephone to her lap, and her coffee table, which was filled with medications. From that day on, we stopped conducting interviews in her bedroom for moving from one room to the next had become too risky. Anabel greeted me with a few "hellos" and "goodbyes" and "Praise the Lords," but overall, she remained noticeably quiet. Mrs. Melnick was eager to talk. She wasn't sure how many more interviews we'd be able to have. "I am progressing," she said and started to cry. Her legs and abdomen were strikingly swollen. Her right arm and right leg had become increasingly harder to control. Nadia had to help her take showers. At night she couldn't lift her leg to get into bed. And she started to lose control of her bowels. "My stools just shot out, and I was mortified, and Lena cleaned the whole bathroom down," she said. She would watch a movie and an hour later, forget all about it. Only a week earlier, she had the ability to fold clothes, but the day I saw her that seemed like an unmanageable task.

The thought of not seeing her children ever again devastated her. Whom would they call when they needed help? Would Paul finish his culinary training without her emotional and financial support? Would her "helpless" husband John, who was so used to being taken care of, be able to carry on?

"He just found out that there was a filter in the dryer!" she exclaimed. She feared that Mr. Melnick would languish, although she also acknowledged Anabel's ability to give him support. The parrot was especially attached to her husband. "Right now, I think how much more I should have done through the years," Mrs. Melnick went on. "I will even think about when I was a little girl that I was cruel to somebody. And it flashes back. I will even think of that, and I think, 'I wish I would have been a better person.' Oftentimes I think of that, but without depression. I am not browbeating myself, because I did do some nice things, too. But I wish I would have done more nice things, even as a child. I think how my God loves me, and he is so alive to me, and I know he is going to forgive me for these things, but I just wish. . . ."

Nadia

Over the next few weeks, Mrs. Melnick's bowel incontinence became a regular problem. When getting up in the morning, she often defecated on the floor. Although she agreed with Sue that stool hardeners were likely to cause the even more serious challenge of constipation, she hoped there was an alternative solution to the situation. Sue, who did not have an answer, started feeling inadequate as a nurse. She began to experience Mrs. Melnick as someone who seemed to want things Sue couldn't offer and who rejected things she could. When it came to her personal hygiene, for example, Mrs. Melnick declined Sue's offers to help. Emotionally, Sue found herself disengaging from Mrs. Melnick. She turned her attention to technical matters, such as the provision of needed medical equipment and the identification of people who would be able to stay with Mrs. Melnick once she started requiring round-the-clock care.

Nadia still saw Mrs. Melnick five days a week. She had gotten to know her well, and she liked her. Yet the intensity of Mrs. Melnick's dependence on her made her uncomfortable. She found Mrs. Melnick intrusive. Mrs. Melnick seemed to want to know everything about her. She asked to meet Nadia's children, but Nadia gently declined. She explained that it would be emotionally taxing for them to interact with dying patients and exhausting for Nadia herself to keep answering their questions about death. Mrs. Melnick understood and apologized for her request. "My job sucks the life out of me," Nadia said to me. "Then I don't have it to give to my kids, and I don't feel like reading with them, I don't feel like playing with them, because I have given all my guts to Katie or so-and-so all week. It becomes stressful to me going to Katie every day, every day, every day. I need a break from her. I started to feel like the attachment is getting greater, and when she emphasizes how she depends on me, and that her comfort level is only there with me as far as personal care, that gets to me. I feel like she is depending on me too much." On her days off, Nadia felt tortured by the idea that Mrs. Melnick did not shower. At the same time, she recognized a side of Mrs. Melnick to which few others were privy. It was a vulnerable side, a scared side, that was trying to gain minimal control over a horrifying and uncontrollable situation. "It is like knowing that a Mack truck is going to run over you and watching it come toward you," Nadia said. "Can you imagine the intensity of that?"

The Bed

At the beginning of February, Mrs. Melnick reported that Pat, a childhood friend from Ohio, was going to take care of her during her final days. Pat, she said, would help her smoke when she was no longer able to hold a cigarette. "I am totally addicted," she laughed. "I will have withdrawals if I stop smoking, and I have enough troubles. I don't want withdrawal."

An electric hospital bed was delivered to the Melnicks free of charge and was placed in Mrs. Melnick's bedroom, next to her queen-size bed. Mrs. Melnick was alone when it arrived. Its sight upset her. "Once I am in the hospital bed," she told me in tears, "I know for sure it is down, down, down. That is a big turning point." Wendy, the hospice social worker, spent a visit discussing with Mrs. Melnick what this new development meant to her. Lena joined that conversation, too. Mother and daughter admitted that the hospital bed symbolized the imminence of Mrs. Melnick's death. The first time Lena saw it, she sat across from it in shock and sobbed. Soon after, she was joined by her father, who put his arm around her and wept for the first time himself.

"Boy, Does This Suck!"

No one had expected Mrs. Melnick to make it to February. Valentine's Day was just around the corner. In acknowledgment of her mother's second victory, Lena replaced the Christmas tree ornaments with red hearts. Mrs. Melnick was happy and thankful for being alive, but she cried frequently during our meetings. Her bowels continued to move unexpectedly. Accidents took place on a daily basis and required Lena to clean up. Her incontinence was degrading to Mrs. Melnick. Together with the arrival of the bed, she added it to the milestones of her decline. Still, she said, "I have never questioned 'why me.' I just accept what is happening day by day. Look, the doctors said I would not be here. I just put my faith in God, and I am here. God knows. He wrote the book. He knows the beginning and the end. He knows why I'm here. God has his reason for the bowel movements, too."

Lena was less accepting of the situation. She saw Mrs. Melnick's cancer as an "unseen monster" that was robbing her of her dignity. She was overwhelmed by her mother's rapid deterioration. A stalwart woman had, right in front of her eyes, transformed into a fragile cancer patient with a "cabbage patch" face, no hair, a distended belly, flaccid skin, and feet that looked like "balloons." Although Lena's resentment toward her mother remained unabated, she noticed that caring for her had brought her into a new position—one in which she felt protective of Mrs. Melnick and wanted to make sure that her departure from this life would take place in peace.

By the beginning of March, Mrs. Melnick's face had swelled up further, her eyes looked sunken in dark circles. Her lower legs showed signs of mottling. "There is no other word for it," she said to me, while taking slow and shaky puffs on her cigarette, "I am waiting to die. I am not going to get better, I am getting worse, and there is less and less I can do. I am waiting to die. That is it." "She is really, really, really scared," Paul told me after one of his visits back to Lancaster County. "I could just see it in her eyes. Her favorite saying now is, 'Boy, does this suck!' She never talked like that before. Then you have to crack up. She says, 'One of these days I would like to wake up and this is all a nightmare. It has to be a dream.' I just laugh and say, 'Yeah. Unfortunately, it is not.' I tell her, 'You always were brain dead, and now it is true,' and she laughs. When I come here it seems like she cries more because I ask her a lot of questions, like 'How do you really feel?' and she will say 'Okay.' I will say, 'Bullshit! Tell me. I want to know.' Then she will cry."

March was an exhausting month for everyone. Mr. Melnick and the three children hoped that death would come soon. Mrs. Melnick was tired of waiting. Our interviews became slow and scattered. She told me that she couldn't think, even though she made every effort to answer my questions. She felt weaker and drowsier each day. She stopped taking showers because she had lost the strength and motor skills they required. She got sponge baths instead, which she saw as a precious alternative, for she wished to stay clean until the end. The problem with her loose bowels slowly resolved itself. Now she was constipated and had to cope with abdominal cramps and pressure. Enemas did not always work. She reported hemorrhoids, more pain, scalp itching, thrush, and a possible vaginal infection, but with the help of treatments, she asserted that she was adjusting well. "It is very important to me to adjust," she said softly. "I don't want the disease to control me. I want to control the disease."

"I Stay in with My Honey"

On the third week of March, Lena took her father's place at the dry cleaner. This allowed Mr. Melnick to stay home. He lifted Mrs. Melnick in and out of chairs and then retreated to a quiet world of his own. No one knew how he was feeling. He spent many hours in the living room watching television or interacting sweetly with Anabel. He rarely participated in conversations with visitors and, at times, even failed to acknowledge their presence. I never invited him for an interview because he seemed uncomfortable when I paid attention to him. One time, in the middle of my conversation with Mrs. Melnick, she turned to him and asked, "John, do you want to say something? How are you feeling now with it getting closer to the time? You know, how do you feel about death? It could be only two more weeks and I could be dead, but how do you feel about that?" He replied that he didn't like it at all. That was the end of the discussion.

His response, albeit short, at least revealed that he understood his wife's prognosis. This seemed like a departure from earlier times when his reactions suggested that he questioned the severity of Mrs. Melnick's illness and resented her requests for help. Sue, Nadia, and Wendy had all felt worry that he would not be a compassionate caregiver. But now, to their surprise, they saw him changing. First, he started emptying Mrs. Melnick's commode. A few days later, he began lighting her cigarette. And when I saw him, he was getting ready to rub lotion on her head. "I have not been out in I don't know how many days," he said. "I stay in with my honey." "I am still in shock that John is doing all this," remarked Mrs. Melnick later. "He never did that. I was starting to feel, you know, my kids love me, they are close, and my husband is still cold and then, all of a sudden, he is just wonderful. I think he is finally realizing that this is happening, but it is more than that. He just never did those things for me."

In anticipation of Easter, Lena decorated the Christmas tree with paper eggs and flowers. She was tired and distraught and wished that her mother would die soon because she couldn't stand to see her suffer any longer. She felt more love for her now than ever before, she said to me. But she also worried. She didn't think Mrs. Melnick would be able to let go without acknowledging her mistakes and making peace with the people she had hurt.

"Prescription for K. Melnick—Please Knock"

Paul and Carl arrived together to see their mother on April 4. Mrs. Melnick opened her eyes briefly and with a glassy stare asked Lena to close the store and stay home. A quiet tension filled the house. Mrs. Melnick's breathing was uneven. She went through moments of apnea. Her knees were mottled, and her urine output had decreased. Nadia spent her visit washing Mrs. Melnick's face and moistening her lips. She told Mrs. Melnick goodbye. "I thought about how I would like to say it," she reflected later. "Katie," she said, "the time may be coming soon, and I just want you to know that I feel very fortunate to have gotten to know you, and I really feel that we have become special friends. Even though I have to maintain a certain professional level, I consider you someone that I would have loved to be friends with, even if we had not met under these circumstances." Then she left.

An uneasy quiet fell upon the Melnicks again. Suddenly, Mrs. Melnick opened her eyes. "I am going to Hell!" she shouted. Her voice was startlingly loud. Lena heard it in her bedroom. Mr. Melnick ran to her side and reassured her that she was a good person, that she was not going to Hell, that she had done many good things over the years, that there was no reason to worry. But Mrs. Melnick insisted she knew better. With the few words she could utter, she asked for a Catholic priest to absolve her of her sins. The priest arrived within hours. He spent some private time with Mrs. Melnick and left. "I felt fortunate to be part of everything," said Lena when she recalled that day. "My mother apologized for things she said way back when, and how she had such a problem with alcohol. She knows Jesus Christ is her savior, but I guess with the brain tumor she got too confused." Soon after the priest's departure, Lena called hospice to report that her mother was seeing angels.

April 5 was the first day that Mrs. Melnick could not get out of bed. She was surrounded by Mr. Melnick, their three children, and Pat, her friend from Ohio who had arrived a few days earlier to help. In the afternoon, she started to moan. Assuming that she was in pain, Paul and Lena bolted out of the house to pick up a prescription for more morphine. When they got to the drugstore, they found a note on the door saying, "Prescription for K. Melnick—please knock." "Boy, is that nice," Lena remembered thinking. "They close the store, but they realize how bad we need the prescription. They are going to let me get it. That is really nice of them." She knocked, feeling happy but also nervous, because she didn't quite understand what was happening with her mother. The pharmacist came to the door looking solemn.

"Hi," Lena said, showing her checkbook. "I am here for my prescriptions for Katie Melnick."

As she started to write the check, the pharmacist shook his head.

"What happened?" Lena asked. "You don't have the morphine or what is the matter?"

"No, no," the pharmacist replied. "We got a call ten minutes ago that you are not going to be needing it anymore."

Lena stood stunned. "She died?"

"I think so," the pharmacist said, his eyes welling up with tears.

Mrs. Melnick had taken her last breath minutes earlier, lying next to her neatly folded prayer blanket. Pat reported that her death was peaceful. "Paul and I were not meant to be there," Lena told me later.

The Melnicks were in shock. They cried. They wailed. They held each other. They called Nadia, who came to the house immediately. Lena gave Nadia a gift that her mother had bought for her. It was a small porcelain vase. With it came a card from Mrs. Melnick, which Nadia recalled "just moved me because it was almost as if she was talking to me, her words, that she was glad to have had me for a nurse and how she appreciated me."

Mrs. Melnick's body looked exhausted. The black bags under her eyes and her dry, wrinkled skin communicated that she had struggled. Nadia compared her to a traveler who crossed the Sahara Desert and died. When the undertaker arrived, the Melnicks withdrew into a bedroom. They didn't want to see Mrs. Melnick's final exit. As he carried her body out of the house, they heard a loud, "Bye-bye, Melnick!" It was Anabel.

"There Were Just Too Many Memories"

Mrs. Melnick was cremated. Her funeral was attended by about 25 people, including Sue, Nadia, Wendy, and two other personal care nurses from hospice.

Anabel sat in the Melnicks' car. Tearful, Mr. Melnick asked Wendy for a follow-up bereavement visit. Then he and his family took off for Maryland to deposit Mrs. Melnick's ashes.

At the end of April, Mr. Melnick and Lena were back at work. They told Wendy that their trip gave them consolation because it reunited them with old friends. What they found most difficult was returning home. Everything in their apartment reminded them of Mrs. Melnick. The empty, overstuffed living room chair startled them. They wanted to move out. But they also announced that they no longer needed bereavement visits. They thanked Wendy for her help and gave her three gifts from Mrs. Melnick—one for herself, another for Sue, and a third for me. "It is like she's still alive," said Paul with a chuckle when I spoke to him a few weeks later. "I was going to get a pair of shoes for the funeral, and I was thinking, 'Oh, I'd better get a nice pair or she is going to bitch. I don't want to go home and face the music.' And it was like, 'Wait a minute! She isn't there! That is why I'm going to get the shoes.' I was laughing. She was probably laughing too, saying, 'You idiot! I have really got you trained!'"

In May, the Melnicks closed the store. It had been an unprofitable business, full of painful memories. They were happy to get rid of it. Then father and daughter parted ways. Mr. Melnick traveled to Georgia to spend the summer with his brother. Lena stayed in Lancaster County with Anabel. She was eager to spend more time with her new boyfriend. Her father advised her to move to a new apartment, but she couldn't find anything as affordable as their own. Adjusting to a new life was difficult, she said. And she continued,

> Oh, I miss Mom so bad. I do. I know she is in a better place. I understand it was her time. God took her and I understand that, but it hurts so bad. Everywhere you look I see her glasses, her cream, her shoes, or her clothing or something, and it is just difficult. My dad and I were so used to taking care of her, it is still instilled in me: I have got to get home—I don't know what I am going to do, but I have got to do something. My dad was a real wreck for a while. It was bad. He broke up a lot. I never saw anything like that. He could not stay in the business. There were just too many memories.

Five months after Mrs. Melnick's death, Lena still had dreams that her mother was alive and cured. Her mother's closet emitted a smell of smoke. She went through all the clothes and gave many of them away. The one thought that uplifted her was that her mother had made peace with her before she died.

"That made me feel so good because I wanted so badly, so desperately, to be close with her, and she just could not become close with any woman. I felt like I was on cloud nine. I was like, 'Thank you so much,' and I am crying, and I was saying, 'I love you so much, you have no idea,' and she was like, 'I know, I know.'"

Lena and her boyfriend got engaged in July. A month later, Mr. Melnick announced that he had bought a house in his brother's neighborhood in Georgia. Lena felt abandoned, but she was also relieved that her father had started a new life. His brother had always been a good friend to him, and the closeness between them comforted her. "I hope he is not thinking he can run away from the memories or the emotions, because they are going to come haunting back," she remarked. She wished she could ask him about his feelings, but she knew that he was too private to handle such a question.

"I cannot imagine my life without my dad now," Lena said to me. "Not at all. One day he had a very rough morning, and we both cried together, and I was holding him, and we were holding each other and just talking, and he said, 'I love you.' He said, 'Thank you.' He said, 'I thank God for you.' He said, 'I don't know what I would do without you,' and it made me feel really good. When you don't hear things and then you do, you are like, 'Wow.'"

Authors' Comments

Katie Melnick did not fear death. Or that is what she said. "I could die to-morrow," she announced, "and I will be at peace because I know where I'm going. I'm going to Heaven. I'm going to be with Jesus." Her deep and abiding Christian faith, the very first subject she introduced when we began the interviews for our project, gave her profound equanimity at the prospect of her death. But she had many fears about the process of dying, which she enumerated poignantly in one of our conversations. When would it happen? When would she lose her independence? Her conscious awareness? Her modesty? These unknowns filled her with dread. Hospice and palliative care workers can play an important role to assuage such fears by providing straightforward information—at the level and pace desired by the patient—about what typically happens, physically and cognitively, in the last weeks, days, and hours of life, especially in deaths from diseases like cancer with a relatively predictable trajectory. The brochure "Gone From My Sight," by

Barbara Karnes, is one very popular resource that hospice programs frequently share with patients and families.[1]

As we observed in the narrative of Stanley Gray, Mrs. Melnick's intense focus on her faith in God was a mixed blessing for her caregivers. On the one hand, it enabled her to speak about dying with a frankness that her hospice team appreciated and made some aspects of their jobs easier. Indeed, all of Mrs. Melnick's caregivers were, like her, White, church-going Christians. This cultural homogeneity—while it could lead to misunderstanding and marginalizing of some patients, as we commented in the case of Shamira Cook— in this case underlay an immediate bonding between caregiver and patient. Talking about God and faith was a readily available lubricant to smooth the hours of caregiving and companionship that hospice provided and that are a hallmark of this narrative. On the other hand, Mrs. Melnick's preoccupation with God, as well as her repeated assertions that she would go to Heaven may have built a protective distance between her and her caregivers, who may have missed opportunities to detect and address aspects of her past that tortured her and that greatly complicated her daughter Lena's efforts to be close to her as she died.

Might Mrs. Melnick's overt religiosity have been too readily available? Mrs. Melnick had a history of alcoholism, and her children, especially Lena, still carried traumatic memories and resentments from her parenting. Mrs. Melnick herself expressed regret for cruel things she had done "as a little girl" and wished she had been a better person—a reference to memories of her childhood that may well have been a displacement of guilt and shame at the actions of her older self. Indeed, close to the time of her death she cried out in terror that she was going to Hell and asked for a priest to absolve her of her sins. Lena found this to be a healing moment, as it led her mother to apologize for her hurtful behavior. We might wonder whether this turning point might have occurred earlier and in a less urgent and more transformative manner with the help of sensitive interventions from the hospice team, had they been more attuned to hidden aspects of Mrs. Melnick's life.

Overall, the hospice team expended enormous effort in trying to manage Mrs. Melnick's increasingly distressing symptoms. And they offered hours of tender and compassionate personal care that may have supported, if not facilitated, the soothing comfort that Mr. Melnick was able to give to his wife at the end. Nadia Lantz, the personal care nurse, visited five days a week and became Mrs. Melnick's trusted, indispensable confidante. This took its toll, however. "This job is sucking the life out of me," she said at one point, going on to detail how draining it was to have Mrs. Melnick so dependent on her. She struggled to set limits, and urgently needed a break. Palliative care workers are at risk for "compassion fatigue" and burnout as the demands of increasingly complex nursing functions that they share with other health providers are coupled with the expectation that they engage closely and empathically with their patients' complex and sensitive end-of-life issues. The COVID-19 pandemic, as Anna Towers described in the opening chapter of this book, brought caregiver stress out of the shadows and onto the front pages of our daily newspapers.[2] It is a topic of serious and ongoing professional concern.[3,4]

References

1. Karnes B. Gone from my sight: The dying experience. 2008. https://bkbooks.com/products/gone-from-my-sight-the-dying-experience?variant=36961181171868. Accessed November 13, 2021.
2. Wei E, Segall J, Villanueva Y, Dang LB, Gasca VI, Gonzalez MP, Roman M, Mendez-Justiniano I, Cohen AG, Cho HJ. Coping with trauma, celebrating life: Reinventing patient and staff support during the COVID-19 pandemic. Health Affairs. 2020;39(9):1597–1600.
3. Mills J, Wand T, Fraser JA. Exploring the meaning and practice of self-care among palliative care nurses and doctors: a qualitative study. BMC Palliat Care. 2018;17(1):63. https://doi.org/10.1186/s12904-018-0318-0.
4. Moreno-Milan B, Breitbart B, Herreros B, Olaciregui Dague K, Coca Pereira MC. Psychological well-being of palliative care professionals: Who cares? Palliat Support Care. 2021;19(2):257–261.

19

Susan Mulroney

A Private Matter

Narrated by Patricia Boston

Susan Mulroney had always considered herself a very private person. She had many friends and a caring family, but all her life she prided herself on being very independent and in control of her own affairs. She never liked to burden family or friends with her problems. When she was diagnosed with advanced cervical cancer at the age of 47, she did not talk much about it to anyone. During the next few months, she remained stoic in the face of her illness and tried to continue with her life normally, as though nothing eventful had taken place. But chemotherapy did not work, and she felt increasingly tired, physically weak, and unable to cope on her own.

Not wishing to burden family members, Susan chose to be admitted to the Palliative Care Unit, where her condition rapidly became worse. Her physical symptoms were controlled, and she seemed comfortable. But no one could tell how she was coping emotionally with the knowledge that she would soon die. When people tried to talk with her, she usually found them intrusive. Ten days following her admission to the Palliative Care Unit, she died. Except for one close friend, no one knew much about how she had felt or what the last few months of her life had been like.

A Private Life

Susan Mulroney was a schoolteacher. Born in Montreal, she was raised by parents of Irish descent and lived in an English-speaking area of

Montreal. In her early twenties, she married Richard Gratton, a wealthy businessman. She loved children, and it would have given her great joy to have been a mother. But Susan and Richard did not have any children. After some years the couple began to have marital difficulties and Susan filed for a divorce. Richard remarried. Susan did not, although she met many potential suitors.

In the years following her divorce, Susan threw herself more heavily into her career. She enjoyed teaching in the early grades of high school, and her activities at the school helped to alleviate the sadness of not having children of her own. She became active in school policy and administration. After further study in curriculum development and special education, she became an independent education specialist.

With the extra qualifications came an increase in her salary, which enabled her to afford comfort and beautiful things. Following the breakup of her marriage, she moved to a large, spacious penthouse apartment in a green area of the city. She loved her apartment with its panoramic views. On a clear day she could see mountain peaks as far as one hundred miles away.

The apartment was a refuge of peace and solitude. Though Susan had family and many friends, women and men, she liked living alone. Had she met "the right person" she wouldn't have been averse to the idea of remarriage. She met a few men with whom she could go to the theater and concerts, but there had been no single person she wanted to be with for a lifetime. As the years passed, she couldn't imagine not being able to go home to her own place. She always felt peaceful there. Many of the things in her apartment she had collected on her vacations abroad: porcelain china figurines, delicate wood carvings, and many fine pieces of Eastern artwork, tapestries, and crocheted work.

Susan did have a few special people in her life—her sister Judy and her friend Jack Peterson. Judy was 18 years Susan's senior and had always felt protective toward Susan. When the girls were growing up, their mother was ill with multiple sclerosis. She was often unable to care for the two girls as well as she would have liked. Judy had always looked out for Susan, making sure she got to school on time and helping her with homework, as well as making meals. "I was more like the mother in the home," Judy recalled to me. Over the years, the two sisters joked about what would happen when they were older and Judy became ill and infirm. With such a great age difference between the two women, they assumed Judy would be the one "to go first."

Susan had anticipated looking after Judy in her old age, saying to her laughingly, "I'll take care of you when you get old and you're in a wheelchair."

For a while, when their lives took different paths through marriage and careers, the sisters saw less of each other. Susan had married a businessman and Judy, a lawyer. Later, when both sisters were divorced, they renewed their bonds from childhood. "It was as if we were like schoolgirls again," Judy later recalled. On their vacations together they went mostly to Florida and Barbados in the winter, but also to Africa, India, and Southeast Asia. Once they went on safari.

Despite all the time together and all the trips and outings, there were, Judy said, "limits to how far people could go into Susan's private thoughts. I always knew when I should stop questioning her about something, when what we were talking about was off limits."

The person in whom Susan felt she could confide most of all was Jack Peterson, a colleague at work. The two worked together as teachers for 20 years and saw each other daily. If Susan was facing some dilemma in her teaching or with a colleague, she could talk to Jack, knowing that nothing she told him would be taken any further. It was a "real friendship," Susan told me. Jack later recalled,

> I respected her need for privacy. But it was what you could call a real, honest, good type of relationship. I could say anything to her, and she would say anything to me. I would say I knew most details. If she had a man friend and wasn't sure about the relationship, she'd feel okay about talking things through with me. I think in a way, she felt safe with me. We were pals in every sense of the word.

Susan believed she had led a healthy life. She never smoked. She might have had the odd glass of wine at a restaurant for dinner, but she wasn't someone who sat at home and drank alone. When she cooked for herself, she enjoyed healthy food, vegetables in season, and a lot of fruit. She was active in sports and loved bicycling. On a good day in the spring or summer she could cycle up to 20 miles, she told me, without "taking so much as a second breath." When the weather didn't permit bicycling, she took long walks or a jog in the countryside. Even in winter, in temperatures of minus 15°F, she thought nothing of bundling up in her parka and boots and taking a long, brisk walk. Susan was rarely sick.

"You Could Have Told Her It Was Stage IV, and She Would Have Said, 'Stage IV Out of What? Stage X or Stage XI?'"

I was not able to ascertain precisely when Susan first noticed some unusual symptoms. The first anyone else knew of them was when she mentioned to Jack that she was having pains in her lower back. At the time, Susan had simply joked, "I'm just getting old." She also told Judy about the pain, saying it was because she was "getting too close to 50."

Susan had other symptoms as well, but she didn't tell anyone. She did say once that she didn't feel herself, but did not go into detail. Sometimes when Jack visited her, Susan appeared to be preoccupied with medical books, especially gynecological books. He thought that was odd, but Susan had a curious mind and loved to read. Then she began to frequent medical bookstores and health clinics where she could get the latest information on gynecological illnesses. By then, Jack felt "something wasn't right" because she seemed so single-minded about this kind of information. But she did not go to see a doctor. Looking back, Jack thought that Susan must have had a clear idea that "something was very wrong."

In December 1994, Susan did at last consult Dr. Jean Paul, her gynecologist. He examined her and took a Pap smear. One week later, his secretary telephoned and asked if Susan could see Dr. Paul at his office regarding the results. The pap smear was reported as Stage IV, which meant that she had cancer in her cervix. When Dr. Paul told Susan this, she accepted the news calmly. She was not a medical person, so it was not immediately clear to her what it meant. Jack's wife, Rita, however, was a nurse and she knew what a stage IV pap smear meant: something was seriously wrong.

Rita did not want to interfere in any way, but she thought that stage IV must mean that the cancer was already at a very advanced stage. Jack recalled,

> When Susan got the news from Dr. Paul, it seemed funny that she never went through any crying fits or anything. She seemed to accept everything. It was, "Okay! It's business as usual." She seemed to accept everything easily, almost too easily. In many ways, I don't think she knew what stage IV meant. You could have told her it was stage IV and she would have said, "Stage IV out of what? Stage X or stage XI?" She'd never been exposed to anything medical in that sense.

Dr. Paul urgently referred Susan to Jacob Lieberman, a surgical oncologist, who immediately ordered tests to determine how far the cancer had spread. It was very advanced. Dr. Lieberman told Susan that he would do all he could to arrest its growth, and Susan began chemotherapy. Some weeks later, she received radiotherapy externally and internally to the uterine cavity. When she told Judy that she had cancer and was getting it treated, Judy was frightened. Susan had led such a healthy life! Why her?

Judy would have liked to have asked more questions, and perhaps have a chat with Dr. Paul. But her only function was to accompany Susan to the chemotherapy clinic for treatments, and there were to be no questions asked. As she later recalled,

> I would sit and wait with her while she got to see the doctor and when she went for blood tests. She always seemed to be handling it. Sometimes she'd be irritable when she was getting the blood tests because we'd sit and wait and wait and wait. But she wouldn't talk about it. Sometimes she'd say, "That's it, I'm not waiting anymore," and I'd almost have to sit on her, and I'd say, "No, no. We need to wait." Then she'd go in to see the doctor and I'd have to wait outside. She never ever mentioned what he said, and I never asked.

Susan had a way of changing the subject very quickly if one asked questions she was not prepared to answer. As Jack said, "She'd tell you right off, 'I don't want to talk about it,' and she'd immediately go on to something else. You could try to bring her back, but then she'd get irritated and clam up altogether."

"I Am Going to Die"

Susan underwent radiotherapy and chemotherapy throughout most of 1995. During this period, she tried to continue with her life as though very little of any real consequence were happening. She loved to go shopping and buy clothes. Sometimes she'd go downtown and "spend every cent she had on a new dress." She still wanted the social life she had enjoyed before with her sister. She went to restaurants and movies and acted as if nothing were wrong. She continued to bicycle, walk, and jog. Sometimes she called Jack and Rita to ask if they wanted to go for a few hours of biking. Rita Peterson was not much for biking, so Jack would go. They would bike for miles.

Yet her condition worsened. She developed increasing pain in her back and legs and sometimes had sharp cramps in her abdomen. She had less and less appetite, even for her favorite foods. Sometimes she would eat a meal and immediately feel full and sick after it. Even a bowl of fresh fruit was difficult to digest. Sometimes it was easier just to vomit what she ate.

In November Dr. Lieberman informed Susan that there was no further treatment for her cancer. It was possible that one of the oncology surgeons at the hospital would be able to suggest another option, but from Dr. Lieberman's standpoint, there was "nothing at all." It was now just 10 months since Dr. Paul had first broken the news.

On November 20, 1995, Susan came into the hospital's surgical ward for further assessment. The surgeon, Ernest Simpson, explained to her that, surgically, there was nothing to be done. The tumors had spread to her bladder and bowel. Dr. Simpson was patient but direct, probably because Susan was that way herself. As Jack later said to me, "She expected you to lay things right on the nose, no messing around."

It was at this time that Susan told Jack about her condition. "I am going to die," she said. Still, she did not talk about her feelings. She was matter-of-fact, concerned with the practicalities of what she needed in the way of night clothes and toiletries in the hospital. When she was in the hospital, she talked about the activities on the ward, the person in the next bed, or something minor or inconsequential a particular nurse or doctor had said. Jack recalled,

> At times, you felt you were walking on eggs. Because she wouldn't feel comfortable if you pushed her on any piece of information she gave you. What she told you, that was her choice to make. And if I ever pushed her on how she felt about something, she'd back off. And then I'd end up feeling uncomfortable that I'd put her in that position.

Cold White Walls and White Coats

As Susan's symptoms rapidly became more acute, Dr. Lieberman and Dr. Simpson referred her to the Palliative Care Service for more specialized management of her pain and discomfort. They thought she would also need greater emotional support than the surgical team was able to provide. Dr. Gillian Webster, of the Palliative Care Service, noted the gravity of her condition. Susan was thin, her abdomen was full and hard on palpation, and she had skin edema. She was experiencing mid-back and epigastric pain, nausea, and vomiting. She was uncomfortable from constipation as an immediate result of the tumors' pressure on her bowel. Her red blood count was low, and she had reportedly been vomiting "coffee grounds" during the previous 24 hours, a sign of gastrointestinal bleeding. There was a risk of major gastrointestinal hemorrhage.

Gillian set up a medication plan with comfort and pain relief as her ultimate goal, prescribing the following: omeprazole 40 mg orally every four hours for epigastric pain; prochlorperazine 10 mg by mouth or rectum three times daily, and dimenhydrinate as needed for nausea and vomiting; morphine 5–10 mg orally every four hours and nortriptyline 25 mg orally every four hours for pain; and, for constipation, docusate and bisacodyl.

Gillian also explained the nature and goals of the Palliative Care Service and the various options that were available. Susan could stay on the surgical unit, she could be transferred onto the Palliative Care Unit (PCU), or, if someone could take care of her, it was possible she could go home. Susan needed to think about this carefully. There was no denying that she needed full-time care. But she would much rather go home and be alone. Besides, it was Christmas time. She could not imagine what it would be like not to be in her own home at Christmas. Judy offered to move in with her if she wanted to be in her own apartment, but Susan kept saying, "I don't want to be a burden to anyone." Judy told me later, "It wasn't a burden. It would have been a gift to care for her." But she also remembered that, during the past year when she had tried to care for Susan at home, she had always felt "a bit in the way."

Susan felt that the surgical unit was "cold" and "sterile." It was generally noisy with the bustle of daily clinical activities. There was no view to speak of from her window, and when she looked around she saw "cold white walls and a lot of people in white coats—all very white!" During the day the nursing station was noisy and intrusive. The PCU sounded "nice and quiet." She had heard there was carpeting rather than linoleum on the floors. She told Gillian she wanted to go to the PCU.

At this point I received a call from Gillian, who had learned that Susan was interested in being a participant in our study. She was, she had told Dr. Webster, "first and foremost a teacher." If it would help other caregivers and medical staff to learn from her experiences, she would like to be involved.

Our first meeting took place in the surgical unit. The unit was brightly decorated with silver tinsel streamers, balloons, and colorful posters announcing holiday parties. There was an atmosphere of busyness, energy, and healthy noise about the place. Everything seemed to be in motion. People called out "Merry Christmas!" to one another. As I passed the nursing station to get to Susan's room I wondered how she must be feeling in the midst of all this buoyancy. Would she be thinking about Christmas?

Her room was depressing and cold. On the wall was a polished plaque, stating that the ward acknowledged the memory of a deceased benefactor. Seen vaguely in the midst of massed flowers on the windowsill and the white and blue draperies, the plaque gave me an eerie feeling of being in the antechamber of a funeral home. I couldn't imagine wanting to stay here knowing I was going to die. Susan smiled as she greeted me. Then she stared straight ahead, hardly making any eye contact. Despite her frailty I noticed how attractive she was and that she looked much younger than her age. She had short, cropped, dark hair; clear, unwrinkled skin; and pale blue eyes that had a soft, innocent, wide-eyed stare.

"I am just waiting around here now," she said. Her words were clipped. I thought she sounded nervous and frightened. "I think it will be a little nicer [on the Palliative Care Unit]. It will be quiet, and people will have more time." She was sitting upright in bed, propped up by several pillows. She looked pale and her skin had a slight yellowish tinge to it. She wore a dark green velvet housecoat. Was she cold, I wondered? She said she liked to keep her housecoat on for getting in and out of bed. "I'm sick," she said, "but not so sick I can't do things for myself." She knew her diagnosis and that her cancer had advanced to a point where her doctor could offer no further treatment. But, she said, "I'm not ready to give up yet. I'm not sure how long I've got. There are still questions to be answered. I'm not ready to give up; now I have to work harder to get past the hurdles."

It was not clear to me exactly what those hurdles were to Susan, but she still seemed to retain hope that her life would carry on. She asked Dr. Webster, who had come with me on this visit, if the oncologists could look into the possibility of more treatments. Later that day, Dr. Lieberman came to see her. Gently, he reiterated that there was nothing more the team could offer surgically or through radiotherapy. Perhaps Susan already knew the answers Dr. Lieberman would have for her. But, as she told Jack later, "I had to be sure that everything possible has been done, even if I am dying."

Christmas Time

On December 7, 1995, shortly after our first meeting, Susan was transferred to the PCU. It was Christmas time, and yes, she did think of that, she told me when I came to see her on the unit. It was a holiday she loved. She would have liked to have been at home, but not if someone had to be there to take care of her "like a child." "I like to be alone at Christmas," she said, "to enjoy it in my own way."

The PCU was decorated for the holidays, not only for Christmas but also for Hanukkah. At the entrance there was a large menorah with candles on one side and a brightly lit, tinsel-decorated Christmas tree on the other. Notice boards advertised choir services and Christmas and Hanukkah concerts. At the holiday tea that day, the music therapist and her group sang carols and Hanukkah songs. This made Susan think of the children at her school and their caroling. She loved to decorate the classroom. Right now, the children would be making greeting cards and papier maché toys to give as holiday gifts to their families. "It was magic for them!" Susan said. As Susan and I talked, I couldn't help feeling uncomfortable, perhaps a little guilty, at my own Christmas at home with a caring family. I also loved Christmas and its music. I thought of the concerts I planned to listen to and remembered that on this very same evening I would hear a live performance of Handel's *Messiah* in one of Montreal's most beautiful churches.

Susan had always delighted in giving presents to Judy's two young grandchildren. She loved them both as her own. She asked Judy to buy some of their favorite toys and to put them under the tree at their home. Even if she could not be there to see the children unwrap their gifts, it would give her pleasure just to think about them on Christmas Day. It was hard for me to imagine why Susan had chosen to be transferred to the PCU instead of being at home at Christmas with her sister who could help care for her. But each time I visited her she reiterated that it was the right decision.

After five days on the unit, Susan looked more ill and pale. Now she looked directly at me, wide-eyed, when she spoke. I thought there was honesty and dignity in her gaze. "I know I am going downhill," she said to me. "Maybe I don't have long to go, but I will still fight as long as I have breath in me." She did not elaborate on these feelings, though at times I wished I could press her to do so. But, fearing she would find further questions intrusive, I held back.

Over the next few days, she talked about the changes that were taking place in her body. It took greater effort to get up alone and go to the bathroom. She had difficulty keeping down food and would sometimes vomit right after a meal. The dimenhydrinate that Gillian Webster prescribed did help to stave off the feelings of nausea, however. She was now receiving morphine 5–10 mg every four hours for the pain in her back. Sometimes she dreamed a lot or fell into a half sleep. Gillian had explained that this could be a side effect of the morphine and suggested that the regular dosage be reduced to avoid excessive drowsiness and perhaps the disturbing dreams. Susan tried this. For a while she felt comfortable and clearer in her mind.

Only the light, padded footsteps of the palliative care team broke the tranquility of the ward. Susan appreciated the nurses. What was most important to her was to feel comfortable and to have someone there to help her when she needed to vomit. Barbara, her primary nurse, did this and had special ways of easing her back and the pain in her stomach, such as arranging the pillows under her knees as she lay in bed. She also felt more comfortable if she lay in certain positions. This way she needed less medication. Susan also liked Barbara because she "didn't pry."

To Barbara, Susan seemed very stoic and strong on the surface. But there was something about the way she was coping that made Barbara feel very uncomfortable. She commented to me,

> The more I interacted with this patient, I had the feeling she was frightened and alone. I felt a lot of tension, and that she was dealing with a lot of feelings about having come on our unit. She has some family support and good friends, but there is more there, and I feel I need the time.

She worried that she did not spend as much time as she would have liked with Susan, to allow an opportunity for Susan to talk if she needed to. Several people had died within the past five days, and there was a shortage of staff on the unit, which made it harder to provide one-to-one care. With this type of work, Barbara said, one needed to have time beyond the usual nurse–patient ratio in the general health system. People who are dying need nursing time.

But it was hard to talk to Susan. Denise, one of the volunteers on the unit, resolved to spend time trying. But, Denise told me, "she talks in short sentences and there is a long pause before she will say something. She says that her sister will have a hard time with her being on this unit. She says she is fine, but I wonder if she is the one who is having a hard time. She says that coming on the unit is like 'a slap in the face.' She doesn't want to elaborate."

Jack said that Susan had a way of closing her eyes and pretending sleep or tiredness if she wanted to end a conversation. Sometimes she would start to retch or cough and ask the person to return later. Susan often found that easier than "to be so blunt as to tell the person to leave." Although she did feel tired or nauseated, it was also a way of avoiding difficult topics.

Susan told me that she wanted to be as helpful as she could with our research project. "It is important for education," she said, and education and learning were important for everyone. But she needed to think about things on her own, too. "I need to feel I'm independent and for that I need my privacy," she said.

All the Key People

As Christmas drew near and Susan's illness seemed to worsen, more and more people came to visit. Richard, her ex-husband, sometimes came and sat on the sofa in her room, but they didn't talk very much. Susan would lie for long periods, apparently awake but with her eyes closed. Richard would sit deep in thought, looking out the window onto the bustle of the city below. His face looked sad. He did not feel like talking to me, either. The whole situation was sad, he said.

Judy brought in stuffed animals, flowers, and orchids, which she knew her sister loved. The flowers' scent filled the room. Their bright blue, pink, and purple colors seemed to give brightness and voice to a place where no one was talking. Judy would sit at the foot of her sister's bed. When Susan appeared to be asleep, Judy would tiptoe outside into the corridor, where she would cry helplessly. I met her there at one of these times. She looked exhausted. "I can't believe it," she said to me. "Everything has happened so fast. She's so young. I always thought I'd be the one to go first." It was especially hard, she continued, because Susan had never really talked about how ill she was. Surely, she had known for some time that the cancer was serious. They had not talked, and Judy hadn't really been aware of the seriousness of it all, until now.

When Susan did open her eyes and acknowledge someone, it was usually when Jack was there on his own. A few days earlier, a pastoral care worker had stopped by to visit and suggested that Susan write a journal of her thoughts and experiences. Susan liked that idea and asked Jack to help. He brought in a tape recorder so Susan could dictate her thoughts, which she felt comfortable doing with Jack. But after a few days she felt too tired and weak.

Dr. Webster visited several times a day. Susan lay in bed peacefully and quietly, covered by knitted quilts and soft toy animals. She rarely spoke, and, when she did, she would often drift in and out of sleep in the middle of a thought, which was clearly distressing to her. She was slipping into a coma.

Gillian considered offering her some intravenous hydration, which can sometimes help to reduce a patient's confusion in the last few days of a terminal illness by balancing the electrolytes. Except for ice chips and lemon swabs that the nurses were using to moisten the inside of her mouth, Susan had taken no fluids by mouth. The decision was a difficult one. Susan now looked peaceful and comfortable. A short time later, Barbara reported to Gillian that Susan had passed melena stools, which meant that she was undergoing a gastrointestinal hemorrhage. Gillian concluded now that intravenous hydration would not be helpful.

Now all the key people in Susan's life had assembled in her room or in the small kitchen down the hall. Her brother Edward, and his wife June, had just arrived from Vancouver. They were shocked and angry. Edward felt some information was missing and asked whether the cancer had been picked up late because his sister ignored some early warning signals and did not seek medical attention in time. All of Susan's family struggled with the idea that she was now dying of an incurable cancer. Only Jack said he was taking things well. "I think it has been easier for me," he later explained. "We were close friends, and even if she didn't tell me everything, I was more prepared. Susan did confide in me a lot."

Susan never came out of her coma. A few days before Christmas she died in the presence of Judy, Jack, and Rita. She had been a patient on the PCU for just 10 days.

"I Have Not Lived My Life That Way, Why Now?"

People were not sure if Susan would have liked a formal religious ceremony at her funeral service. Throughout her illness she never expressed her religious beliefs to anyone. She had described herself to me as "not an especially religious person." She had been baptized a Catholic, but she disliked overt displays of religiosity. She did talk to the pastoral worker on the PCU, but expressed little interest in talking about God or religion, nor had she expressed interest in receiving the Last Sacraments. "I have not lived my life that way, why now?" she said.

While her family wanted to respect her beliefs, they decided that a Catholic service would be the most fitting, since she was a baptized Catholic. A requiem Mass was held in the small parish church near her home where she had lived for the past 20 years. Richard, her former husband, attended with his wife Alison. Judy came with her children and grandchildren. Richard's mother was there, as were Edward and June. Susan's funeral was attended by the many friends, colleagues, and students whom she had taught and who had come to know her over the years.

Jack also attended the funeral, taking a seat with Rita at the back of the church. "I guess I didn't really see myself as legitimate family," he recalled. Jack felt touched and gratified when Judy made a special point of inviting both his wife and him to sit near the front of the church with the family. Still, it didn't feel right. It was an odd feeling, he told me. He felt he had known Susan Mulroney like his own sister. But that was then; it wasn't his place to intrude now. "I'm not family," he said.

Judy

At first, in the days immediately after the funeral, Judy felt fear and a sick feeling in her stomach. She didn't feel afraid of anything in particular, but rather a pervasive sense of being "nervous," as if something were suddenly going to happen. It was hard to imagine that she couldn't just pick up the phone and talk to Susan, to ask her to go shopping or perhaps to go for a drive on a sunny day.

As the weeks passed, Judy's sense of loss, "the big hole," did not diminish. The funeral was over, and everyone had gone home. There were fewer telephone calls. She could still go over to her son's house and babysit her two grandchildren. But everything seemed so empty, and the emptiness seemed to get worse instead of better. There were days when Judy felt she "just couldn't go on." She tried to keep busy with her young grandchildren. Although other things kept her busy, as well, sometimes it was hard to concentrate on what anyone said. It was hard, she said, to concentrate on other people's lives when there was so much going on in your own mind. Sometimes, Judy would try to find solace by taking out a photograph of her sister. But that gave limited comfort, for after Susan learned that there was no cure for her illness, she destroyed whatever personal papers and photographs she could find. Because she was "a private person," Judy explained, "she didn't want anyone intruding on her private life after she was gone."

She wondered why Susan had not talked about her illness. Why had she not told her own sister when she knew that she didn't have long to live? "If only I had known the truth," she said to me, "I could have done something.

I feel let down, cheated. How could I have not known that things were so bad?"

What had Susan been thinking, she wondered? How much had she been informed about her disease? Susan did not have a husband or children. There was Jack, but surely as a family member, Judy should have been consulted.

She also felt let down by Edward. He was their only brother. Why had he not taken more of an active role during Susan's illness? "He didn't bother with her for the whole year," Judy said to me. "And rather than hurt her or get her upset, I never said anything. I just told her that I called him and told him she was sick. He had called a couple of times and when finally, at the end, when Dr. Webster had suggested I should call him right away, it took him three days before he got here." Judy paused, and then continued, "Anyway, he was here for the funeral and for a few days after that. But he never got involved in her illness."

Still, Judy went on, people couldn't help what happened. It's nobody's fault. "You can't go on blaming people," she said. "I feel angry that she could not have lived longer, but most of the time now I think, what was there that anybody could do? There wasn't anything!" She reached for a tissue and cried. "I'm like this a lot of the time," she said after a moment. "I miss her. I still can't believe it. I just can't believe it."

Judy did not see the need to seek professional help for her grief. The palliative care bereavement services had called to see how things were. They were very kind, but she did not want to see a bereavement counselor. What could anyone do? "I lost both of my parents and I've been through a divorce. It's something I'll have to get over," she said. "They say it takes time."

Jack

Jack Peterson also struggled. He still felt he was in an odd position, for he was a close friend, but not a family member. He had suggested a lawyer who could help with Susan's estate, but it was clear that Susan's brother, Edward, wanted her will to be settled in a way that would ensure the best legal arrangement for himself and the family. It was better that the family hired "a good investment counselor."

Still, Susan had been a close, dear friend. Sometimes Jack went over in his mind those last days on the PCU. The memory was so vivid, he told me. He could still see Susan lying there, dying in the quietness. Sometimes he wondered if she could hear anything in those last hours of her life. He thought about what Dr. Webster had said when Susan appeared to be unconscious: "If you talk to her, she will be able to hear; if you say something she will hear." But Jack had not talked to her at that moment. As the last days came and people drifted in and out of the room wanting to say goodbye, Jack still wondered if Susan would have heard anything.

Another thing that sometimes puzzled him was why Susan had not received intravenous feeding in those last hours before she died. Perhaps "it wasn't medically correct" to give people intravenous feeding when they were dying, he said to me. But should people still not be treated? "I would think that someone who is in palliative care who's having difficulty eating should continue to receive intravenous feeding," he continued. "She was not eating at all, maybe a few sips of water before she went unconscious. I didn't think she'd get more radiation or chemotherapy or anything, but I say to myself, if the disease is going to kill me, okay fine. But say a person who's dying has an infected finger; I still say that the antibiotics should be given, even if the person is dying."

As the months passed, Jack was often plagued with thoughts that maybe he should have encouraged more of a dialogue with his friend. He said,

> I still get those nagging doubts about whether I should have talked more about the fact that she was dying. We had known each other for so many years and had been through a lot together. Should I have pushed it? Maybe yes, maybe no. But I console myself by saying, well you know, if she really wanted to talk about it, she would have. She didn't. I think it was more important for her to go out for lunch and have a laugh. But still, you have those little doubts.

Six months after Susan's death her family was still trying to cope with their loss. The estate was still in the process of being settled. Judy made a point of contacting Jack and Rita and asked if Rita would like to have Susan's collection of Spode china figurines. She knew that Rita loved to collect china and remembered Susan talking about it. It was right, she said, that "Rita should have the Spode."

Jack told me he was touched by Judy's offer. He also spoke to me about "the bigger picture." He believed strongly in an afterlife. He knew that his friend had not been a practicing Catholic, but he held on to his own strong faith and told me of his "personal assurance that there were spiritual rewards beyond this life." He then said to me, "It's easier when you have a faith and you're very sure of it. I believe Susan has gone to a better place than this. Christian faith tells us, there's something beyond and the person has gone to a reward, a reward of something better."

Authors' Comments

Some people appear to cope with a terminal diagnosis alone and prefer not to talk about their feelings. Susan Mulroney was such a person. Throughout this narrative, she showed herself as a very private person; the extent to which she understood the gravity of Stage IV cervical cancer when it was first diagnosed, and the feelings she had, are not clear. Her desire for privacy prevented her from talking about her diagnosis to family members or to people who might be considered close to her, such as her friend Jack or Jack's wife Rita, who was a nurse.

Susan did try to read medical books to find out the latest research on gynecological illnesses. But she was alone in her task of pursuing this information. Perhaps Ms. Mulroney could have benefited from professional counseling outside of her immediate circle of family and friends. She may have been more comfortable talking privately to a psychologist, a palliative care social worker, or counselor who appreciated the challenges of exploring difficult or painful topics and who would have offered confidentiality

Ms. Mulroney's friend Jack felt that he had known Susan like his own sister, at least in the context of having a long-standing work relationship. And even though she had chosen not to talk about her illness, there had still been many times when she had shared significant life events with him. Yet, Jack didn't appear to see himself as having any special place Susan's funeral. He sat in the back row of the church with Rita, not wanting "to intrude" by joining Susan's family at the front of the church. It is clear from his comments that he felt he was an outsider. "I guess I didn't really see myself as legitimate family," he recalled. He neither expected nor felt entitled to social sympathy or any public support.

In the literature on grief and bereavement, Jack's situation is recognized as *disenfranchised grief*, which has been defined as "grief that results when a person experiences a significant loss and the resultant grief is not openly acknowledged, socially validated or publicly mourned although the individual is publicly mourned."[1] The term came into currency during the AIDS epidemic of the 1980s and 1990s, where it described the plight of previously unacknowledged or unknown partners of gay men who died of the disease.

Susan's sister Judy grieved Susan's death intensely. As time passed, Judy's grief did not diminish, and she questioned over and over why more could not have been done for Susan's illness. She was angry toward Susan, the doctor, and her brother. She found it hard to concentrate on anything other than her loss. Things seemed to get worse rather than better. There were times when she felt she "just couldn't go on." Six months after Susan's death she was still trying to cope.

Judy's grief appeared different from the type of grief most people experience after the loss of a loved one. It was continuously present over many weeks and months, and it affected all of her thoughts and activities. When grief is prolonged like this, and accompanied by the symptoms we witness in Judy's case, the person may be considered to suffer from *complicated grief*: a clinically significant condition which (a) deviates from normal grief (according to cultural norms) in the time course and/or intensity of grief symptoms (separation distress, difficulties accepting the loss and moving on) and (b) is associated with impairment in significant areas of health and social and occupational functioning.[2] While Judy initially declined grief support, she might have accepted some help in the longer term or in the context of follow-up care had it been available.

Grief and bereavement care is still only sporadically provided in Canada, and it depends on the policies and available resources of individual health authorities. Many Canadian palliative care centers and hospice associations offer bereavement packages to families. There are also community volunteer organizations that offer bereavement support groups in some locations.

For me as an interviewer, this case was a difficult challenge. I had to respect Susan's privacy, and I was committed to conducting an interview that her comfort level would allow. I felt we were learning from Susan, and yet I wondered if there wasn't more to be learned. Sometimes after leaving an interview, I felt a sense of helplessness, that perhaps we could never really communicate. I was struck by the detachment that existed between us, particularly in me. I felt very much the intruder, often thinking that I had no place in this very significant piece of this person's life. I tried to think how I could become closer to her, and yet, at the same time, it seemed that Susan wanted the distance—at least from me, a stranger—because, after all, I was a stranger.

References

1. Doka, KJ. Disenfranchised grief in historical and cultural perspective. In MS Stroebe, RO Harrison, H Schut, and W Stroebe, eds. *Handbook of bereavement research and practice: Advances in theory and intervention.* Washington, DC: American Psychological Association; 2008: 223–240.
2. Eisma MC, Stroebe MS. Emotion regulatory strategies in complicated grief: A systematic review. Behav Ther. 2020;52(1):234–249.

20

Costas Metrakis

"It Was Not a Peaceful Death"

Narrated by Patricia Boston

It was unusual for the palliative care team to see someone like Costas Metrakis, a 58-year-old man who had only recently been diagnosed with terminal illness, on the Palliative Care Unit. Usually, the people they cared for, and their families, had time to absorb some of the anguish and turmoil that accompanies the news of a fatal illness. For the Metrakis family there was no time. From the date of his diagnosis of incurable cancer of the stomach to his reluctant admission to palliative care was a period of only two weeks. The whole family felt numbed. They could not accept palliative care. "It is a place where they send people to die," Elie Metrakis, the patient's wife, said. Reluctantly, recognizing that help for Mr. Metrakis's symptoms would be available on the unit, the couple agreed to be transferred there from the medical ward. After only three days on the unit, despite his burdensome symptoms, Mr. Metrakis asked to go home. The team mobilized the support they could, and Mr. Metrakis went home on a weekend pass. As soon as he came back to the unit, he insisted on returning home again. Four days later he was dead.

A Healthy Life

Costas Metrakis was born in Lebanon of Greek parents. He was the oldest of six children in a close-knit family. The family moved to Greece when he was young, and his parents died soon thereafter. Mr. Metrakis married in the 1960s, and he and his wife Elie moved to Canada. Most of his family remained in Greece, but one sister, Sophia, moved to Canada at about the same time. She lived close by in Montreal. Sophia was especially close to Mr. Metrakis. He had been like a father to her after the death of their parents.

Mr. Metrakis lived with his wife and children in a wealthy, English-speaking suburb of Montreal. Although their small, two-story home was comfortable, it stood out in rather simple contrast to other ornate and stately homes of the neighborhood. Their three children (two sons, aged 21 and 17, and a daughter, aged 15) all lived at home. Mr. Metrakis's first love was his family. They had built their lives in Montreal and had become immersed in the local Greek community. While they did not profess to be deeply religious, they regularly attended services at the local chapel.

Mr. Metrakis was a professional artist. He spent much of his life on the road exhibiting his work, but, as Mrs. Metrakis recalled, he missed his family when he was on the road. He would call home late at night to see how everyone was doing. His wife and children anticipated his calls and would stay up late waiting for the phone to ring.

Late in September 1995, Mr. Metrakis started experiencing frequent episodes of heartburn. For a few months he ignored the discomfort, attributing it to eating the wrong kind of food. The symptoms persisted, and, in May 1996, he consulted his family doctor, Dr. Luc Gorges. A gastroscopy was normal, so he was sent for an upper gastrointestinal X-ray. This test was also normal. Mr. Metrakis was instructed to relieve his heartburn with an antacid.

His symptoms continued. He continued to take antacids, but by now he had developed frequent episodes of vomiting, which got progressively worse. He was able to eat, but then 10 to 15 minutes later he would vomit. Mr. Metrakis was becoming weak, and he noticed that he had lost 15 pounds. In mid-November 1996, Dr. Gorges sent him for further investigations, and he had a computed tomography (CT) scan of his abdomen. He was now vomiting continuously and was unable to keep down any food. On November 28, weak and dehydrated, he went to the hospital emergency department, where the CT scan report was located. It showed metastatic disease to the abdominal cavity with ascites. Although there was no obvious primary tumor seen, a lesion of the stomach was suspected. Lying on his cot in the emergency department, Mr. Metrakis was not yet aware of these results.

The Medical Ward

He was admitted to the hospital with the diagnosis of gastric outlet obstruction. The doctors suspected a gastric tumor but wanted further studies. The resident doctor who had seen Mr. Metrakis in the emergency department wrote in the chart that the medical team, rather than the surgeons, would continue to follow Mr. Metrakis "as the case is mainly palliative." He was not a candidate for surgical treatment of the tumor. Already the medical team was expecting the worst.

Mr. Metrakis shared a room on the medical ward with three other patients. He occupied a bed near the window, and Mrs. Metrakis and Sophia made it as cozy as they could with flowers and photos from home. The windowsill became congested as more and more bouquets and plants were added to its tiny space.

By the time Dr. Gorges came to visit him in the hospital, Mr. Metrakis had been informed of his diagnosis: advanced gastric cancer. The two men agreed that Mr. Metrakis should get a complete picture of his options, and Mr. Metrakis was seen by many physicians over the next few days. The medical oncologists could not offer any curative treatment, but they were willing to offer experimental chemotherapy for palliation.

It was a difficult decision. Mr. Metrakis was still trying to face the fact that he had stomach cancer, and he needed time to think. Two days later, he agreed to the experimental treatment. The next decision was how Mr. Metrakis was going to be fed. His stomach was full of tumor. It was possible to insert a feeding tube into the small intestine, a procedure known as a jejunostomy. Mr. Metrakis agreed to this, but he was still numb from the course of events.

When Mr. Metrakis went into the operating room to have a jejunostomy tube inserted, things did not go smoothly. The surgeon called the medical oncologist to the operating room. He had found an extensive spread of the cancer involving most of the small bowel and the abdominal cavity. The jejunostomy could not be done, and the surgeon now felt that experimental treatment would probably be of no benefit either. The medical oncology team agreed and told Mrs. Metrakis that a palliative approach, emphasizing comfort rather than prolonging life, was her husband's only option. Mr. Metrakis knew nothing of this, as he was still asleep following the surgery.

When he woke up, he was confronted with a breathtaking transition. Within a space of two weeks he had gone from thinking of himself as a healthy person with indigestion to being terminally ill with only a few weeks to live.

Palliative care was not an acceptable option to the Metrakis family. Dr. Mary Thompson, the first palliative care consulting physician to visit Mr. Metrakis, later recalled to me,

> When I arrived. I found a man who looked physically not too bad, except that he had gastric outlet obstruction and he was very, very scared. And we already knew from the scans that there was a lot of intra-abdominal disease. His sister and wife were totally denying the situation and were telling me that we hadn't read the tests right, and they would get others because we didn't know what we were talking about, and they would get their own Greek physician involved because we were wrong. His wife asked me, "Can't they just take out his bowel and clean it off and then put it back in?" And I was trying to tell them, "Well, I'm sorry. This is what it is."

Sophia was devastated. She couldn't bring herself even to talk to Dr. Thompson. When Irene Clermont, the palliative care fellow, came to the medical ward to talk to the family about the role of palliative care, Sophia told her to leave the room. "Why does everyone come and tell him he is dying?" she said. "It is depressing for him. Okay, we know he is sick. But people don't have to keep telling him all the time."

Sophia angrily demanded to know why no one had discovered Costas's cancer when there was still time to do something about it. "Why didn't the doctors find the tumor before?" she asked Irene. "You know that he had an ultrasound in the summer, and they didn't see anything. How could they have not seen anything? The doctors tell us that the tumor is everywhere now, but why didn't they see it when they did the ultrasound? All they did was give him Maalox and send him home!" She wept with anger and grief.

Irene tried to explain that sometimes gastric tumors develop very fast. She suggested that perhaps Mr. Metrakis's tumor had been too small to see when he had those tests. She said that Mr. Metrakis's tumor had been very aggressive and perhaps it had spread quickly. She promised to come back to the medical ward each day to see what she could offer to alleviate Mr. Metrakis's symptoms.

Elie Metrakis couldn't understand why the doctors needed to tell her husband the truth about his diagnosis. When I spoke with her about this later, she told me,

It was crazy when we were told that he had only one month to live. I asked the doctors not to tell him. It made me so mad. He was afraid of dying, and I didn't want him to know. But the doctors said it was the policy of the hospital. It is a hard thing to know you are dying. It would have been better if he didn't know.

Elie told Irene that her husband had always been "scared of dying." He had always disliked flowers and candles because "they reminded him of death." If he had not been told, he would never have suspected he was dying, she said. He might have suspected that things were bad and that he was very sick, but not that he was dying.

Different Messages

Mr. Metrakis's difficulty in making decisions was not only due to the speed of events or to his state of shock, also but to the fact that many physicians had become involved in his care and each one had his or her own point of view. The family was continually bombarded with different messages within a short period of time. Some physicians discussed palliative treatments and symptom control, while others talked about chemotherapy and surgery. Dr. Gorges had at first led the family to believe that there wasn't *anything* wrong. When Mr. Metrakis was in the hospital, Dr. Gorges had told them that, even if it was cancer, there was a lot that could be done. So the family kept hoping. Then, another doctor told them that Mr. Metrakis had only one month to live. The family called Dr. Gorges, who told them that was impossible; there were *so many* things that could be done, including feeding Mr. Metrakis through a tube. Then, after Mr. Metrakis's laparotomy, all the doctors, including Dr. Gorges, seemed to agree: the situation was hopeless.

Within a few days, Mr. Metrakis developed symptoms of total gastric outlet obstruction. He could not keep any food down at all. It was now necessary to hydrate him intravenously. The medical team asked the palliative care consultants to transfer Mr. Metrakis to the Palliative Care Unit (PCU). When the palliative care consultant Dr. Thompson came to the medical ward to make her assessment, she quickly saw how highly charged the situation was. The family was barely ready to consider any kind of palliative care involvement; they were certainly not ready for Mr. Metrakis to move physically to the PCU. Dr. Thompson told Mr. Metrakis that because he wanted to continue his IV hydration and vitamins, he should stay on the medical floor. In the meantime, she added, she would stay involved to help keep him as comfortable as possible.

That weekend, John Langley, another palliative care physician, was on call. A friend of his who also knew the Metrakis family had called John, expressing concern about Costas. The mutual friend knew about the PCU and wanted the palliative care team to be involved in the case. When John went to see Mr. Metrakis, he was asleep, so he spoke with Elie. He encouraged the family to come to the unit and offered to give Elie a tour. As John later explained to me, it was routine for the Palliative Care Service to show the unit to prospective patients and their families "as a way of defusing any anxiety about [it] being a 'death house.'"

As far as Dr. Langley could tell, Mrs. Metrakis seemed to like the general layout of the unit, the patients' rooms, the kitchen, and the large, home-like lounge. He thought her response to the tour seemed "very positive." He was wrong. As he later heard, Mrs. Metrakis had been upset "about any number of things" after her tour, though he did not know exactly what had upset her.

Within the palliative care team there was disagreement on what immediate actions to recommend. John Langley was under the impression that the family wanted to move to the PCU and felt it would be helpful to them. "We just have so many more resources to be helpful," he commented to me. "I mean, that's our job. Time after time the ward does make a difference and it happens very quickly over a few days, very few days. I was just hoping that might be a catalyst in some ways for him, and for them." At the same time, John knew that the family was in tremendous turmoil. "I'm quick to realize," he continued, "that the relationships and the care in other settings, on other wards, is often exemplary and that you have to be careful in moving somebody to [the PCU], that you're not interrupting the most helpful relationship they have, which is with the nurse who's giving them chemotherapy, or the cleaning woman who always comes in to see them in the morning, or whatever."

For her part, Dr. Thompson felt that such a move was premature. The family had made it explicit to her that they wanted a cure. Mr. Metrakis had asked for anything that would prolong his life. When he heard about palliative care, he had said, "All I can say is that I am a fighter, and I will fight this all the way." Mrs. Metrakis was also looking for treatment. She was urging the medical team to add vitamins to her husband's intravenous nutrition.

The nurses and physicians on the medical ward were also in conflict about whether Mr. Metrakis should go to the PCU at this time. Excerpts from the notes by several different members of the multidisciplinary team further illustrate the conflicts.

> We believe that it is not possible to treat him effectively and that the care plan should be palliative. Too somnolent to discuss with patient at this time. . . . Patient and family reluctant [to agree] to PCU transfer because of hydration issue. . . . Family reluctant to stop IV hydration because it would shorten his life. Gave info re: PCU and possibility of going home. . . . Wife and family not ready to see IV discontinued. Not ready for PCU. . . . I believe the patient would do best in PCU . . . . For psychological reasons the patient should stay on the medical ward. . . . Condition is not improving. Would do best in PCU.

After a week of discussions, Mr. Metrakis decided to move to the PCU. On November 29, Dr. Clermont wrote in the chart: "Discussed palliative care goals. Patient agrees to transfer but to discuss with his family." In an attempt to help the family with this transition, Dr. Langley was asked to see the patient once more. After his discussion with Mr. and Mrs. Metrakis, they were willing to accept the transfer. It was December 1.

The Palliative Care Unit

At 6:00 P.M. that evening, Dr. Clermont was rushing to see her last patient of the day before going home. She had just finished her formal admission of Mr. Metrakis to the PCU, including a careful physical examination and a conversation with Mr. Metrakis, and had written her notes in the medical record. As Irene passed Mr. Metrakis's room on her way to the elevator, she was stopped by Mrs. Metrakis and Sophia. With a worried look, Mrs. Metrakis told Irene she needed to talk to her. Irene asked if it could wait or was Mr. Metrakis having some trouble settling onto the ward? Mrs. Metrakis said, "It's just a quick question." Irene paused and waited. "Everything's okay," Mrs. Metrakis said. "It's just that we heard people come here to die."

Dr. Clermont knew this was not going to be a short conversation. "Well, yes," Irene said, "I guess some people come to this ward to die. Other people come to this ward for pain control. Some people die here, but some people also go home from here. Who told you that people come here to die?"

Mrs. Metrakis and Sophia answered in unison, "People on the other ward."

"The doctors?" Irene asked.

"No, no," Sophia said. "The families of the other patients in our room."

Mrs. Metrakis said, "I thought this is where they send all the patients in the hospital who were going to die."

"Actually," said Irene, "patients die on many wards in the hospital. They don't just send all the dying patients to one ward. This ward is a very special ward where people can come and have specialized doctors take care of any symptoms they are having and make sure that they are comfortable."

"Oh," Mrs. Metrakis responded, without much conviction.

Irene was watching Elie closely now. "Did you think they were sending Mr. Metrakis here to die?" she asked quietly. Mrs. Metrakis nodded tearfully. "That must have been terrible," Irene added.

There was a long moment while Dr. Clermont waited for Mrs. Metrakis to regain her composure. Then Irene put her arm around Elie's shoulder, saying, "We want to help Mr. Metrakis to be comfortable and for him to spend as much time with the people he loves as possible."

"We need to get him home," Mrs. Metrakis said. She stood silently for another long moment. "I'd better get back to my husband," she said. "I've been away for quite a long time."

"I Want to Go Home Now"

I met the Metrakis family soon after their arrival on the unit. Mr. Metrakis's single room was much larger than the area he had occupied in his four-bed room on the medical ward. There were reclining easy chairs for family members and visitors, and there was enough space to set up a folding cot. But the room wasn't as colorfully decorated as the windowsill Mr. Metrakis had in his corner of the room on the medical ward. In place of the bouquets and plants were a few faded flowers. Despite the get-well cards, mementos, and drawings that Mrs. Metrakis pinned onto a cork bulletin board on the wall, the atmosphere in the room was somber.

When I entered the room, Mr. Metrakis lay motionless on his side, his face turned toward the door. His bed, with its crisp white sheets, seemed freshly made. Several large, puffy pillows surrounded his body, one comfortably tucked in behind his back, another positioned underneath his right arm. Though the room was quiet, Mr. Metrakis was clearly awake. His dark eyes were wide open; they followed me as I walked toward his bed. Still, I felt the need to whisper. "How are you?" I asked.

"I want to go home now," he responded. "I want to go home to see my children. This is no place for children."

It seemed like an effort for him to talk. He took long pauses between each sentence, carefully choosing his words. But he ignored my suggestion that we stop talking for fear of overtiring him. "When they give me something to stop vomiting, I can go home to my children," he went on. "My wife will take care of me there."

Elie was sitting in a chair facing the foot of the bed. She seemed able to concentrate only on her husband, staring at him for long periods whether he was asleep or awake. Sophia sat at one side of her brother's bed. She was very tender in her interactions with him, often stroking his hair or caressing his arm, but to me she looked very angry and distraught. When I introduced myself, she didn't smile. Her dark eyes seemed to look through me, almost accusingly. But, along with the rest of the family, she did agree to participate in our project. Mrs. Metrakis didn't seem as openly angry. I thought she was frightened, perhaps still stunned at hearing her husband's diagnosis. Although I could not be certain, I had the sense that the two women rarely talked to each other. There was little eye contact between them, and I seldom saw them seek solace from one another. They did not embrace or hug each other. Once, when Elie had come out of the room to talk to Dr. Thompson, Sophia followed behind her and abruptly started interrogating Dr. Thompson about her brother's progress as if Mrs. Metrakis were not there.

By the time Mr. Metrakis was transferred to the PCU, he had many severe symptoms: intractable vomiting, nausea, persistent hiccoughs, and abdominal pain. Medical management of these symptoms was very difficult. When Mrs. Metrakis described the situation to me, she related that her husband was never comfortable. "He continued vomiting and hiccoughing," she told me. "All the time vomiting and hiccoughing. It was so frustrating."

Despite the severity of these symptoms, the family requested that Mr. Metrakis be discharged home almost from the moment he arrived on the unit. It was not unusual for patients to leave with short-term passes, for a weekend or longer. Sometimes patients would be discharged home for a while and return to the unit when and if they felt the need. However, this particular request on the part of the Metrakis family presented extraordinary nursing and medical challenges. Mr. Metrakis still had a catheter draining from the surgical incision in his abdomen. He was receiving subcutaneous hydration by a process known as hypodermoclysis, which provides hydration without the use of an intravenous line. He was hooked up to a syringe driver to receive subcutaneous steroid medications and octreotide to alleviate his vomiting and abdominal pain. Oxygen would also be required as his condition deteriorated. In addition, he was very weak. As one member of the team recalled to me later, he was "vomiting, sometimes without relief, and when he wasn't vomiting, he was sleeping. I thought he was dying."

Mrs. Metrakis still felt that her husband would be better off at home. He was "sad" on the PCU. Whenever the children came to the hospital to visit, the whole encounter was upsetting. She would set his bedroom up on the first floor of their home with a commode, she said. She would hire a private nurse for nights. She would learn how to regulate the syringe driver and give injections. She would learn to insert the small needles under his skin that were providing his fluid intake via hypodermoclysis and would monitor them and reinsert them if necessary to keep them functioning properly.

The next day, Mrs. Metrakis changed her mind. Now it seemed to her that Costas was too sick to come home after all. Over the next three days, the intensity of Mr. and Mrs. Metrakis's desire for him to go home fluctuated with the intensity and severity of his symptoms. If they were not controlled, he wanted to stay in the hospital; if he was doing well, he wanted to go home. Finally, everyone agreed to try to get Mr. Metrakis home for a weekend. It would be a trial, to see if it were possible for him to stay at home for a longer period.

In addition to their desire to accommodate Mr. Metrakis if at all possible, the team felt that time at home was important because the family, especially his children, were having a difficult time talking about Mr. Metrakis's illness. It was too painful for Mr. Metrakis to talk to them about his diagnosis, so they did not even know the true seriousness of their father's condition until his admission to the PCU. Since it didn't seem likely that the children would visit while Mr. Metrakis was in the hospital, a weekend at home might help the family as a whole to come to terms with what was happening.

When Irene Clermont told Mrs. Metrakis that they would try to help them get home, Mrs. Metrakis smiled. It was the first time anyone on the team had seen her smile.

Home

On December 4, 1996, three days after being admitted to the PCU, Mr. Metrakis went home. Dr. Clermont called him two days later. Mr. Metrakis said he felt well and wanted to stay at home for two more days. Irene offered to make a home visit. When she arrived, she was led upstairs to the master bedroom. Mr. Metrakis was lying in bed. Mrs. Metrakis was sitting on the bed next to him. Irene sat near Mr. Metrakis on a small stool. Mr. Metrakis said he had had a lot of vomiting, but still, "it is better at home. I've built up this house all of my life. My kids are here, and my wife is here all of the time." He had a lot of good memories. He could be more relaxed. When the children were home, they would come to his room and talk about what they did during the day. They had a lot of visitors, too, Elie said, which was good, though her husband did get tired. It was hard to ask them to leave, for these were friends who had worked together for 30 years.

Irene could see that Mr. Metrakis was comfortable at home, but Mrs. Metrakis did not seem as comfortable. She seemed insecure managing the complicated medical treatments, though she was handling them well. The palliative home care nurses were not visiting because Mr. Metrakis was technically still an inpatient, home on a pass. The family could telephone the PCU ward nurses if they had a question. Mrs. Metrakis had some nursing support from the community health center but relied mainly on her family for support.

Everyone was "Okay," Mrs. Metrakis said. "We all do our things, and everyone acts as if nothing is wrong."

Irene was worried by this remark. "Something *is* wrong," she said to Mrs. Metrakis. "Mr. Metrakis is sick."

From Mrs. Metrakis's point of view, however, that was not the issue. She wanted to maintain hope for a cure at all costs. It had been upsetting for her that in the hospital the doctors kept telling them that he had only a month to live. They kept saying, "There is no hope. There is no hope." But, Mrs. Metrakis said, "I have to hope."

Four days later, Mr. Metrakis returned to the PCU. The doctors tried to control his persistent vomiting and hiccoughs, but the medications often made Mr. Metrakis drowsy, and this was unacceptable to the family. After one day, Mr. Metrakis asked if he could return home again. Another four-day pass was arranged, with the understanding that Mr. Metrakis would stay at home permanently if at all possible.

His physical condition was rapidly deteriorating. He had now developed a fever and was increasingly short of breath. Dr. Thompson suspected he had developed pneumonia. He still had a catheter draining from his laparotomy incision. But Mr. Metrakis wanted to go home. The team believed it was important to prepare Mrs. Metrakis for the fact that he would likely die there, and soon. Irene Clermont spoke with her the next day.

"How are you feeling about going home?" she asked.

"Good," Mrs. Metrakis replied. "I think it will be okay. It's just the vomiting."

Dr. Thompson had consulted a gastroenterologist to see if he could perform a procedure that would involve inserting a tube to drain her husband's stomach through the abdominal wall, thus preventing the vomiting. Irene asked Mrs. Metrakis if she had spoken to the gastroenterologist.

"He told us there is nothing he can do," she said. "The cancer is all over the stomach and prevents him from putting the tube in, just like they had said before at the surgery."

"Well, I guess that means that we will have to continue to adjust the medications to see if they will help," Irene said. She paused briefly. "I want to talk to you about some difficult things now. Would that be okay?"

"Yes."

"I want to know if you have thought about what to do if Mr. Metrakis dies at home. If you keep him at home, it is possible that he may die there."

"I don't want to think about it."

"Do you think Mr. Metrakis has thought about it?"

"Yes, I know he has."

"What has he been thinking about?"

Mrs. Metrakis's voice broke. "If he dies, he wants me to burn him and then scatter his ashes in Greece," she said, looking away and trying to keep her composure.

Irene waited several moments before speaking again. Then she said, "It's very difficult to think about losing someone that you love. I can see that you love Mr. Metrakis very much, and I know that he loves you, too. It is hard to lose such a good friend."

"Yes," Mrs. Metrakis said in a whisper.

"It Was Not a Peaceful Death"

The next morning the PCU nurses gave Mr. Metrakis a bath, washed his hair, and went over his medications one more time with Mrs. Metrakis. The community health agency and the palliative home care service had been informed that the patient would need to be followed at home. Mr. Metrakis went home with his wife and Sophia by ambulance. It was Thursday, December 12.

On Monday, December 16, Mary Thompson made a home visit. The palliative home care nurse had not had a chance to visit because of the intervening weekend. When Mary arrived at the house, Sophia opened the door looking very upset. She led Mary to the bedroom where Mr. Metrakis was lying semicomatose and breathless on the double bed. He was vomiting very frequently. It was obvious to Mary that he was dying. Mrs. Metrakis was hovering near the bed, anxious and tearful. She had not slept for days and looked exhausted. At one point she looked up at Mary and said, "He has not drained much from his abdominal catheter. Could it be that his cancer has disappeared?"

Dr. Thompson said that the only important thing to do at the moment was to make her husband as comfortable as possible. She suggested morphine for his shortness of breath and for any pain he might be experiencing, and chlorpromazine suppositories to calm him when he became agitated. Then Mary took Sophia and Sophia's husband into the kitchen. Sophia had barely looked at Mary since she had arrived. But now Mary felt compelled to tell her that her brother was dying.

"How long will it be?" Sophia wanted to know.

Mary said it was hard to say for sure, that she had seen things go on like this for several days sometimes. Because Mr. Metrakis was struggling to breathe, looked fearful, and seemed to be in some pain, Mary recommended maintaining the dose of morphine. Sophia looked uncertain, but when they came back into the bedroom Mrs. Metrakis agreed that her husband should sleep if that was the only way to control his discomfort. However, she asked Dr. Thompson if Mr. Metrakis could be given his intravenous digoxin (heart medication) since he had not had it yet that day. Mary explained gently that the digoxin would not be helpful at this time. She felt that the best intervention would be to maintain the patient's comfort and to allow him to relax and sleep. As Mary was preparing to leave, Mrs. Metrakis was tearful but seemed accepting of Mr. Metrakis's weakened state. Speaking through her extreme fatigue, she told Mary, "I want to take care of him here throughout the night." Mary told her that she was doing a tremendous job.

Mr. Metrakis died a few hours later. Mrs. Metrakis called the funeral home and arranged with them to remove her husband's body. Later, she told Dr. Thompson she thought he had been in a lot of pain at the end. Mary believed that Mr. Metrakis had died with a great deal of fear and "angst," but she did not think that he had been in a great deal of physical pain, at least relative to many other deaths she had witnessed. She was upset to think that Mrs. Metrakis would retain this impression. Still, she could not be absolutely sure, and, in any event, she reflected later, "it was not a peaceful death."

"It Feels Like He Has Gone on a Trip"

Mr. Metrakis was well known and well loved by many people, and most of them were in shock at the suddenness of his death. There was a very large attendance at the funeral. Then it was Christmas time. The holidays were very difficult for the family—it seemed that they would never end—though Mrs. Metrakis said later that the constant stream of visitors helped the time pass. Friends kept up a steady supply of food and gifts and kept the family company.

Marian, a bereavement counselor with the Palliative Care Service, made several telephone calls to Mrs. Metrakis over the next several weeks. Though Mrs. Metrakis was always polite, Marian had the feeling she did not really want to be called. When Irene Clermont called, however, Mrs. Metrakis seemed glad to have the chance to talk, even though there were also times when messages went unanswered.

In one conversation with Irene that took place in February 1997, Mrs. Metrakis told her that the family was going to the cemetery every day to light a candle at Mr. Metrakis's grave. (She made no reference to her husband's request to have his ashes scattered in Greece, and we have no other information that helps resolve this apparent inconsistency.) Mrs. Metrakis said they were still wondering, still trying to piece together the events of the past year. "We continue our routine," she said, "but it is an adjustment for everyone. We keep thinking he is coming back. It is like he is away traveling. I keep thinking he will call at night, like he used to, when he was working and traveling. It feels like he has gone on a trip."

Months after Mr. Metrakis's death, the family still insisted that he should not have been told the truth about his prognosis. Mrs. Metrakis was still upset that the doctors had told him that he was dying. Why did they have to do that? He had always been terrified of everything having to do with death and dying. If they had not told him, he never would have suspected things were that bad. It just didn't seem fair, she told Dr. Clermont. She had thought there was a cure for cancer. Now she knew this was untrue.

Later that month the PCU held a memorial service. Both Mrs. Metrakis and Sophia attended. By coincidence, the service took place on Mr. Metrakis's birthday. Sophia brought a picture of her brother, taken when he was in his twenties. She sobbed during the ceremony, but Mrs. Metrakis looked detached and distant. The last time Marian called her on the telephone she said she was fine and that "everyone is coping." Marian was not convinced, but left the door open in case Mrs. Metrakis should want to talk to her at a later time.

Authors' Comments

How do patients hear what is conveyed as "bad news"? When the medical oncologist told Elie Metrakis that a palliative approach emphasizing comfort was the only option rather than prolonging life, the family's reaction appeared to be one of fear and disbelief. It is clear that the Metrakis family were not able to accept the rapid transition from their belief that Costas was relatively healthy—with merely a case of indigestion—to his being terminally ill with only a few weeks to live. This affected communication with the palliative care team, as well. Normally, palliative care physicians have time to allow the family time to absorb the fact that the chance of cure is remote or even impossible. Indeed, one of the reasons patients with advanced cancer have been disproportionately represented in hospice and palliative care programs is the "fit" between the typically slow, but progressively deteriorating course of the disease and the philosophy of open communication and psychosocial support while patients and families gradually absorb the bad news. In Costas Metrakis's case, however, events had been proceeding much faster than the palliative care team was used to.

Elie Metrakis and Sophie, in particular, were unwilling to accept the various test results and wanted the doctors to treat Mr. Metrakis in spite of the news that his cancer was inoperable. Clearly, at that point, the family could only think of a cure, and they wanted Mr. Metrakis to remain on the medical ward where he could continue having intravenous therapy. Moreover, the family was receiving many conflicting messages from various multidisciplinary sources. At that time, if he was transferred to the PCU, intravenous therapy would not have been continued. Today, more than 20 years later, there is now more flexibility in the palliative care approach, and intravenous therapy, transfusions, chemotherapy, and antibiotics may be offered if the patient wishes. We cannot know whether Costas Metrakis's distress and that of his family could have been lessened, given the rapid progression of events. But perhaps a simultaneous model of care that included both active treatment and palliative care would have been helpful.

Elie Metrakis was angry when the doctors told her husband he only had one month to live. As she put it: "I asked the doctors not to tell him. It made me so mad. . . . But the doctors said it was the policy of the hospital. It is a hard thing to know you are dying." We discussed the issue of truthful disclosure of diagnostic and prognostic information in the Authors' Comments for the narrative of Sadie Fineman, including the cross-cultural aspects. The Metrakis family lived in a Greek community and participated in traditional Greek cultural and religious activities. Elie Metrakis's acute reaction to the doctors who told her husband that he was going to die would likely have stemmed from the traditional values they practiced as a Greek family. While it is unlikely that all Greek families will choose to have the truth withheld, and many will prefer to know the full facts and circumstances of the patient's illness, cultural values and mores may differ depending on the community and individual preferences. It is important for palliative care providers to consider these possibilities.[1] In my role as the interviewer, having been witness to the events surrounding this family's painful reaction to the bad news, I wondered later whether we as care providers should not reconsider how we convey information to the patient. Mr. Metrakis may have wanted to know (although we have no details on this), but Mrs. Metrakis would now retain the memory that her husband had died knowing fully that he had a terminal cancer diagnosis, something he had dreaded all of his life.

Recent Canadian literature has called for a "rebranding" of the language and understanding of palliative care for physicians who make referrals to palliative care. The language of "palliative care" often translates in patients' and families' minds as "a place to die." As Elie Metrakis said to Irene Clermont: "It's just that we heard that people come here [the PCU] to die." Dr. Clermont was able to rephrase the purpose of the admission to palliative care to include pain control, and this appeared to offer some reassurance. It is not clear that any difference in terminology could have alleviated Elie's fearful response, but the newly emerging models of palliative care that are now communicated to patients often include survival as a possibility, albeit with full awareness of the reality of mortality. This dual reality is character-ized as "hoping for the best but planning for the worst."[2]

References

1. Mystakidou K, Parpa E, Tsilila E, Katsouda E, Vlahos L. Cancer information disclo-sure in different cultural contexts. Support Care Cancer. 2004;12(3):147–154.
2. Hawley P. Barriers to access to palliative care. Palliat Care. 2017:1–6. Published online February 20.

21

Joey Court

Death of a Child

Narrated by Yanna Lambrinidou

The death of a child is a relatively rare event in medicine. Joey Court was born with an unusual and invariably fatal medical disorder. His parents anticipated Joey's death from the first year of his life but tried their best to treat him as they would any other child. Nine years later, they made the difficult decision to stop his life-prolonging treatment and called on hospice for palliative home care. To their surprise, Joey lived another five months. This narrative is about a family coming to terms with a child's death. It touches on several themes in pediatric hospice care: the decision to terminate aggressive treatment, the anticipation of an unnaturally premature death, the grief and bereavement of family members of all ages, and the question, "why?"

"Joey Recognizes Us and His Grandparents"

I remember vividly the first time I drove into the Courts' driveway. It was a hot summer day in August 1996, and I was nervous. All I had heard about Joey, the elder of two sons, was that he was a nine-year-old boy who had the mental capacity and motor skills of a three-month-old baby. Joey was unable to hold his head up. I had difficulty imagining what he looked like or how I would be able to interact with him. My arrival was announced promptly by the family dog, Coco, a Labrador retriever whose dark brown coat had inspired his name. Behind him appeared Amanda Court, a thin White woman in her early thirties whose warm smile did nothing to hide the dark circles under her eyes. Mrs. Court welcomed me into the house and introduced me to Mike, her four-year-old son, who leaned against her shyly and smiled. She then led me to the den.

Joey was lying on the sofa, his head propped up with pillows. Mrs. Court spoke to him sweetly. She told him my name and allowed me to stroke his cheek. Joey had the face of a nine-year-old—thick black hair, brown eyes, sparkling teeth, and a sweet smile. His body, however, weighed only 28 pounds. He looked fragile, bony, pale. He wore diapers. His feet were kept warm with tiny socks. I greeted him like I would a baby. Staring straight ahead, he waved his arms. "Joey recognizes us and his grandparents," explained Mrs. Court. "He knows voices. He does say about six things." But only she and her husband could understand him. Mike interpreted his brother's arm movements to mean, "Let's play!" Quickly, he placed his miniature hockey figures on Joey's chest and moved them slowly to give him the opportunity to watch. I couldn't tell how well Joey could see this.

The demands of Mrs. Court's life seemed so taxing that I was surprised by her willingness to participate in our study. Mrs. Court worked part-time as a recreation center administrative assistant. It was through her employment that she received health insurance. Joey required round-the-clock physical care that fell almost exclusively on her: liquid medications, frequent turning, and constant supervision to prevent him from sinking his face in his pillow and suffocating. His father, Brian, looked after him in the evenings. During the day, he worked 12–14 hours in the maintenance department of a large housing complex. Mike seemed starved for attention. He begged his mother to play with his hockey figures and join him in an interactive ice hockey video game. When Mrs. Court was too busy, he often refused to eat or demanded to be spoon-fed just like his brother.

Although I didn't interview Mrs. Court that day, I got the sense that she looked forward to the opportunity to talk. She seemed eager to spend time alone with me to speak more openly about her situation. With a shaky voice, she told me that in the nine years of his life, Joey had suffered more than any child deserves. And because of the rareness of his disorder, he had been experimented on as well. Mrs. Court would never forget the day when she planned to give Joey his first haircut. She stepped out of his hospital room for a short break, only to come back and find his head shaved and pierced with intravenous needles.

On my way out that day, Mrs. Court remarked that our time together had already helped her. Sharing with an interested listener had been a relief.

"He Does Not Walk, He Does Not Sit Up, He Does Not Do Anything on His Own"

Our second meeting lasted nearly two hours. Mrs. Court and I sat on the living room sofa while Joey napped in the adjacent den. Mike was in daycare, Mr. Court at work, and Coco sprawled in front of us. I asked Mrs. Court to tell me about Joey. She said that she and her husband had always wished for a big family. As a sports fan, she laughed, Brian had wanted enough children for a football team. Early on, however, Amanda had managed to talk him down to four. With their first child, Mrs. Court had the "perfect pregnancy." She ate well, gained the right amount of weight, and exercised. She experienced no complications, and when Joey was born, he looked healthy. But he couldn't keep his food down. On the fourth day of his life, his physicians discovered that he was missing a kidney, and a significant portion of his small intestine did not function. In recounting Joey's first surgery, which lasted approximately five hours, Mrs. Court began to cry. "It just makes me think of the way he was so little, and he really had a hard life," she said as tears rolled down her cheeks. After removing the nonfunctioning portion of his intestine, the surgeon announced that the baby was likely to die. If he were to survive, however, he had a good chance of leading a normal life. Joey survived. But he spent two of the first twelve months of his life in the hospital. Until his second year, he was fed intravenously.

When Joey reached six months, Mr. and Mrs. Court thought the worst was over. They were wrong. One day Joey stopped breathing. The emergency room doctor informed them that he was having seizures. He diagnosed Joey with a rare congenital disorder that usually limits children's life to two or three years. The message Mrs. Court took away was, "Your child is never going to walk, never going to talk, never do anything. You are going to have this vegetable child for as long as he lives."

"We know now that he has done a lot more than they told us he would ever do," Mrs. Court asserted. "I mean, they told us, 'We have to tell you the worst of what could happen,' even though they could not tell us exactly what was going to happen. He reaches out to Daddy when Daddy is there to hold him, and it was kind of neat every time he did a little thing like that. That was a big boost to us, to say, 'This child is not as bad off as they said he was going to be!'" Mrs. Court paused and lowered her voice. "But, he kind of is. He does not walk, he does not sit up, he does not do anything on his own. He will always be like a baby."

Joey never learned to chew. His diet consisted primarily of puréed foods and thickened liquids. He had difficulty keeping his food down. He could not expectorate the copious mucus that accumulated in his nose and throat. He required frequent suctioning and nebulizer treatments. He had bouts of aspiration pneumonia. Trips to the hospital were routine. In his first year alone, his medical bills approached $200,000. Although Amanda's insurance covered a large portion of this cost, and the state of Pennsylvania contributed as well, the Courts ended up paying what for them was an exorbitant amount of out-of-pocket funds. It took them six years to settle a physical therapy bill that had accumulated over a seven-month period. Ironically, a few weeks after Joey's fifth birthday, someone notified them about a medical assistance program that covered children with Joey's condition—but only for the first five years of their lives. The idea that most of Joey's medical expenses could have been covered with public funds exacerbated the Courts' frustration. It seemed that unless there was a crisis, Joey's health providers didn't volunteer information about agencies and resources that could help them.

When Joey turned three, the state did pick up the cost of his diapers, and several agencies paid for expensive equipment to facilitate his care. A wheelchair, a special car seat, a body brace that enabled him to sit up, and a special feeding chair were only a few of the supplies that the Courts acquired.

"He Really Does Understand This!"

Babysitters were intimidated by Joey's medical needs. Even his grandparents avoided staying alone with him. For the first few years of his life, Mr. and Mrs. Court assumed the sole responsibility for his care. But when Joey reached the age of three, they enrolled him in a school for children with disabilities that offered free physical therapy, sensory stimulation, and recreational activities. Joey loved school. He was mesmerized by different sounds and fulfilled by the individual attention he received. In the evening, he spent time with his father. When Mr. Court came home from work, he gave Joey a bath and held him on his lap for hours. The Courts built a swimming pool in their back yard and bought their son a floating bodysuit that kept his head firmly above the water. They didn't take vacations, but the Make-A-Wish Foundation offered them a week-long trip to Disney World. "[Joey] loved the rides," recalled Mrs. Court. "The only part he got scared at was when all of a sudden, we started shaking, and there was a big fire at the side of us, and you were supposed to feel like you were in an earthquake, and he reached over and grabbed onto my arm. You know, to us that was like, 'Oh my gosh! He really does understand this!'"

Dr. Heather Willis, the Courts' family physician, was always struck by how Brian and Amanda ascribed thoughts and feelings to Joey. "If you heard [Amanda] talk, you almost thought that Joey was a mildly disabled child," she remarked. "I don't know if it was denial, or if it was subtle things that she would respond to because of being with him so much that the rest of us would not see. I don't know. I think Mom was really alert to those subtle ways that he was responding, and the rest of us weren't."

When I asked her what she thought about the Courts' approach to Joey's illness, she said,

My personal feelings are pretty mixed. Because you see the use of resources on someone who does not have a good prognosis—he is really terminal, but you don't know *how* terminal. But we had to admit him to the hospital a few times with high-tech sort of care to get things going again. On the one hand, that makes you feel like, "Why are we doing this?" but on the other hand, you see the parents' involvement with the child and their inability to let go and you think, "No, we can't crush the hope that they have at this point."

Heather experienced a challenge: how to help the Courts come to terms with the likelihood that further attempts to prolong Joey's life might do more harm than good without seeming to force on them unwanted or unacceptable decisions. "I guess there just seems to be a time when they are ready," she continued. "I think you have to say a few things, like 'this is terminal,' and at times you have to point out that your interventions are uncomfortable for the child, and you have to point out that the child is suffering. At some point the family will have to catch on that, yeah, they are suffering and that prolonging things isn't in the best interest of the child."

The Courts worried about Joey every minute of the day. Still, they wanted a second child. Although the results of their blood tests remained inconclusive, they did not seem to suggest that Joey's disorder was genetic. Mike was born in 1991, when Joey was five. It took the Courts a year to lose their fear that their second child was sick as well. Only after repeated assurances from his physicians did they stop interpreting the rapid movements of his eyes as seizures.

"My Gosh, I Can't Help Him Anymore!"

Like both of his parents, Mike grew up to be protective of Joey. He played with him, talked to him, hugged him, and kissed him, and watched carefully when his mother and father tended to Joey's needs. He learned to wipe the sputum off his brother's face, rearrange the pillows under his head, and cover his feet with a small blanket. When Joey developed aspiration pneumonia, Mike rejected his own food. And when Joey's pneumonia required hospitalization, Mike missed his brother terribly. But he missed his parents, who spent much of their time at Joey's bedside, even more.

During one of Joey's hospitalizations, Mike told his mother that he wanted his brother's illness. This way, he said, he would get his parents' attention. After one of Joey's worst bouts of pneumonia, during which he had such a severe reaction to an antibiotic that he almost died, Mike began to yell. "I think that was his way of coping," Mrs. Court remarked, "but that is hard on the family, because when he is acting up like that, I mean we are already stressed out, and now—oh, my word!—we have to handle this child, too!"

Mrs. Court asked Joey's case worker if Mike was eligible for psychological help, only to be told that he was too young. Mike was only three, and the mental health agency involved with the Courts did not offer counseling to children under six. Amanda tried to give her younger son more attention. Still, she said to me, "I think Mike's life is really centered around Joey's. It is almost like he does not have a life of his own, because whatever we do as a family is centered around Joey. [If we have a trip planned] and Joey can't go, or Joey is having a bad day, we have to tell Mike, 'Sorry, we can't go today.'"

As time passed, Joey became harder to handle. Although he was only 28 pounds, his body grew longer. Transferring him from one position to another became challenging. Starting in January 1996, Joey's pneumonias began to show signs of resistance to antibiotics. For a period of four months, the Courts made weekly trips to the hospital. Then Mrs. Court fell sick. High fever and a severe respiratory infection kept her in bed for a week. A letter from her employer announced that because she had used up both her medical leave and vacation time, her position at the recreation center was in jeopardy. If she were to lose her job, she would also lose her health insurance. This would drive the Courts into bankruptcy. Mrs. Court didn't have the strength to fight. She hoped that her employer would show enough compassion to accept her back when she recovered. Her employer did accept her back. Mrs. Court returned to her part-time job with relief.

At the end of April 1996, Joey's medical team told the Courts that they were running out of medications to treat Joey's pneumonias. To prevent him from aspirating his food, they suggested inserting a percutaneous endoscopic gastrostomy (PEG) tube into his stomach. Such a device would allow the Courts to feed Joey without requiring him to swallow. After serious thought, Brian and Amanda turned down the offer. They knew that Joey was terminally ill and had long outlived his prognosis. At nine years old, he was one of the oldest children with his disorder. Even if he survived the operation, they questioned whether the PEG tube would prolong his life enough to justify additional suffering. Even with the PEG tube, Joey was bound to develop more pneumonias from aspirating his saliva.

To Mr. and Mrs. Court, the battle was over. "You kind of feel helpless," Amanda said. 'My gosh, I can't help him anymore!' You have helped from [when he was little] to nine years old, and now all of a sudden, 'Oh my gosh, I can't do anything!'"

When news traveled that Brian and Amanda had decided to put an end to their son's life-prolonging treatments, some of their friends and members of the network that supports children with Joey's condition stopped talking to them.

Hospice

Mr. and Mrs. Court wanted Joey to die at home. Given the high frequency of his pneumonias, they expected to lose him in a matter of weeks. They asked Dr. Willis for a referral to hospice. In an effort to protect him from unnecessary infections, they withdrew him from school. To keep him limber, they arranged for biweekly home visits from his physical therapist. They told the hospice admission nurse that all they wanted was symptom control for Joey, emotional support for Mike, and hospice volunteers so that Amanda could go to work.

For Mike, hospice offered the Illness Support Group within their children's program, "Coping Kids." Twice a month, the group met to explore through play the experience of living with a terminally ill person. The minimum age for participation was five, but Sally Walters, the group's coordinator, agreed to accept Mike, who was four and a half at the time. Sally, a serious yet energetic and playful individual, had a long phone conversation with Mrs. Court, which led her to the conclusion that Coping Kids had the capacity to help Mike and that Mike had the maturity to work with older children.

For Joey, hospice provided three volunteers: Amy Rymes, Jessica Austin, and Martha Diamond. All women in their fifties with children and grandchildren of their own, they agreed to watch Joey on Mondays and Fridays. But Mrs. Court worked three days a week and needed one more person for Wednesdays. Hospice was unable to find a fourth volunteer. Joey's case worker advised Mrs. Court that she was eligible to apply for a mental health grant, which would cover weekly nursing visits. Mrs. Court submitted an application immediately. Mr. Court got permission from his employer to stay at home one day a week. This solution was temporary and conditional, however. To make up for his lost hours, he promised to work on weekends.

"Can I Do This?"

"I must say that the first time I went [to the Courts'] I was frightened," said Amy Rymes, in a warm, confessional tone. "You know, I thought, 'Can I do this?'" Ms. Rymes looked after Joey for five and a half hours every Monday. She fed him, gave him his medications, turned him over, changed his diaper, and read to him. When he cried, she soothed him by calling his name. His cooing enthralled her. "When he sat on his chair," she noted, "his legs just hung limp, and we put a hassock there so that his feet could prop on that a little bit. But if you ever worked with a ventriloquist or saw a ventriloquist who had a dummy, that is how their legs hang, you know, and I thought how different he is, and yet he is so lovable even though he is not giving you the love back or the hugs. But he needs you. When you dried him, it was like putting a diaper on a little skeleton. There was nothing there. Nothing at all." Ms. Rymes' greatest fear was that Joey would choke during her shift and die before his parents were able to get back.

Jessica Austin volunteered on Friday mornings, between breakfast and lunchtime. She was thankful for that because she had heard that feeding Joey was a challenge. The care Joey received from his family touched her. Every time she entered the house, she watched as Mrs. Court sat next to her son, stroked him, and told him goodbye. Mike carefully covered the lower part of Joey's body with a blanket before taking off for his grandparents' house. Inspired by the affection, Ms. Austin decided to talk and sing to Joey herself. Her favorite song was "Jesus loves me, and Jesus loves you, and Jesus loves the little children of the world." She had a feeling that Joey liked that song, as it made him smile.

The first few times Martha Diamond took care of Joey, she sang songs to calm him down, brought bells to get his attention, and wore bright clothes to stimulate his vision. But when she didn't see a response, she stopped trying. She reflected,

> My feeling was, "Why are we trying so hard to stimulate him? It is nearly over." That may be a bad attitude, but that is the way I thought. Why are we trying to make him progress when he is really regressing? It is too frustrating to me with no results and so little response. Maybe the baby activity in a larger body bothered me. I think maybe it did. You know, you look at them and you think, "Well, it should not be this way," and, "They should be eating and swallowing." I don't know. Maybe it was a mental thing in there about how infant-like his eating was for his looks and his size. I don't know.

"All Right, Start to Detach Yourself"

Joey never left his mother's thoughts. The idea that his death was imminent terrified her. The day she found the milk in the cupboard and the cereal in the refrigerator she knew that her stress had caught up with her. She told Claudia James, the hospice social worker, that her life felt like a roller coaster. Joey's ups and downs and the constant level of tension at home were also taking a toll on Mike. Her little one had grown more hyperactive and disobedient. When he missed Coping Kids, he yelled, broke rules, and slept poorly. One time, he stripped himself naked in the presence of a hospice nurse. Another, after a long day of misbehaving, he looked at his father and said, "I know I was bad, Daddy, and I did not mean to be today, but I have things on my mind that are bothering me."

In the middle of June, after more medical crises, the Courts decided, with Dr. Willis's support, to stop administering more antibiotics. Maggie Laslett, Joey's hospice nurse, advised them to prepare for a respiratory crisis and encouraged them to make use of the morphine that had been prescribed to minimize the experience of breathlessness if suctioning and nebulizer treatments did not seem to help. Joey began appearing sleepy. The involuntary twitching of his eyes and the stiffening of his body looked like he was having more seizures. His congestion and dyspnea worsened. He developed fever. During her shift one day, Jessica, the hospice volunteer, noticed that he was extremely pale, coughed frequently, and had difficulty breathing. "I had a quick prayer," she told me. "'Dear Lord, don't let this child die while I'm here with him.'" She then gave him a nebulizer treatment.

The month of August unfolded no differently than June and July. Joey had good days and bad, and so did his family. When September came along and Mike started daycare, the Courts were devastated by the fact that Joey wasn't going back to school. Mrs. Court said,

> You always expect your children to outlive you. We always knew that this could happen and that he was sick, and he has almost died I don't know how many times. So we have been to this point, but never to the point where now he is not going to school this year. And now hospice is here—it is real final. It is like, now we are there. But it seems like he always keeps pulling out of these bad spells, and I think that is just as hard. It is almost like, if he was going to be sick and get sicker and that was going to be it and this was going to be over with, I think it might almost be easier than the ups and downs.

Mrs. Court seemed to have reduced her interactions with Joey to matters relating to his body. In our conversations, I found it almost impossible to get a sense of who Joey was to her—what she loved or would miss about him. Her references to him were strictly medical. She, herself, alluded to the distancing. "As he gets sicker," she said, "I think I withdraw myself more away from him, only because I am preparing myself for what is going to happen. Now that hospice is here you are like, 'All right, start to detach yourself,' only because it is going to be hard in the long run."

Mr. Court seemed to be moving in the opposite direction, displaying greater and greater attachment to his son. During Joey's last hospitalization, he did not leave his side. And at night, when he returned home from work, he extended the time he spent with him. Joey showed deep affection for his father. Lovingly, Mrs. Court called him a "daddy's boy." When he heard Brian's voice, he whimpered and begged. "Do you want Daddy to hold you?" Brian would ask sweetly, "Is that what you want?" And when he picked Joey up, father and son seemed in peace.

Mike

In September, Mrs. Court found Mike to be especially "clingy." He had just started preschool and for the first time was spending weekdays away from his grandparents, who had served as his daytime caretakers during the first few years of his life. At night he visited his parents' bed for comfort. He asked if Joey was going to die. Mr. and Mrs. Court never hid from him the seriousness of his brother's condition, but they also didn't know how to talk to him about death. Although Mike used the word himself, they weren't sure what he meant by it. "Does he really understand that once Joey dies, he is not going to be laying on the sofa anymore?" Mrs. Court wondered. She told her son that when people pass away their spirit goes to heaven. But after watching a burial on television, Mike couldn't understand why the coffin was placed in the ground. The contradiction disturbed him.

Amanda and Brian

Mrs. Court always spoke fondly about her husband. When I asked her about Joey's impact on their relationship, she told me that, if anything, Joey's condition had strengthened it. She and Brian stood on a solid foundation, she said: their love and commitment were unshakable. When Joey was born, they knew that their struggle was going to bring them closer, and it had.

Amanda took care of Joey's medical needs in the daytime, and Brian looked after him early in the morning and at night. Before work, he fed him breakfast, dressed him, carried him from his bedroom to the den. After work, he bathed him and held him on his lap. They had silently agreed on a division of labor in which Brian was responsible for Joey and Amanda, for Mike. "When we plan to go somewhere, just for a picnic or to visit [Brian's] mom or dad or whatever," Amanda said, "Brian will automatically pack Joey's backpack, food, diapers, whatever we need, and I will automatically make sure what Mike needs. I will often say to Brian, 'Do you have Joey's stuff together?' and then I will say. 'I have all of Mike's stuff together. Now we are ready to go.'"

Amy Rymes

Ms. Rymes, the hospice volunteer, grew more and more attached to Joey. She explained that her experience had taught her a big lesson about compassion. She had come to recognize that although Joey was different from other children, he was lovable. He adored his family, liked some foods and disliked others, enjoyed sounds, loved being rubbed on the face, and took pleasure in tossing his arms. Sometimes his physical therapy sessions enabled him to make new movements. The time she saw him throw one leg over the sofa made her laughed. She found Joey beautiful. She noticed that when he slept, his black hair shone. He was always clean, and every Monday he was dressed in a T-shirt she had given him. It featured a colorful rainbow with the words, "I am a possibility."

"My Name Is Mike, and My Brother Joey Is Sick"

Sally Walters, the coordinator of Mike's support group, was impressed with the little boy's growth. Mike was the youngest child she had worked with. When he first joined the group, he was so "terribly, terribly, terribly shy" that he rarely spoke. He tried his best, however, to participate in every activity, including the ones that required writing. Mike did not know how to write, but he agreed to draw instead. He looked up to a 13-year-old in the group, and, week after week, made a point of sitting next to him.

In the children's Illness Support Group, Ms. Walters didn't dwell on death and dying. Aware that some children held hope for their loved ones, Sally was careful not to dishearten them. At the same time, she felt that children like Mike benefited from an environment in which their relative's illness was acknowledged. "Mike has really come along and, I think, grown and has a better understanding of the fact that his brother is sick," she said. "[He] is now able to say, 'My name is Mike, and my brother Joey is sick.'" Sally had the feeling that Mike would miss Joey because Joey was his most captive audience. She knew that Mike liked to include his brother in his play, even though he did all the talking.

"He Just Got Real Ill and Just Couldn't Take It No More"

Friday, September 20, was Joey's 10th birthday. On September 16, Mike announced that he was ready for Joey's party. Brian and Amanda followed him in singing "Happy Birthday," but Joey was weak and lethargic. He struggled to breathe. Mike unwrapped his brother's presents. They included sweat suits from their grandparents, bibs from the hospice volunteers, and shoes from Brian and Amanda.

Three days later, Mike yelled at his mother all the way back from preschool. A note from his teacher explained that his class had held a funeral for their deceased hermit crab.

When I called the Courts on September 30, I was surprised to hear Mr. Court answer the phone. On weekdays, he was usually at work. I asked him about Joey. "It was a little rough yesterday," he said calmly. "He just got real ill and just couldn't take it no more. He just fell asleep. So he is gone." Mrs. Court came to the phone a few moments later. "I can't say we weren't expecting it," she said. "But it's still a shock." She explained that Joey never recovered from his last respiratory crisis. She kept giving him morphine as instructed by Maggie, but on Sunday he didn't open his eyes. He stopped breathing a few hours later. "It was quick for him though, so we were glad for that," she said. "He did not lay there and struggle or anything," she continued. "He just stopped breathing."

Mike didn't seem to understand what had happened. He cried at first, because he saw his parents crying, but then he went back to playing. Mrs. Court suspected that Joey's death would become more real to him at the funeral, where he would see Joey's casket lowered to the ground. She said that she herself felt "pretty good." She then added, "I think it will be worse later on."

Hospice nurse Colleen Stone told me that the day of Joey's death was her saddest day with hospice. Ms. Stone knew the Courts, for she had visited them a few times in place of Maggie. On the morning of September 29, she was on weekend duty. Mrs. Court called hospice to report that Joey had died. When Ms. Stone arrived to make the official pronouncement of death, she found Mike running excitedly around the living room. In the den, Amanda, her siblings, Brian's siblings, and all four grandparents sat in a circle, crying. Brian picked up Joey and held him in his lap while Colleen listened to his heart. Then he handed him to the person next to him, stood up, hugged Colleen, and sobbed. Everyone took turns cradling the deceased boy. Coco went around the room resting his head on the leg of the person holding him.

Brian's mother was startled by the coolness of the corpse. "Get me a blanket, because Joey is cold!" she exclaimed, before realizing what she had said and discreetly laughing it off.

More visitors filed in. At the door, Mike kept announcing that Joey had gone to heaven. A few times, he said that Joey had died. But every now and then he turned to his mother and asked, "Is Joey going to live with us, Mom?" Until the arrival of the undertaker, almost four hours later, Mike kept himself busy with his toys. When he saw the hearse, he broke into tears. His parents assured him that he would see Joey again at the viewing. The undertaker brought Joey's body into the living room. Everyone watched quietly as Amanda picked her son up and placed him gently on the small bed. Her lip quivered. The undertaker covered the body with a sheet, and one by one, the 30 visitors kissed Joey goodbye. Brian, Amanda, Mike, and Colleen all stepped out to see the hearse leave. "We waited," Colleen told me, "until we could not see the car anymore."

"Joey Is Dead, But I Am Not"

The Courts spent the morning of October 1 at the funeral home. They dressed Joey in one of his new sweat suits and placed his feet in his favorite sneakers. By the time of the viewing, they were exhausted. "You almost feel like there are no more tears," Mrs. Court recalled. As friends and relatives paid their final respects, Mike was busy drawing pictures and laying them at the foot of the white coffin. He had a new teddy bear, which he named "Joey Bear."

The next day at the cemetery, relatives, friends, church members, co-workers, health providers, schoolteachers, and hospice staff formed a long line to greet Mr. and Mrs. Court. The two were cordial but emotionally flat. Mike was excited. Proudly, he ran to his support group leader, Sally, and showed her his bow tie. Sally picked him up and told him that he looked swell. Mike beamed. He then placed his hands on Sally's face and said, "Joey is dead, but I am not." Before she knew it, Sally found herself in front of Joey's casket. Mike wanted to show her the drawings he had made for his brother. He told her that Joey was going to take them with him to heaven. He then casually lifted Joey's head and rearranged the pillows.

When Mrs. Court saw Amy, the hospice volunteer, in the mourning line, she introduced her to her father and told him that she was indebted to her for her help. Without the support of hospice, she said, she would have not been able to work. Looking back at her experience with Joey, Amy told me, "I got more in return than I ever gave." Still, Amy didn't look forward to working with another dying child. She said that her visits at the Courts' had exhausted her, not because she worked hard, but because she was constantly on edge.

Heather Willis

During Joey's five months with hospice, Dr. Willis lost almost all contact with the Courts. In retrospect, she regretted that she hadn't called them for updates or offered them her support. She also wished that she had stayed in closer contact with Joey's hospice nurse, Maggie. She said,

When hospice comes in, they take over, you know. That is good, and they take over with all the little details of managing the patient's comfort and things like that, and then I will get a message on my desk that hospice would like a change in medicine, or this, or that, and that is fine. But I feel a lot less in touch than when [Amanda and Brian] were coming to me for the management. I wouldn't mind talking to a hospice nurse more. You know, they are sensitive to the doctors and their time and things, and try not to bother us during hours, but maybe some of us would like to be bothered.

From her ten years of work with Mr. and Mrs. Court, Heather had grown close to them. She attributed Joey's longer-than-expected life to the extraordinary care they gave him.

"It Is So Hard That He Doesn't Need Me Anymore"

A week after Joey's funeral, I went back to visit Mrs. Court. Mike was in preschool. Mr. Court was at work. The living room was filled with flowers. Amanda remarked that even though she had expected Joey's death for ten years, she found it extremely painful. The finality of his absence horrified her. Now she realized that her husband had done the right thing when he kept taking photographs of their son. Six albums were filled with shots from the first until the tenth year of his life. She relished looking at them.

Because Mr. Court worked long hours, he had not had the opportunity to experience his son's subtle, day-to-day decline. Joey's death had caught him off guard. Now he walked aimlessly through the house, wondering what to do with himself. He skipped breakfast because he missed feeding Joey. For Mrs. Court, not having to care for Joey added so much free time to her day that she didn't know how to fill it. "I am just so used to being busy," she said, "that now I go to relax, and I get right back up and do something. I think to myself, 'Brian will get home from work,' and I will think, 'Oh my gosh! I had better run to the store quick'—or here or there—'because tomorrow I can't, because I have Joey!' And then I think, 'No, I don't have to do that now.' If Mike says, 'Mommy, can we play this?' I will look at what time it is, thinking, 'What does Joey need?' or 'Do I have time to do this quick?' I am so used to Joey. It is so hard that he doesn't need me anymore."

She told me that what kept her strong was her conviction that Joey was at peace. "We know that he is not suffering," she said, "and I think that has helped us to handle it. This might sound odd, but when the undertaker came to get him and I put him up on the bed, he had a smile on his face and he looked so peaceful, and the undertaker kept that smile on his face for the viewing. Normally they would close the mouth completely. We said it was a comfort to us, and everybody who was at the viewing said, 'Oh my gosh!' It was an overwhelming feeling of peace."

Joey was buried in a nearby cemetery. The Courts visited him daily. Mike took flowers to his grave, and on his way to school he stopped by with his mother to tell Joey, "Good morning." Mrs. Court told me that ever since he had received his new teddy bear, Mike acted like Joey was still at home. "By the next day," she said, "he was play-acting that [the teddy bear] was Joey. He was feeding him breakfast the next morning, burping him, and then he laid him on the sofa before he ate. When Mike got up the morning of the funeral and I said, 'What do you want for breakfast?' he said, 'Oh no, Mom, I can't eat breakfast yet. I have to feed Joey.' When we go by the grave, he keeps asking me, 'Mom, is his body still there, or did the rest of him go up to Heaven?'"

"My Name Is Mike, and Joey Died"

In the middle of November, Mrs. Court looked the most rested I had seen her. The dark circles under her eyes had faded, and she seemed relaxed. From two tranquilizer pills a day she was now down to a half. The money she and her husband had received from relatives had helped pay off a significant portion of Joey's outstanding medical bills. But Mrs. Court was still concerned about Mike.

Mike was now five years old. He had been having diarrhea for several days, bit his nails, and acted out in all the ways he knew irritated his mother. When Amanda refused to feed him like a baby, he didn't eat—a behavior he had adopted when Joey was sick. At dinner the night before, Amanda resorted to a favorite game to hurry Mike through his meal so that they could be on time for church. She pretended they were in a race to see who would finish first.

"Mike, I beat you!" she called out. "All right, Mike, I'm done!"

"Well," Mike replied, "I am going to beat Joey because Joey is not done yet."

Mike's new Loss Support Group was a lot bigger than the Illness Support Group, with an average of 20 children per session. Tracy Torres, a soft-spoken volunteer, recalled, "You could tell he was frightened to be there. I would sort of coax him a little bit to stay with me, and I would sit beside him and, even then, I could tell he was still afraid, and he just did not say much at all." Tracy made a point of staying close to Mike at every meeting. When it was his turn to introduce himself, she spoke for him. Within a few months, Mike became more open. He giggled and laughed with the other children. He participated eagerly in group activities. And he started to speak for himself. "My name is Mike, and Joey died," he said at the beginning of every meeting.

As Christmas neared, Mike began singing songs about Joey's life in heaven. On the weekends, on the way to ice hockey practice, he made his father drive by the cemetery to pick his brother up. "We keep reinforcing to him that Joey is always with him, and I think that is just his way of grasping that—to think that he has to drive by to get him," said Mrs. Court. Mike would fasten his brother's seat belt, talk to him quietly in the car, and bring him to hockey practice for luck. He worried, however, about how Joey was going to celebrate the holiday. The small Christmas tree his aunt placed on Joey's grave gave him some consolation.

Mike was concerned about Joey's body. Was it all in heaven? Was some of it in the ground? His parents' answer was always the same: that it was his soul that had gone to heaven and that Joey had a new body now, a healthy one like Mike's. A day or two later, Mike would ask again: What happened to Joey's body?

The Courts received fewer Christmas cards that year, and the families who used to send them photographs of their children now sent only a card. "They think it is going to hurt our feelings or something like that," Amanda said to me, "because they still have their child, and we don't. But I don't look at it that way. I want to see how they are growing." With their own card, the Courts included a photograph of Mike and one of Joey, taken two weeks before he died. Amanda told me that it meant a lot to her when people talked openly about her boy. She appreciated every sign that he was remembered.

Joey as Memory, Joey as Spirit

Four months after Joey's death, Mr. and Mrs. Court joined hospice's Loss of Child Support Group. Mrs. Court recalled that when she first started attending the meetings, she cried on the way there, cried while there, and had a headache all the way back. Now she looked forward to going. She still cried sometimes, but she also laughed and shared her thoughts. The meetings were drawing her closer to Brian as well, teaching her things about him she didn't know. Once, in a discussion about personal bereavement rituals, Mr. Court shared that, before going to bed and upon rising in the morning, he made a point to touch Joey's door. "I didn't know that!" Amanda exclaimed laughingly. "I knew he was close to Joey. I saw him go by. But I never—when he said that, it was funny, because I did not know he was doing that!"

Mike continued to pick Joey up on his way to hockey practice. When he played well, he attributed it to his brother. When he didn't skate fast enough, he asked Joey to push him harder. "He is so cute," said Mrs. Court, "because he is so little. [The other kids] are all like 6, up to 12 to 14. He is the littlest guy, and he doesn't even always understand where he is supposed to be. The coaches told Brian that they can tell that his heart and soul is really in there. He goes around and signs autographs for people already. Even for the undertaker! [Mike] says, 'I am going to go to college, probably in Michigan—to Michigan College—and then I am going to play for the Hershey Bears, and then I am going to play for the Colorado Avalanche.' And it is so odd to us because our kids were so different. We knew Joey would never have a future, and here is one who is planning this huge future. It is so odd. It is almost like we had kids at complete, total, last points on the spectrum."

At the end of April, Coping Kids carried out a memorial service to commemorate the death of the children's loved ones. The service opened with a brief welcoming introduction by a young member of the Loss Support Group. "Good evening, everyone," said the boy at the center of the stage, "my name is John Balch. Welcome to the Coping Kids memorial service. Tonight is a night to talk about our most special memories and the love we always will have for people who have died." The children lit candles, sang hymns, and played a song that one girl dedicated to her deceased mother. Then, one by one, they walked toward a large box they called a "treasure chest." Each child announced their favorite memory of their departed loved one and deposited an artistic rendering of this memory in the chest.

When it was Mike's turn, Tracy asked him if he wanted her help to describe his memory. Mike said he did. "Mike's memory that he treasures is about his brother Joey," Tracy announced into the microphone. She then turned to Mike. "And what do you want to say it was Joey's favorite thing to eat?" she asked. "Applesauce!" Mike said loudly. He then placed his drawing into the treasure chest: a big smiley face, smeared with yellow lines.

"Joey Pulled the Sun Up, Making It Nice"

The last time I saw Mrs. Court was in August 1997. She looked happy, rested, and tanned. The family had recently returned from a trip to Canada. Having that break was superb, she said. Far away from the physical reminders, she hardly thought about Joey. But when they arrived back home, the house felt empty. The quietness in Joey's room startled her. The next time Amanda and Brian attended the Loss of Child Support Group, Amanda cried all the way through. "Now I am okay again," she said to me. "It was almost like, when we were away, we did not deal with anything, and when you come back, it is like reality hits again—almost like you're starting all over. But it does not take that long to get back to where you were. You just kind of backslide for that short time."

The Courts decorated Joey's grave regularly with flowers, wreaths, wind chimes, and objects that symbolized religious and national holidays. Mike still talked about Joey, but not nearly as much as before. On a windy day at Coping Kids, he drew a picture of a child, reproduced here, with an ominous circle in front of its face. He announced that this was his big brother who was blowing the clouds. When it rained, he claimed that it was Joey who brought the water, and at sunrise he once said, "Joey pulled the sun up, making it nice." He had stopped waking up in the middle of the night, and he no longer needed to drive by the cemetery several times a day. When he felt sad, he talked more about his feelings. He told his parents that he played hockey for Joey. One day, he said, he was going to dedicate the Stanley Cup to him.

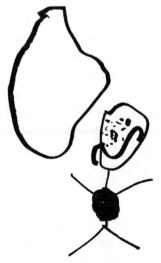

Mike Court's drawing from "Coping Kids."

Mrs. Court continued to browse through the family photo albums. She searched in Joey's closet for things she had tucked away years earlier. When she came across Joey's baby book, she opened it to the page where parents record the milestones of their child's growth. She looked to see if there was a space to mark Joey's death. There was none.

Authors' Comments

Children are not supposed to die, in wealthy countries at any rate, a point bluntly reinforced for Amanda Court when she saw there was no place in Joey's baby book to record the date of his death. Children in wealthy countries do die, of course. Not only are global levels of preventable infant and child mortality grievously high and marked by vast, socially determined racial and wealth disparities, but many childhood deaths result from noncommunicable, often non-preventable diseases as well, such as cancer, metabolic and neurological disorders, heart disease, and congenital disabilities. For these latter conditions, the specialized field of pediatric palliative care, which was in its infancy at the time of our research, has grown apace. Recent textbooks survey the state of the art in clinical practice,[1,2] and there is an active research agenda,[3,4] including a call for focused investigation into the needs of children with chronic, progressive disorders of the type that afflicted Joey Court.[5]

In Joey's case, the hospice team had precious little to do at the bedside. This was due in part to the nature of Joey's condition. He had been terminally ill from birth, and his parents had become quite adept at the demanding routines of his care. Amanda Court's extraordinary competence and devotion to Joey's every need seemed to render outside help almost superfluous, as the hospice nurses and volunteers all discovered at one time or another. This did not mean, however, that Amanda failed to appreciate outside support. She was physically and emotionally exhausted by the rigors of nonstop nursing, which were aggravated by her and Brian's determination to treat Joey as a "normal" child while trying to nurture the growth and development of their younger son, Mike.

Hospice's greatest and most impressive contributions to this case occurred away from the bedside, in the bereavement support groups for the Courts. The relative rarity and "unnaturalness" of a child's death intensifies parental grieving.[6,7] Hospice of Lancaster County's extensive bereavement services were in many ways ahead of their time, as institutional recognition of the importance of supporting grieving parents has only recently become widespread.[8,9] Amanda and Brian entered their support group at Hospice of Lancaster County emotionally devastated, exhausted, and in need of healing. They emerged as providers of support to others and found this transition to be part of their own healing. Mike flourished in the Coping Kids program. Indeed, this narrative captures rich and moving reactions of a young griever, a member of a demographic group that is often invisible to caregivers, whether the dying patient is a child or an adult.[10–12]

The changes in social welfare policies in the United States since we carried out our research—especially the Affordable Care Act (ACA) and the Family Medical Leave Act (FMLA)—would have greatly reduced the financial burdens and stresses of Joey's illness had they been in place for the Courts. As it was, Amanda and Brian faced enormous out-of-pocket healthcare costs and worried that their caring for Joey was jeopardizing their employment, which was the source of the limited health insurance coverage they did have. The ACA has decoupled the availability of health insurance from employment. And the FMLA, though it does not grant *paid* leave and applies only to private-sector employers with more than 50 employees, at least protects the job of someone caring for a seriously ill family member for up to twelve weeks a year. A troubling aspect of the narrative is the fact that the Courts *could* have received public assistance for Joey's care for the first five years of his life, but they did not learn of this until *after* Joey's fifth birthday.

Why did none of Joey's professional caregivers make the Courts aware of this source of support? In reflecting on this question, we first must recognize that the narrative of Joey Court tells two overlapping stories. One is of hospice workers offering palliative care for a dying child and his family. The other is of parents seeking and providing healthcare for a child with profound disabilities. Looking at the narrative through the lens of the second story, several features stand out strongly. They might be brought into focus with the question, "What—and who—did people see when they looked at Joey Court?" Heather Willis, the Courts' family physician, commented, "I think Mom was really alert to those subtle ways that [Joey] was responding, and the rest of us weren't." Heather's comment introduces a thread that runs through the narrative: whereas Amanda and Brian, who watched every one of Joey's movements and cherished every sign that Joey was connected to the world, saw a real person and value in him, bonded with him, and did everything they could to keep him alive, many others saw in Joey little more than a hopeless cause and a drain on both the family and the healthcare system.

This spectrum of perceptions was embodied in the varied reactions to Joey on the part of the hospice volunteers and nurses as well as the nature of the care that each provided. It was remarkable how some saw beauty in this child as Amanda and Brian did, while others, whose gaze was more clinical and detached, could not see the point of keeping Joey alive, a view that even those who grew close to him eventually came to share. Is it possible that one of the reasons medical and nursing staff routinely failed to inform the Courts about financial assistance options was that they, by and large, had written Joey off?

The intersection in our narrative of end-of-life care with the status of disabled people in our society is a contested space that is being negotiated prominently in the public sphere today, not least because of the pressures to ration life-saving treatments during the COVID-19 pandemic.[13] For example, *Not Dead Yet*—a national, grassroots disability rights group that opposes legalization of assisted suicide and euthanasia "as deadly forms of discrimination"—views policies for advance directives and surrogate decision-making as dangerous vehicles for end-of-life determinations by individuals who are incapable or unwilling to see the lives of disabled people as inherently valuable.[14] In other words, what appear to many able-bodied people as self-evidently desirable forms of self-determination are deemed threatening by people with disabilities who fear—legitimately—that the quality of their lives is routinely and systematically underestimated, if not dismissed outright.

Ironically, the Courts themselves, after years of tireless advocacy for Joey's very life, were subjected to the harsh judgment of friends and members of the network for children with Joey's condition over their own long-deliberated, painful decision to end their child's life-prolonging treatments. How easy it is to strike a righteous pose; how complex to live with life's powerful bonds, doubts, and ambiguities.

References

1. Wolfe J, Hinds, P, Sourkes B, eds. *Textbook of Interdisciplinary Pediatric Palliative Care*. Philadelphia: Saunders-Elsevier; 2011.
2. Hain R, Goldman A, Rapoport A, Meiring M, eds. *Oxford Textbook of Palliative Care for Children*, 3rd ed. New York: Oxford University Press; 2021.
3. Steele R, Bosma H, Johnston MF, Cadell S, Davies B, Siden H, Straatman L. Research priorities in pediatric palliative care: a Delphi study. J Palliat Care. 2008;24(4):229–239.

4. Feudtner, C, Rosenberg AR, Boss RD, Wiener L, Lyon ME, Hinds PS, Bluebond-Langner M, Wolfe J. Challenges and priorities for pediatric palliative care research in the US and similar practice settings: Report from a pediatric palliative care research network workshop. J Pain Symptom Manage. 2019;58(5):909–917.e3.

5. Bao D, Feichtinger L, Andrews G, Pawliuk C, Steele R, Siden HH. Charting the territory: End-of-life trajectories for children with complex neurological, metabolic, and chromosomal conditions. J Pain Symptom Manage. 2021;61(3):449–445.e1.

6. Darlington AE, Korones DN, Norton SA. Parental coping in the context of having a child who is facing death: A theoretical framework. Palliat Support Care. 2018;16(4):432–441.

7. Morris S, Fletcher K, Goldstein, R. The grief of parents after the death of a young child. J Clin Psychol Med Settings. 2019;26(3):321–338.

8. Morris SE, Dole OR, Joselow M, Duncan J, Renaud K, Branowicki P. The development of a hospital-wide bereavement program: Ensuring bereavement care for all families of pediatric patients. J Pediatr Health Care. 2017;31(1):88–95.

9. Schuelke T, Crawford C, Kentor R, Eppelheimer H, Chipriano C, Springmeyer K, Shukraft A, Hill M. Current grief support in pediatric palliative care. Children. 2021;8(4):278.

10. Bugge KE, Darbyshire P, Røkholt EG, Haugstvedt KT, Helseth S. Young children's grief: parents' understanding and coping. Death Stud. 2014;38(1-5):36–43.

11. Dowdney L. Children bereaved by parent or sibling death. Psychiatry. 2008;7(6):270–275.

12. Webb, NB. The child and death. In Webb, NB, ed. *Helping Bereaved Children: A Handbook for Practitioners* (3rd edition). New York: Guilford; 2010:3–21.

13. Guidry-Grimes L, Savin K, Stramondo JA, Reynolds JM, Tsaplina M, Burke TB, Ballantyne A, Kittay EF, Stahl D, Scully JL, Garland-Thomson R, Tarzian A, Dorfman D, Fins JJ. Disability rights as a necessary framework for crisis standards of care and the future of health care. Hastings Cent Rep. 2020;50(3):28–32.

14. Not Dead Yet. The Resistance. https://notdeadyet.org/. Accessed November 14, 2021.

22

Paula Ferrari

Another Triumph of the Spiritual Over the Practical

Narrated by Patricia Boston

Paula Ferrari was diagnosed with amyotrophic lateral sclerosis (ALS), an incurable degenerative motor neuron disease that leads to progressive weakness of the muscles in the extremities and trunk. For the next three years, Paula lived with ALS. When she was admitted to the Palliative Care Unit, she was no longer able to eat or swallow on her own. Paula knew that these changes would take place and that her disease would progress until she wouldn't be able to breathe alone. She knew that many others suffering with ALS would have given up and tried to seek physician-assisted suicide if it were legal and available (as it was not in Canada at that time). But for Paula Ferrari, to seek help to hasten one's death was an act of total self-deprivation. Death, she insisted, is an integral part of our being and existence. To undergo the experience of dying, regardless of the physical suffering it entails, is our ultimate lesson of life. Experiencing suffering offers a unique opportunity to know about ourselves and who we are in our spiritual existence. Paula did suffer physically. But she stood firmly by her beliefs and never wavered. For her caregivers on the Palliative Care Unit, Paula Ferrari seemed to have mastered the extremes of living with a fatal illness.

Life Before Illness

Paula Ferrari was born in Philadelphia. She was raised by Italian parents and lived there until she married her husband John, an American citizen. When

John got a job teaching chemistry at a Montreal university, the Ferrari family moved there with their young family. They had four children—two sons, Franco and Greg, and two daughters, Rosa and Rita.

After some years of raising their children together, things started to fall apart for the Ferraris. The marriage was strained by conflict over financial affairs, and Paula and John each wanted to pursue very different life goals. They decided to separate.

Shortly after arriving from Philadelphia, Paula enrolled in a master's degree program in philosophy. She began to study seriously the spiritual and philosophical questions that had confronted her over the course of her life. Following her marital breakup, she worked as a hospice aide, then as a Roman Catholic chaplain, and finally as a professor and teacher of religious philosophy. She became actively involved in scholars' groups concerned with the relation between religion and spirituality and became known for speaking out publicly on religious political issues. She was a poet, artist, musician, and philosopher, never tiring of speaking about her religious beliefs.

In the pursuit of deeper spiritual understanding, Paula traveled to Italy. She wanted to renew herself within the context of her Italian roots, to reflect on who she was, and to learn her ancestral language.

It was not only her Italian heritage that led her to return to her parents' homeland but also her childhood faith of Catholicism. For a long time she had formally accepted her faith in the teachings of the church, but she constantly wrestled with psychological and spiritual questions.,

She embraced the monastic life at the Villa Benedictine monastery in the solitude of the Italian mountains, where she explored the various dimensions of her experience—her roles as a mother, wife, feminist, and academic—and how she could relate them to her own spirituality. It was a happy life, she later recalled, and a life where she gained much insight. As she practiced the monastic rituals, she began to reconcile her life experience with her spirituality and found a sense of inner spiritual freedom among the nuns and the life they led.

The Diagnosis

In my dreams, I travel a lot, walking, talking and guiltily smoking cigarettes. There's nothing I can do for myself. Like an infant, I depend on others to survive. I have entered a merciful, if sometimes frustrating, world.

While she was in Italy, Paula Ferrari fell. It wasn't a very noticeable or serious fall, but later she told me that she thought it was odd, since she hadn't tripped over anything, and this had never happened to her before. After returning to Montreal, she found that she often stumbled and tripped, seemingly for no reason. Sometimes she needed to hold onto a piece of furniture to keep her balance. Six months after she returned from Italy, Dr. Sean O'Leary, her family doctor, suggested that she undergo a series of tests. When he had the results and informed Paula that she had Lou Gehrig's disease, she couldn't believe it was true.

Lou Gehrig's disease, or amyotrophic lateral sclerosis (ALS), involves a pervasive and inexorable loss of function. Insidiously, the patient experiences a gradual loss of the use of arms, legs, bladder, and bowel. Swallowing becomes difficult, and ultimately the capacity to breathe diminishes, resulting in death. Paula Ferrari's tests showed an extensive degeneration of the muscles in three limbs.

Paula's first reaction was hopelessness and despair. "I screamed a lot," she said, recalling this time much later. "The thoughts of losing my children and not living long enough to know my grandchildren were painful," she said. "It was excruciating to me." But it was not only the thought of losing her loved ones that pained her: "I was now forced to mourn the loss of my body," she said. "I was forced to lose control of who I was as I had always known myself."

Coping at Home

[John] said, "Don't worry, I won't die—
I'll take care of the kids."
He nearly died this year of cancer,
but I believe him.
We used to be married.
Now he enters my room in the dark
to speak from his heart,
or sit up and watch
'till I fall asleep.*

---

* These lines, as well as the lines at the beginning of subsequent sections, are from poems Paula Ferrari wrote on the Palliative Care Unit.

As she found it harder to walk, Paula moved out of her large home into a small one-bedroom flat in a working-class Italian neighborhood in the west end of the city. The flat was on the ground floor, so she wouldn't have to manage stairs. It was also immediately adjacent to the small, traditional Catholic church, Our Lady of Mercy, where she had sometimes attended Mass. In some ways, she told me, this move continued the spiritual journey she had made the year before, though the life of the neighborhood in which she now lived was very different from the solitude of the Italian mountains and the monastery.

Paula found a comforting innocence in the day-to-day life of the neighborhood. The community was not large, stretching about six blocks to a highway. From her window, she could see children playing hockey on the streets and women sweeping their front steps or scrubbing the driveway. On a windy day, she saw rows of men's shirts, socks, and underwear strung on clothes lines between the houses. There were a few stores, and a local bakery which sold large, flat, fresh-baked loaves by the hour, as well as large, ornate, multitiered wedding cakes. In the daytime, the stores were frequented by black-shawled, elderly women. At night, they became a quick stop for men to buy cigarettes on the way to the pool hall. Most of these men were craftsmen, skilled laborers, or factory workers. Tomatoes and sunflowers filled the tiny front yards in the late summer months. For a few dollars, some of the men rented small allotment gardens from the city that were close to the railroad tracks or at the edge of the neighborhood and produced plentiful crops of fruit and vegetables.

Paula's daughter Rita recalled that the apartment had wall-to-wall books, almost up to the ceiling, and her mother had read all of them. She could read in German, Greek, Latin, and Italian. Sometimes she'd have three or four books going at once.

Paula Ferrari had lived alone for many years before her illness, and although she loved people and parties, she was happy being alone. Rita said she thought her mother was quite content with her reading and her cat. But as it became increasingly difficult for her to walk, it was becoming impossible for her to manage alone. One of the children stopped by each day to visit and see if they could help—perhaps cook a meal or offer their mother an arm for a walk outside. However, these visits were becoming insufficient, and, after a family meeting, John decided that the best thing to do would be for him to move into the flat and help with Paula's care on a full-time basis.

The move did not seem unnatural to John, even though they were divorced. The couple had kept up a close friendship, and, in some ways, he still loved his former wife. From John's perspective, the only thing they had ever quarreled about was money. The marital breakup had not been bitter, though the couple had pursued different paths. John had met a new woman friend, and Paula had thrust herself into her work on religious philosophy. When John learned about Paula's illness, he thought it best to end his new relationship to devote his time to Paula.

For a while, things went well. John did as much as he could: cooking, laundry, driving Paula to appointments, generally trying to help with whatever she needed. But just a few months after he had moved into Paula's flat, John began to feel ill himself. When he consulted his doctor, he learned he had malignant lymphoma. "It was hard on everybody," he recalled to me. "Our kids then had to take care of the two of us."

Caring for their mother became a major commitment for the four children. They took daily shifts, so that Paula wouldn't be left alone. Franco recalled,

> It was a full-time job, though I'll never regret it. For the longest time I had wanted to travel, but while she was sick, I never felt comfortable leaving the city for more than two weeks. I felt like, what if something happens? Or, I'm throwing the workload onto my brother and sisters. Because it was a shared workload between us four. So there was that sense of responsibility, and also the sense now that this was precious time with my mother and I shouldn't be taking off, seeing the world or whatever. So all of our plans were put on hold.

"Hey, I'm Sick, Too, You Know!"

Some months following Dr. O'Leary's initial diagnosis, Paula's muscles were rapidly deteriorating. She had increased spasticity of her elbows and knees, and there was a marked change in her overall muscle ability. She could no longer walk without the aid of a cane or without holding someone's arm. Rita, Rosa, Greg, and Franco were coming daily to share the tasks of Paula's daily toilet care and shopping.

Meanwhile, John's condition stabilized. While in the hospital, he had undergone extensive chemotherapy and was now in remission from his cancer. He felt a bit neglected, even slightly resentful. With all the attention focused on Paula, he felt he had been forced to carry the burden of his own illness alone. He loved his family, but he wanted to say, "Hey, I'm sick, too, you know!"

John tried to understand that his children were already heavily involved in Paula's care. It was not easy to get outside nursing help. They could get up to 35 hours of home help in a week, but this wasn't enough for a person who needed care 24 hours a day, seven days a week. Somebody needed to put Paula to bed, take her to the bathroom, and help her with every part of daily life. Her children took turns helping her every night, but they felt a lot of stress, and it came out. John recalled,

> The kids would get angry with each other. They just were at their wits' end, you know, because they could come over, there was a schedule, but occasionally someone would mess up. It didn't often happen, but there was stress. You had to be there that night or at a certain time, and that was it.

"Well, This Is the Last Step"

The children were finding it increasingly difficult to cope with the daily physical demands. Sometimes when agency nurses called in sick, by the time a replacement arrived at the house, Mrs. Ferrari had lain in bed until 1:00 in the afternoon. Occasionally, Rita or her siblings would call their mother's house and get no answer. When they arrived, they would find her in bed, with soiled bedding that had to be changed. They worried about having to leave their mother's door unlocked so people could come in to help her. "So it was a constant worry," Rita explained to me, "and I think it was also a big burden, especially when my sister became pregnant, and we were only three, and there was a third night that we had to sleep over and then the next day you get up and go to work. [So we agreed she had to go to palliative care] and it was sad because it was like, well, this is the last step."

Paula could also see how quickly her disease had progressed and how difficult it was for everyone to manage at home. She saw that everyone was tired. She knew it was time, and she was ready to go to be cared for at the Palliative Care Unit (PCU). She knew that her disease would progress and that it would not be long before she would completely lose the use of the muscles in her limbs. She would lose the use of muscles in her hands and fingers, and eventually she wouldn't be able to breathe on her own.

Paula thought at the time that she didn't have long to live, perhaps a few months.

She thought about death and what it was going to be like to be dying. But these were peaceful thoughts, for she felt an enormous love for God, and felt a security—anticipation almost—and joy in herself that everything would be well. She told a friend, "As we lose control over our lives, we gain the ability to learn a unique lesson of life and perhaps to become closer to God."

Some months before, Mrs. Ferrari had written to Dr. O'Leary, making it clear that she did not want to be tube fed or be kept alive artificially on a respirator. It was not that she wanted to shorten her life—quite the contrary. Dying was "the ultimate experience." It had "something to teach," she said later. But she wanted to be nursed and cared for in as natural a way as could be done. She knew of the care at the PCU, and, from her own hospice work caring for men who were dying from AIDS-related complications, she knew what the philosophy of palliative care entailed. She was not afraid.

In many ways. Mrs. Ferrari remarked to me, this final path on which she was forced to embark had the possibility of becoming "a deep and beautiful time." "Dying had a necessary place," she said. There was something to be celebrated in not succumbing to "the practical," as she put it—in other words, to the desire for medical aid in dying (MAID). Franco later recalled that his mother "really couldn't understand people who asked for their life to be ended before it was time."

Settling into the Routine

> Pink sky and two small lavender clouds.
> A buttermilk wash floods my window.
> Blue sky and green leaves transfigured by light.
> Six o'clock: the nurses turn me over.
> Adriana empties the trash, Ivo vacuums the hall.
> The kitchen courier delivers her menus.

Four days later, Paula Ferrari was admitted to the PCU, under the care of Dr. Sylvie Dupuis. She arrived in a beautiful colored skirt with a purple top. Margaret, an experienced palliative care nurse who was assigned to her primary care, recalled that Mrs. Ferrari "looked like she had done her best to be happy when she came." In Dr. O'Leary's letter of referral, he noted, "The patient communicates by guttural sounds and by pointing at an alphabet board with a mouth pointer." Dr. O'Leary also stated that he was uncertain how long his patient could be expected to live. He reported: "Her respiratory reserves are minimal, and she is choking intermittently, which indicates there is a risk of aspiration pneumonia."

Rita took the week off work because she wanted to help her mother get comfortable and settled. Rita was worried that the nurses wouldn't understand her mother because it was so hard for her to talk. She spent every day working with her mother's palliative care nurse to help her learn her mother's routine. Margaret wondered to herself whether this was such a good idea. "She relies on her daughter so much," Margaret commented to me. "She loves her so much, it could be difficult for everyone after Rita leaves."

Indeed, there were differences of viewpoint and method as to how to proceed with certain nursing procedures. Because Rita and her family had been the main caretakers for their mother, they knew her routines as well as all the unspoken, daily idiosyncrasies that her care involved. For example, Rita had specific ideas on how one person alone could lift Paula back and forth from her bed to the chair. Her own training as a gymnast had oriented her to certain ways of lifting. As the week passed, however, Paula's weakening muscles made it very difficult and dangerous for anyone to lift her alone. The nurses, who had many people to lift and needed to protect their backs, preferred to work in teams, or even to use a mechanical lift, all of which appeared to Rita as intrusive and embarrassing for her mother.

Paula was also very clear on how she wanted to be given care. Though she wanted to accept the new ward routines, and people tried, everyone had a different way of approaching her physical care. She knew what she wanted, and there were many little things she could have said to help the nurses understand her needs. But she could not speak clearly enough to make herself understood. As Margaret later recalled,

She often would break out into uncontrollable crying or laughing, which is part of the disease, but it would be out of her frustration at trying to show us how to put her hands in a certain place; how to move her in bed; how to put her glasses back up on her nose; when just these little things take so long to explain, and she couldn't explain.

The Room

A pot of Basil on the windowsill
hides the white chimney,
the suggestion of Ligurian hills
masks the odour of ashes.
The weather is torrid—
if I fail to pay attention
my basil will wilt, wither, and dry.

I first met Mrs. Ferrari in her room on the PCU. She was sitting in a wheel-chair. Attached to her head was an apparatus that held a pointer, which she used with either an alphabet board or a computer to communicate. When she looked up at me, she raised her eyebrows, then smiled and made gut-tural sounds, her way of extending a warm greeting. She had chin-length, slightly graying, dark hair. Although I couldn't be sure how tall she was, I had the impression that she was not tall and perhaps even a little stocky in build. I thought she looked much younger than her 57 years. Using the pointer, she tapped out a message to me on the computer, slowly, almost painfully, it seemed to me. The computer generated a voice. It was hard to know how her real voice sounded, but her welcome was clear: "I am happy to see you," she said. "Thank you."

Paula's room told me much of what I have since learned about her. It was not a large room and was somewhat dark. Though it didn't have much of a view, it was decorated with things from home, all the things which, Paula said, "bring me joy and memories of all the happy things in my life." Her room became a warm and peaceful haven for caregivers and visitors alike. Even if staff were off duty, it was not unusual for them to drop in and sit for a while. Over and over again, Paula's caregivers' stories described a sense of peace and love that seemed to emanate from that room.

"Her room is warm and peaceful," Margaret said. "You feel you want to stay in there even when the unit is really busy. It's like when you're in there, sometimes you even forget you're working."

This was easy for me to understand. The room was colorful—bright flowers of red and yellow, depending on the season; large green hanging plants; a small herb garden growing on the windowsill. There were paintings of the ocean and woodland scenes, and photographs of Rita, Rosa, Greg, and Franco. A large painting hanging high on the wall, on the right-hand side of the bed, displayed forests, with a pathway between the trees. Mrs. Ferrari said, "I want to walk on the road where I can see. The road in the picture leads to the ocean. When I think of the ocean, I think of smells and seaweed." Sometime later, Rosa told me that Rita had painted the picture while on a special art scholarship in the Philippines. There were also items from times long past: photographs of Paula with her mother and father, old greeting cards with a message of love or encouragement. Old poetry manuscripts lay on a chair or bureau, as well as poems that she was writing now with the aid of the computer and the typing stick.

Relationships and Routines

Someone offers me lunch—
I say, "First the neck brace off."
I try to spell it with a chart and a straw between my teeth,
but he mistakes "collar off" for "colour of"
and offers me a spoonful of orange.
It is a very little problem compared with others'.
They've offered to double my "Prozac."

The demands of Paula's care were becoming greater and greater. Four months after her admission, Margaret's nursing record reported

Patient needs total care, needs feeding at all meals; oral hygiene needed, drools and has dysphagia [difficulty in swallowing]. Patient presents a risk of aspiration when eating.

The record included other complications of the disease: Paula had become constipated and uncomfortable; she had problems choking when given both fluids and solid foods; and skin rashes were appearing all over her body. At times Paula had trouble sleeping at night; it was sometimes 2:00 A.M. before the night nurse found her asleep, even though she was taking sedatives. Sylvie Dupuis prescribed scopolamine, a medication that helps to dry out mouth secretions and that can reduce the risk of aspiration, and docusate to reduce the constipation. She also prescribed chloral hydrate, a mild sedative that helped Paula sleep.

Sylvie's record indicated increasing flaccidity of Paula's limbs. Now at least two nurses were needed to help lift her onto the commode beside her bed or into her wheelchair. Rita visited most evenings and Greg, Franco, and Rosa came two or three times a week. They also tried to help lift their mother. Everyone tried to use Rita's technique of pivoting her onto the commode. It could be difficult, because sometimes her head and neck would be in danger of dropping forward if she wasn't positioned carefully. She was fitted with a large, wide, gauze-covered foam collar to give her neck a little support. But it was uncomfortable and itchy.

After she had been bathed and dressed and given her usual morning care, Paula liked to sit in her wheelchair facing the door to the hallway. Here she would write her thoughts with her straw and alphabet board. She was thrilled when she got a computer that recorded the typed message through an electronic voice system. Sometimes she wrote short letters to friends or family, but when she had the energy, she spent much of her time composing poetry—about her day-to-day life, small moments of her hospital routine, memories.

She loved to watch people and would delight in a small happening on the unit, seeing the color of a volunteer's blouse or the way the sun would light the colors in a nurse's hair. Although she enjoyed the many visitors who came to see her every day, there were times when she would have liked more solitude. The nurses put a sign on her door that read, "Meditating. Please do not disturb." But it was still very difficult for Paula to protect her privacy. People felt they needed to go in and check on her, and always left the door slightly ajar.

Paula needed to be fed every mouthful of food, which had to be soft in texture and cut up into tiny bits. This required care and delicacy, because her choking spasms appeared without warning. The daily record showed that she was choking more despite medication to try to prevent the spasms. It usually happened after meals, which meant that there was an increasing risk of aspiration pneumonia.

These were emotion-filled, difficult days. Paula had become used to talking by guttural sounds and by expressive facial movements such as raising her eyebrows, closing and opening her eyes, frowning, or smiling. When she couldn't say what she needed, she would become distraught, crying and screaming, and then even more distraught because she could not wipe away her own tears. Sometimes, when I went in to sit with her, she would look sad and forlorn. I had read that ALS sometimes results in pseudobulbar tearfulness, but I couldn't always be sure what she was thinking. Dr. O'Leary had reported that she had had similar symptoms at home and was receiving fluoxetine, which helped to stabilize her emotional state.

The volunteer, Jean, first met Paula one evening during suppertime when she was going around the unit to see if anyone needed help with their meal.

She noticed that Paula could not feed herself, so she began to feed her the soup that was waiting on the tray. It was not so easy. Jean described the scene to me.

I was feeding her her soup. She began to pause and looked up at me as though she didn't want the soup. So I stopped feeding it to her. But then she cried out and motioned that, oh yes, she wanted the soup. I saw she was trying to say something else. Then she screamed. Dr. Legare came by at that moment and showed me how to talk to her through the straw and the alphabet board. She pointed to the number 11, and I realized she had been waiting to listen to a special musical concert on the TV on channel 11. Things were fine after that, and she smiled, but I realized what it was like not to be able to communicate. It upset me, and I was kind of drained, exhausted. It was an emotional strain because I wanted so much to help.

And then she tried to spell out two words for me. Again, I couldn't make the two words out. But I just pretended I understood and went on and smiled. But she's nobody's fool and she saw I didn't understand. So I made her spell it out again. So she spelled it and it said, "Thank you." And I was so touched that it was so important to her to say thank you to people who take care of her. I just left at that point and I started crying. It touched me to that point. Later I went back into the room and gave her a big hug. John, her former husband, was there, and he just squeezed my wrist. I've been very attached to her since that point.

Passing Time

Hilvette feeds me.
She was up last night
celebrating Christmas.
Hilvette says every month has a colour.
The colour of July is brown. Like her.

Despite the frustrations, Paula Ferrari settled into a daily routine that Rosa later said she had loved because "it kept meaning and friendships in her life." She would go to Mass in the hospital chapel after getting her care in the mornings, take a nap, and then look forward most days for people to come to visit. There were so many: friends from her neighborhood, or from the small Italian church where she had attended Mass, and from the many charity organizations she belonged to as well as her family. Paula could scarcely talk, but many who came into contact with her, either through an act of caregiving or friendship, felt changed in some way by their encounter with her.

In various ways, she befriended the housekeeping staff, volunteers, nurses, and doctors. Whether it was the person who changed her water pitcher, the volunteer who brought in library books, or the TV repairman, people seemed to know her in some special way. She shared her knowledge of poetry writing and became a teacher to one physician who wrote poetry. One of the volunteers said she had taught him the joy of listening to Bach. She seemed to nurture friendships, old and new, with an energy that far surpassed her doctors' assessment of her medical condition. One of the physicians she had befriended said

> I feel a deep, personal bond and extreme closeness to her. On the one hand, I think she is the closest person to me. I constantly learn from her about myself and my work. And I never feel I am doing the giving. It is as though she is always the one who gives to me. The more I came to know her, it seemed as though she had a most extraordinary gift of looking right into your soul.

Rick, another volunteer, said

> It's hard to put into words. It goes beyond words, because the relationship is not spoken words. She communicates mostly with her eyes and just certain expressions. But there is obviously a tremendous trust that has developed, a real comfort on her part with me. What has developed is that I'm able to get into her head, to finish her sentences. So I try and save her the energy of finishing her sentences. And I have [come] to know how loving, compassionate, and spiritual she is.

Dr. Dupuis noted that in Mrs. Ferrari's case "her medical problems are of secondary importance to her. The first level of importance is really her life—what is going on in her life." Sylvie hadn't experienced this before in a patient with this disease. Most people with ALS had such distressing symptoms that it was all that they could think about. But for Paula Ferrari, it seemed more important to express herself in terms of her own spiritual life.

Mrs. Ferrari did not consider herself religious in a formal sense. Once when I asked about the picture of Jesus that hung at the foot of her hospital bed, she explained that the picture was a "crib picture of the post-resurrection appearances of Jesus." "I painted it," she added. "I painted it in egg tempera. It was fun and I love the theology of it." As if to answer my unasked question, she said, "I do not agree with all of what the church teaches, but I want to be part of its rituals."

Rita, Greg, Franco, Rosa, and John visited the unit regularly. Rita seemed now especially close to her mother and would go every evening to help her write poetry. The poems that Paula wrote now were about love for her children, her life when she was well, memories intermingled with sadness and joy. A particular joy during this period was the birth of her first grandchild. Yet she was worried about Rosa and was sad that she could not be with her for the birth of her child. Her physical problems were less painful to her than this feeling of exclusion.

Looking Forward

The first time we met,
your round dark eyes stared
unable to comprehend what I was.
It was mutual.
I fastened upon the craftsmanship of your parts—
the dimple in your elbow,
the transparency of your skin,
and your eyes—entirely iris!
One day you focused,
you smiled, you spoke
serious sounds, happy and sad.
Every day I see you,
you are newer than the day before.

As the time approached for Rosa's baby to be born, Mrs. Ferrari became more excited. There were periods when she would stare off through the window, worrying whether Rosa and the baby would be healthy and strong. When Rita called and said Rosa was in labor, Mrs. Ferrari spent more and more time in prayer and meditation. She couldn't sleep. Margaret commented that it was as if she were vicariously going through the labor herself.

When the baby was born, Paula said, "We think of life, and of the things we know, and the birth of a child is the greatest thing we know as a miracle."

Rosa named her baby girl Jenny. She asked Rita and John if there was some way that her mother could visit her on the maternity ward and see her new granddaughter. Dr. Dupuis thought it would be a wonderful experience and the arrangements were made. Paula told Jean, "This is a happy day."

Seen through Margaret's eyes, however, it was not the simple visit of a grandmother to see her first grandchild. Paula was not in the role of a grandmother, but more like that of a child herself. As Margaret recalled,

> I came on evening shift and the patient was screaming, crying, and unable to wipe her nose or her drooling mouth. Her husband and son Greg were trying to pull on her heavy coat but were unable to bend her arm. She was using a straw to point to each letter on her alphabet board, but she constantly dropped the straw in frustration. She wanted her shoes, her glasses, the poinsettia on the table, the beads from the drawer, and the bunny rabbit in her gift bag. Her son Greg tried to put the beads on for his mother, but she cried more. "They're for Rosa!" I was literally seeing her fall apart. Greg said, "Come on, Mom, you're supposed to be happy. The baby is born."

Small Kindnesses

> Her gentle hands wash me,
> her fragrant creams soothe my skin.
> His friendly eyes hold me,
> his sentences bind my wounds.

The family worried that Paula's increasing dependency would mean that she would be treated more and more like a child. Sometimes people who didn't know her "talk in a babying way," Rita said. "My mother understands and accepts that everyone means well," she continued, but she wished that those people would remember that her mother was sharp and alert even if she couldn't talk or do anything for herself. Margaret agreed. The palliative care team had talked about this issue in their patient meetings. She said, "I think we all realize that we sometimes have a tendency to baby people when they are physically helpless."

When caregivers spoke of their own feelings of helplessness and inadequacy, it was usually when they couldn't instantly meet a simple request.

Often it was a question of incorrectly perceiving Mrs. Ferrari's request for a pillow to be shifted slightly or to move her hand an inch or two to make it more comfortable. Paula knew they were trying, but these moments were still very hard, and the baby talk (almost unconsciously adopted by the staff at times) would make a hard situation feel even worse.

There were also very rewarding moments. Paula loved the feel of a warm washcloth on her face, her morning sponge bath, and the smell of the creams that the nurses massaged into her flaccid skin. She would laugh and smile when Margaret combed her hair in the mornings. Once Rita cut her hair and restyled it. When she showed her mother her new haircut in her mirror, Paula chuckled, "If it's okay with you, it's okay with me." Rosa made regular visits to her mother's bedside with Jenny. These were happy times. Paula now had no muscle control, and she could not hold Jenny in her arms. Rosa would position the pillow around her so that she could cradle Jenny and feel the baby's body and skin against hers. Sometimes Rosa would hold Jenny's face close to her grandmother's face. Mrs. Ferrari would laugh with loud guttural sounds. One day Rosa said, crying, "She had so much love to give, it's beautiful to watch them together. But I feel sad inside. I know my mother would make a wonderful grandmother." Mrs. Ferrari said of Jenny, "She is marvelous. I can't believe it. I need to pinch myself."

Some other changes were taking place in the family. Rita was considering leaving Montreal to be with her husband, who had recently been transferred to Atlanta. Rita didn't want to leave. Though Paula had already lived a year after coming to the unit, and no one knew how much longer she would live, her condition was weakening day by day. Paula insisted that Rita go to Atlanta. It was important to be with her husband, she said to her. Greg, Franco, Rosa, and John would all be here to help with her care. So Rita left, resolving to come back for a week each month to help with her mother's care.

The Last Days

> I've been wasting my dying
> on frivolous things . . .
> I would suffer for others
> if I suffered at all . . .
> But I'm loved and I know it.
> Can I offer God this happiness?

Christine, the music therapist, knew Mrs. Ferrari well. In the beginning, when Mrs. Ferrari was first admitted and could speak a little, she was up in the palliative care lounge more where there was a grand piano and volunteer musicians gave afternoon concerts. She had even composed a piece of music with her head pointer. When Paula could no longer go to the lounge, Christine would bring one of the volunteer musicians into her room, and they would wheel in a smaller piano. But now Mrs. Ferrari was seriously congested with pneumonia and Christine saw that she was dying. Christine hugged her, wanting to say goodbye. She told me,

> We had a cry and she asked to hear a Beethoven string quartet. The next day I went in and I said, "do you want to hear Beethoven again?" She said yes, and I said, "is it okay if I sit here and listen with you?" And she had some tears, and I would dab them. That was our connection.

"Someone like that, one compares to one's own life," Christine continued. "You come to work, and you are maybe annoyed with children and then you meet with this example of incredible grace in the face of incredible limitations. It was a great learning experience." Christine said that Mrs. Ferrari had somehow connected to what nourished her. "She had humor and faith and she seemed to be living her dying with much more grace and integrity. I am in awe of her."

Over the weekend, Mrs. Ferrari became short of breath, frightened. Sylvie increased her midazolam a little, to allow her a more peaceful sleep. She also increased the scopolamine dosage to try and alleviate the secretions that were welling up in her mouth and throat. When Margaret came back on duty on Monday, she checked the patient list to see if Mrs. Ferrari was there. She was still there.

Caregivers, friends, and family now began to pass by to say goodbye. Some of the staff had gotten to know Mrs. Ferrari very well over the past year, but the family had begun their vigil at the bedside—Mrs. Ferrari had sent for Rita the day before—and the staff didn't want to intrude on these last hours of family time. It appeared that this was going to be a very personal loss for so many—caregivers, friends, and family alike. Rick, the volunteer, wondered if there would be a chance during these hours to have "just one more connection with her before she passed on." He wasn't sure what he would say. "I could always tell her that I care deeply for her and she means a lot to me," he told me. But he didn't think there would be an opportunity to do that, and there was not. Mrs. Ferrari died a few hours later.

Margaret went into the room to comfort Rita, who had been at the bedside at the moment of death. They hugged and talked with each other, and Rita helped Margaret prepare the body. Rita made her phone calls to Franco, Greg, Rosa, and her father, and to the funeral home. Then she started packing up the room. "There must have been at least 25 bags," Margaret said. She wondered to herself whether Rita should wait for her brothers and sister "just so the room looked natural." Rita did wait, though she felt restless and wanted to go.

When John arrived, the head nurse gently suggested that everyone go into Mrs. Ferrari's room for a prayer, the Universal Prayer that the palliative care staff say together when a patient dies. I was there along with volunteers, primary nurses, nurses from the unit who hadn't directly cared for Mrs. Ferrari, and the physicians. Everyone held hands. John stood at the foot of the bed, crying gently. Rita put her hand inside her mother's hand. The pastoral care worker recited the prayer, ending with the words, "Our love goes with her as we now in silence commend her to Your care." After the prayer, everyone made their way out of the room. The staff went back to the routines of the unit and to caring for the other patients. There was a mood of sadness, a great sense of loss. Some of the nurses were putting their arms around one another. Others squeezed hands or said a word of comfort.

As everyone filed out, John said, "I really want to thank you on behalf of my family, for all you have done for Paula. We will never forget you." Somebody else (I am not sure who) said quietly, "Ah, but we will never forget her."

Authors' Comments

In 2000, it was unusual for patients with a non-cancer illness to be admitted to a PCU or be eligible for palliative care. That is not the case at present. A number of life-limiting illnesses are now considered eligible for palliative care, including, for example, cardiovascular illnesses, chronic respiratory diseases, diabetes, end-stage renal disease, dementia, and a range of neurological diseases. Health services researchers are now beginning systematic study of the application and benefits of palliative care in non-cancer illnesses.[1] Gian Domenico Borasio, a professor in the Interdisciplinary Center for

Palliative Medicine and head of the motor neuron disease research group at the Department of Neurology, University of Munich, Germany, pioneered the notion of neuropalliative care precisely because those patients suffering from diseases such as ALS need specific care as their disease advances.[2,3]

There is still no cure for ALS (also known as Lou Gehrig's disease). However, in the past 25 years, the drug Rituzole has been shown to extend life by a few months.[4] Recent clinical trials have shown that sodium phenylbutyrate taurursodiol (PB-TURSO) lessens the decline in function by several months if initiated early.[5]

Paula Ferrari lived for a year on the PCU. It is unlikely under present policies of admission that any patient would have been able to stay on a PCU for this length of time. Some form of institutional care would still have been required, however, once Paula's care requirements increased and exceeded the stamina and resources of her family. Eventually it became a huge commitment for her four children. John, Paula's former husband, agreed to assume the role of major caregiver, but he himself became ill with a life-threatening illness. While caregiver fatigue has been addressed in the palliative care literature, there is a paucity of attention to circumstances whereby the caregiver also becomes seriously ill. As we noted in the Authors' Comments for the Sadie Fineman narrative, caregiver support in Canada is now covered by the Compassionate Care Benefits Program, which offers financial support for up to 26 weeks for the care of a family member at end of life. This form of financial assistance was not available at the time of Paula's illness, but, had it been, it might have allowed for extra help in order to alleviate some of the stress on John. Recent research on family caregivers indicates a greater need for formal recognition of the determinants of poor health and other negative consequences of their performance of this role.[6]

Paula Ferrari really couldn't understand people who wanted to end their lives before their time. She felt that her experience of dying represented "a deep and beautiful time." The narrative exemplifies the need for emphasis on the spiritual and existential domains of patient care. There are cases, such as this one, where people seem to grow spiritually through a life-limiting illness.[7] Without exception, Paula's caregivers perceived her as someone who gave to them. She provided spiritual comfort for many of her helpers, and some sought solace in her mere presence.

At the same time, we wonder: Was Paula Ferrari altogether without spiritual pain? Often, she would cry out in anguish or sheer frustration at not being able to use her typewriter to chat with people, as she loved to do.

The numerous times she found it hard to tell others what she needed often resulted in long periods of crying and sadness. What of her own anguish in these dark periods of helplessness and frustration? Did the comfort and solace Mrs. Ferrari so frequently bestowed on others in fact obscure the need for her caregivers to attend to her spiritual nourishment?

References

1. Quinn KL, Shurrab M, Gitau K, Kavalieratos D, Isenberg SR, Stall NM, Stukel, TA, Goldman R, Horn D, Cram P, Detsky A, Bell CM. Association of receipt of palliative care interventions with health care use, quality of life, and symptom burden among adults with chronic noncancer illness: A systematic review and meta-analysis. JAMA. 2020;324(14):1439–1450.
2. Creutzfeldt CJ, Kluger B, Kelly AG, Lemmon M, Hwang DY, Galifianakis NB, Carver A, Katz M, Curtis JR, Holloway RG. Neuropalliative care: Priorities to move the field forward. Neurology. 2018;91(5):217–226.
3. Brizzi K, Creutzfeldt GT. Neuropalliative care: A practical guide for the neurologist. Seminar Neurol. 2018;38(5):569–575.
4. Andrews JA, Jackson CE, Heiman- Patterson TD, Bettica P, Pioro EP. Real world evidence of rituzole effectiveness in treating amyotrophic lateral sclerosis. Amytroph Lateral Scl Frontotemporal Degener. 2020;21(7–8):509–518.
5. Paganoni S, Hendrix S, Dickson SP, Newman K, et al. Long-term survival of participants in the Centaur trial of sodium phenylbutyrate-taurursodiol in amyotrophic lateral lerosis. Muscle Nerve 2021;63(1):31–39.
6. Ormel I, Law S, Abbott C, Yaffe M, Saint-Cyr M, Kuluski K, Josephson D, Macaulay AC. "When one is sick and two need help": Caregivers' perspectives on the negative consequences of caring. Patient Exp J. 2017;4(1):66–78.
7. Mount B, Kearney M. Healing and palliative care: Charting our way forward. Palliat Med. 2003;17:657–658.

23

Research Methods

The aims of this final chapter of the book are to outline the premises of qualitative research, show the relevance of qualitative methods to palliative care, and explain the specific methods of qualitative research underlying this book. The discussion aims to provide an understanding of ethnographic, narrative inquiry, which was our approach to the experiences of patients, families, and caregivers in palliative care. We outline our rationale for a case narrative study, the ethnographic methods and techniques used to gather and analyze data, the role of the participant-observer, and the ethical issues related to qualitative research in palliative care.

Qualitative Methodology: An Approach to Social Research

Traditionally, research in medicine and the health sciences has been strongly influenced by the biomedical model and research based on the model of the physical sciences, characterized by the manipulation of variables, experimentation, measurement, and deduction.[1-3] Moreover, systematic reviews of evidenced-based medical research have tended to focus on quantitative research rather than on qualitative evidence.[2,4,5] Health practitioners trained in the medical sciences have been exposed primarily to quantitative, experimental methods designed to test hypotheses and seek out universal laws.

In contrast to quantitative research, qualitative methods seek to explore particular settings and experiences and rest on induction and holistic inquiry. Qualitative research can explore in depth various dimensions of the social world, including behaviors and attitudes, values, opinions, knowledge, and experiences. Both qualitative and quantitative methods have much to offer. Whether to choose either method or both in a mixed-methods study depends on the particular research question or issue, the kinds of knowledge that need to be generated, and how the findings are going to be used.[6,7]

Quantitative experimental methods make it possible to measure the responses of large numbers of people within a limited standardized framework and thereby facilitate generalizable, statistical aggregations of data.[1,5,6,8] In contrast, qualitative methods explore questions of meaning and the complexities of human experience.[9] The decision on which approach to employ depends on one's research question and clinical context, as Miller and Crabtree write:

> If the question about one's body, one's life, or power concerns "how many," "how much," "how often," "what size," or numerically measurable associations among phenomena, then a survey research style using the decisions and methods of observational epidemiology is appropriate. If the question asks "if . . . then" or "is . . . more effective than . . ." then an experimental style is reasonable.[1, p. 343]

The aim of research, however, is not always to predict relations or test hypotheses. Questions relating to life experience within a dynamic and changing environment, which are usually concerned with multiple meanings, patterns, and complex human relationships, call for a different form of inquiry. Qualitative methods allow us to explore the social world with the assumption that day-to-day realities are both variable and complex. They enable us to understand everyday experience and how people organize and interpret various aspects of their lives. In qualitative approaches, people in their natural settings are the primary source of data. Qualitative researchers focus on what can be explored and described through questions such as "I would like to understand more about . . ." or "I would like to know more about . . ." or "How does it work that way?"[10, p. 53] They pursue questions of subjective meaning, understanding, and interpretation. Moreover, rather than being separate from the study, qualitative researchers have direct contact with participants. The *researchers* are the instrument of study, and their experiences and insights are central to understanding the phenomena under investigation.[6,8]

As M. Q. Patton points out, "the advantages of qualitative portrayals of holistic settings are that greater attention can be given to nuance, setting, interdependencies, complexities, idiosyncrasies, and context."[8, p. 5] To know how caregiving works in the everyday world of palliative care, for example, we need to know first-hand what actually happens in the daily lives of patients, families, and caregivers—to bear witness to their experience. When we ask how we can enhance the quality of palliative care, we first need to know how caregiving works in the present, what caregivers expect to accomplish through their work, and what their institutions and patients expect from them. Our conviction is that these questions are best explored by delving into the depths of subjective experience. In our efforts to do that, we decided to be with patients, their families, and their caregivers through a very trying period in human life. Being with the people one wants to learn something about is the essence of the qualitative, ethnographic approach.

Qualitative Research and Whole-Person Palliative Care

While the biomedical model of care has provided the means for measuring the patient's biological status, it has done little to foster whole-person palliative care, which emphasizes the intricate and clinically important interactions between body, mind, and spirit. Recognizing that each person is unique and operates within a holistic social and cultural context, the philosophy of palliative care assumes a stance of multiple realities. It acknowledges and values not only the caregiver's assessment of the patient but also the patient's and the family's experiences of illness and care. This stance allows the caregivers' understanding of patients, families, and themselves to change and deepen as situations change.[11-14]

Within this understanding of whole-person care, a focus on personal meaning and on intersubjective knowledge generated through experience are of primary importance for giving good palliative care. There is a strong emphasis on process as well as on clinical outcomes. Care plans are not only based on established scientific models but are also derived from interaction and discussion with the patient and family. Thus, in both qualitative research and palliative care, the crucial focus is on the perspectives and experiences of individuals, which may not always resonate with conventional medical knowledge. Personal experience is valued as a means of understanding what is important or relevant to patients, either in providing care or conducting research. Stories are given primacy because it is the patient's or family's story that supplies the necessary context for clinical interventions. The first task for both caregivers and researchers is to create an atmosphere of trust and mutual respect, suspend predetermined beliefs, and embrace the possibility of conflicting versions of reality.

Qualitative Methods

Participant-Observation

In our fieldwork, we drew extensively on participant-observation. As participant-observers, we conducted our research by entering into the day-to-day lives of the people with whom we worked. This allowed us to observe each patient's physical condition over time, his or her social interactions with family members and caregivers, and the physical settings in which those interactions occurred. We were allowed to witness both formal and informal moments of illness experiences.

The three of us who carried out this fieldwork directly were Patricia Boston and Anna Towers in Montreal, and Yanna Lambrinidou in Lancaster County. During the years 1995–1998, when the research was conducted, Patricia Boston practiced as a nurse-educator and family therapist affiliated with the Department of Psychiatry and the Department of Oncology in the Faculty of Medicine at McGill. Anna Towers initially trained in family medicine and family therapy and was a palliative medicine physician on the palliative care unit at the Royal Victoria Hospital and affiliated with the Department of Family Medicine in the Faculty of Medicine at McGill. Although Anna Towers was a day-to-day participant in the work of the Palliative Care Service, she did not function as the researcher in cases in which she had clinical responsibilities. In those cases where she did have a direct clinical role, Patricia Boston was the observer, interviewer, and narrator of the case. At the time, Yanna Lambrinidou was a doctoral candidate in the Department of Folklore and Folklife at the University of Pennsylvania, where she specialized in ethnographic research methods and cross-cultural studies of healthcare.

As participant-observers we asked questions such as, "How are you doing today?" "What is happening right now?" "What is important to you at this time?" "How would you describe your life?" Our involvement in the lives of dying patients taught us that the experience of dying was only one part of their life experience. Their identities extended far beyond being a patient. They were working people concerned with their jobs or about being unemployed; parents concerned about their children; and citizens engaged in the issues of their communities.

As we participated in patient and family meetings, treatment encounters, and case discussions in patients' homes, in the hospital, and in the inpatient unit of Hospice of Lancaster County, we became part of the social world we were studying, both emotionally and physically. We cried, laughed, helped make beds, and carried groceries. We recorded all these events in detailed field notes. To the best of our abilities, we were able to gain first-hand experience of nuances of communication, nonverbal expressions, and routine caregiving practices. There is no doubt that our perceptions were shaped by our own selective memories and personal interests. Although we could not eliminate the biases of our own standpoint, consistency and repetition of issues and ideas over time within the cases mitigated this effect to some extent.

We must emphasize, however, that we do not consider the narratives in this book to represent either the record of our own subjective states of being during the course of our research or an "objective" depiction of the lives and experiences of the people about whom we wrote. They are, rather, co-constructed versions of the events that took place. To remind the reader of our own part in this construction, we have tried to indicate our involvement in the narratives themselves.

Interviews

Our interviews with patients, families, and caregivers consisted of open-ended, informal, and spontaneous conversations, guided only indirectly by an interview guide that we created at the start of the project. We used this guide as a general and basic checklist of the topic areas we wanted to explore. These areas included the following topics.

For Patients and Families
- The impact of the patient's illness on the patient's (or family member's) daily life and on the patient's and family's overall quality of life
- The quality of relationship and communication between the patient and family and the members of the palliative care team
- The patient's and family's preferences for receiving care at home or in an institutional setting, and the impact of either setting on the actual experience of care

- The personal meaning and significance the subject attaches to the events of the patient's illness, and the emotional and spiritual resources the participant brings to bear on the situation as it unfolds over time.

For Professional Caregivers
- The personal meaning and significance of caring for the particular patient and family
- The quality of relationship and communication between patient and family and members of the palliative care team
- The functioning of the palliative care team in the course of caring for the patient and family
- Cultural and ethical issues arising in the care of the patient and family.

With the consent of interviewees, we audiotaped each interview so we could participate fully and without distractions in every conversation. As the participants drew us into their stories, we asked ourselves questions such as: "What is my sense about the narrative content?" "What have I learned that I didn't understand before?" "What are the things I must now try to learn and understand when we meet again?" "How does my present knowledge compare with our thoughts about this particular case?" "How has my knowledge and understanding changed?" Transcribed interviews became part of the ongoing narrative record. Data collection, transcription, description, analysis, and interpretation proceeded simultaneously. In the case of several patients, family members, and caregivers in Montreal who were French speakers, interviews were conducted in their own language by Anna Towers, who is bilingual. For this book, we have translated all French quotations into English.

Journals

In Montreal, both researchers and caregivers kept journals. In Lancaster, caregivers chose not to do that, for they felt that their already demanding schedule didn't leave time for such an involved activity. Journals were variously referred to as a "diary," a "notebook," or "personal record" and contained personal accounts of insights, preliminary understandings, ideas, thoughts, dilemmas, and decisions made during research and caregiving. For the professional caregivers, we provided a few questions to prompt their journal keeping. These were

1. What thoughts or feelings stand out in your mind regarding the interactions you had today with the patient and family? Were there any particularly meaningful or particularly frustrating incidents?
2. Were there any cultural or ethical issues that you want to comment on?
3. Are there any issues that you wish to record regarding the hospital or the healthcare system in general, as you think it affected the care of this patient today?

In keeping journals, the aim was to capture the present moment while trying to avoid "future recall" as much as possible. We found that personal records facilitated the caregivers' self-reflective process and strengthened their connection to past events during interviews. Our own journals served us in a similar way. They inspired us to reflect, shaped our questions during interviews, and helped us write the narratives in ways that included our own impressions in addition to those of our interviewees.

In summary, the raw data from which our narratives were constructed consist of the hundreds of hours (and pages) of transcribed interviews and similarly voluminous contemporaneous fieldnotes, as well as the formal documentation of caregiving encounters and patient experiences that we extracted from medical records and nurses' progress notes.

Narrative

In the past few decades, the importance of illness narratives to provide meaning, context, and an understanding of the patient's own experience of illness has become increasingly significant for researchers and clinicians in the health and social sciences. A narrative methodology draws on the human tendency to tell stories and search for meaning in personal experience.[15-18] Narrative inquiry examines the lived experience of people's storied lives as they are told to the researcher, and these become a rich source of knowledge and understanding.[19] It has been increasingly emphasized in the medical literature that narratives offer a rich resource for both medical education and clinical practice.[20-23] Life stories, illness accounts, and personal journals are being used as research data in medicine as a means of understanding feelings, experiences, goals, preferences, and needs in illness and treatment.[24-28]

The emergence of the medical narrative has revealed that it is possible to go beyond the traditional clinical case history to understand the course of a patient's illness.

In medical anthropology, the early work of Arthur Kleinman[25] made a significant departure from the conventional clinical case genre. This work reported not only symptoms and pathological processes but also patients' subjective experiences. David Barnard's previous case narrative work has also shown that the illness experience is shaped by the telling and listening to stories over time.[24] Books by Ira Byock, Michael Kearney, and Timothy Quill, which were published around the time of our research, draw on richly narrated personal experience in caring for the terminally ill.[13,29,30] We viewed our research as providing a complement—and in some respects a further development—to their very important work.

Of course, the narratives in this book are *our* stories, told in our voices. In order to transfer the rich, sometimes overwhelming details of many people's experiences into a single narrative, we have had to be selective. We have imposed our sense of theme on experience, which in its pure state has no theme but simply follows the continual flow of life. We have often resorted to devices of narration, scene-setting, and similar features typical of fiction. These narratives are works of fiction in the sense that they are the result of creative, selective shaping processes that are inherent in all storytelling. We do not present them as the definitive, "objective" story, "the way it was." On the other hand, we have tried to be as faithful as possible to what we witnessed, and we have tried to situate our observations and our identification of themes in the larger context of other empirical and narrative research on palliative care.

To say that there are fictive elements in our narratives is not, of course, to differentiate them to any substantial degree from the many forms of narrative that guide medical practice and medical education.[20,31] For, in fact, medical decisions are always rooted in the exchange and creation of stories, which are shaped not only by medical information but also by beliefs, feelings, needs, experiences, impressions, speculations, and perceptions. By acknowledging these fictive elements directly here, and by making frequent reference to our own participation in the cases, we have attempted to provide readers with the information they need to make appropriate critical assessment of the narratives. Our preferred test of the truth value of our narratives is a pragmatic one: Do the experiences we have recorded, and the insights they engender, contribute in any significant way to more empathic, competent, and effective palliative care?

Ethics and Narrative Inquiry

As researchers, we encountered three principal ethical issues: (1) obtaining adequate informed consent, (2) protecting privacy, and (3) maintaining confidentiality within the team and between the team and patients and families. A further ethical issue lay in the challenge for Anna Towers in her dual role of clinician on the palliative care unit as well as that of her role of researcher in our study. Although Anna did not participate in the research process when a patient was specifically under her care, there were times when, as a palliative care doctor, she had responsibilities to care for the entire unit. At these times, when a patient in our study was in distress and asked specifically for help or information, this presented Anna with an ethical dilemma. Reflecting on this issue in the case of Raymond Hynes, she describes her concerns: "I did not want to avoid direct questions regarding prognosis, but I was not Mr. Hynes's physician. I found it difficult to be both a researcher and a physician at this point."

All potential participants—patients, families, and caregivers—received a detailed account of our study's purposes and methods prior to deciding whether to join the study. No patients were contacted for possible inclusion in the research without a prior inquiry directed to them by a member of their palliative care team. Only after learning from that team member that a patient was willing to meet us and hear more about the project did we visit any patients. In our first meeting with patients, we gave them written materials describing our study in detail and discussed with them what their participation would entail. Only with the permission of patients did we contact other family members and ask for their permission to include them in our interviews and observations. We received very few refusals. Two families withdrew shortly after beginning, one out of concern for the emotional nature of the interviews, and one because of the patient's extreme weakness and fatigue.

We were frank in telling all potential participants that our discussions were likely to touch on painful emotions, sensitive family issues, and private experiences. Assurances were given to patients, families, and caregivers, however, that the patient's best interests would always override our research needs. We were prepared to stop interviews, cancel visits, and withdraw from the patient's room at any time. In reality, such requests almost never came. We were also explicit about our plans to publish these narratives and explained that we would do everything possible to disguise personal identities. It was a challenge to tell the participants' stories with honesty and integrity while disguising their identity as much as possible. All names have been changed, as well as other potentially identifying details. We explained to the participants that, despite the disguises, they would undoubtedly recognize themselves in the narratives, though we believed it to be very unlikely that people not connected with their case would be able to identify them.

We assured all patients that what they told us would remain confidential. But to this assurance we made two precautionary exceptions. The first was that if a patient disclosed to us explicit suicidal intentions, we would be obliged to report this to the palliative care team. The second was that if we learned of patient abuse or of circumstances in which the patient appeared to be in imminent physical danger, we would again feel compelled to break confidentialities and inform their professional caregivers. As it turned out, we encountered neither of these situations.

To professional caregivers it was emphasized that we would take note of tensions, disagreements, or resentments among them only if they played a significant role in the patient's care. In some instances, they did. Assurances were given that we would take every measure to protect their privacy and that we would not repeat one team member's comments to another without his or her permission.

In the process of collecting data and writing the stories, however, it has become clear that the formal principles underlying informed consent may not account for the uncertainties inherent in the research process. Even though this study was approved by the institutional review boards and ethics committees of the participating institutions, we became aware that the participants could not fully appreciate at the outset the implications of being involved in this type of research. The dying and their loved ones were asked to reveal important pieces of themselves and to tell us of their experiences of suffering, joy, fear, and pain. We asked them to share moments from the long-forgotten past, presently complicated by life's imminent end. We asked them to reach a level of awareness that, without our questioning, they may well not have reached.

We were always faced with the question of whether or how to proceed when painful memories emerged. After working with us on one case, a caregiver turned down our invitation to participate in interviews concerning a second case. She said that the process of self-reflection had drained her emotionally. Like this caregiver, most participants didn't know what impact our study would have on them when they signed their consent form. Moreover, they didn't know the outcome of their story in advance. They could not know, though they sometimes worried, how their words and actions would be interpreted by the readers of this book.

Despite these risks, many patients, families, and caregivers expressed to us their appreciation for our project. Participants initially volunteered for a variety of reasons. Some felt the project was important for palliative care education and were pleased to have the opportunity to contribute to the improvement of end-of-life care. As one person put it, "It may not be helpful to me personally. I will be long gone. But if my story helps other people to suffer less, then I'd like to help." Another person observed, "I am only a novice in this business of dying but perhaps I can share what I myself am now learning." Some patients joined our study because they liked the idea of taking on an important responsibility and feeling useful at the end of their lives. Other patients craved regular visits by an interested listener. Others saw this study as a unique opportunity to gain posthumous public recognition or to redeem their misunderstood lives and actions, and some people were actually disappointed that we would not use their real names. It was not possible to do this, however, because to do so would have risked exposing the identities of the people who surrounded them.

Several participants told us that they experienced a sense of catharsis in being able to state a personal feeling or opinion. They valued the opportunity to have their perspective heard and, in turn, to learn through their own self-disclosure. Some patients told us that they appreciated the opportunity to rethink their own treatment choices in the process of discussion and reflection. In some cases, they said that the process enabled them to redefine and modify their decisions and desires—an obvious example of the effect of the observer on the observed. As one person put it, "As I talk through the daily events and what is happening, it seems to bring me think of things I had not thought about before. . . . I believe perhaps I am also learning."

We also quickly discovered that our methodology had an important impact on us. Through our work, we were touched by the people who generously allowed us into their lives, and we were changed by them. We learned from them to value highly the things we take for granted and to put our lives into perspective. We each experienced profound moments that will remain forever in our memories. We discovered that there was an element of risk in our work for us as well. We experienced the risk in maintaining relationships with the dying, the risk of loss of closely formed bonds, and the risk that each encounter could challenge our own sense of self and well-being. Palliative caregivers tend not to think of themselves as risk-takers, but it is an accepted part of what they do and is embedded in their everyday care of the dying.[32] In our study, in the midst of our own complacency, we had to think through our own perspectives about care at the end of life. As we witnessed different people's courage and resourcefulness, each one of us, at one time or another, wondered, "Will I cope as well?" or "What will happen when I am dying?" We were forced to reflect on the protected and sometimes controlling nature of our roles as clinicians, researchers, and teachers. As we listened to the participants' stories, there was always an awareness that at any time we could seek refuge behind our identities as professionals or scholars. We would never pretend, therefore, that we reached the depths of the other person's experience. We could leave a painful moment behind; the patients and families could not.

References

1. Miller WL, Crabtree BF. Clinical research. In: Denzin NK, Lincoln YS, eds. *Handbook of Qualitative Research*, 2nd ed. Thousand Oaks, CA: Sage; 2000:607–631.
2. Clark D. What is qualitative research and what can it contribute to palliative care? Palliat Med. 1997;11:159–166.
3. Malterud K. *Qualitative Metasynthesis: A Research Method for Medicine and the Health Sciences*. London: Routledge; 2019.
4. Dixon-Woods S, Agarwai S, Jones D, et al. Synthesising qualitative and quantitative evidence: A review of possible methods. J Health Serv Res Policy. 2005;10(1):45–53.
5. Strange KC, Crabtree BF, Miller WL. Publishing multimethod research. Ann Fam Med. 2006;4(4):292–294.
6. Patton MQ. *Qualitative Research and Evaluation Methods*. 4th ed. Thousand Oaks, CA: Sage; 2014.
7. Braun V, Clarke V. Novel insights into patients' life worlds. The value of qualitative research. Lancet Psychiatry. 2019;6(9):720–721.
8. Patton, MQ. *Qualitative Evaluation and Research Methods*. 2nd ed. Newbury Park CA: Sage; 1990.
9. Polkinghorne DE. Language and meaning: Data collection in qualitative research. J Couns Psychol. 2005;52(2):137–145.
10. Maykut P, Morehouse R. *Beginning Qualitative Research: A Philosophic and Practical Guide*. London: Falmer Press; 1994.
11. Mount B. Whole person care: Beyond psychosocial and physical needs. Am J Hosp Palliat Care. 1993;10(1):28–37.

12. Mount BM, Kearney M. Healing and palliative care: Charting the way forward. Palliat Med. 2003;17(8):657–658.

13. Kearney M. *Mortally Wounded: Stories of Soul Pain, Death, and Healing.* New York: Scribner; 1996.

14. Hutchinson TA. *Whole Person Care: A New Paradigm for the 21st Century.* New York: Springer; 2011.

15. Josselson R. On writing other people's lives: Self-analytic reflections of a narrative researcher. In: Josselson R, ed. *Ethics and Process in the Narrative Study of Lives.* Thousand Oaks, CA: Sage; 1996:60–72.

16. Payne S. Selecting an approach and design in qualitative research. Palliat Med. 1997;11:249–252.

17. McAdams DP, Josselson R, Lieblich A, eds. *Identity and story: Creating Self in Narrative.* Washington, DC: American Psychological Association; 2006.

18. Bingley AF, Thomas C, Brown J, et al. Developing narrative research in supportive and palliative care: The focus on illness narratives. Palliat Med. 2008;22(5):653–658.

19. Clandinin DJ. *Engaging in Narrative Inquiry.* New York: Routledge; 2016.

20. Hunter KM. *Doctors' Stories: The Narrative Structure of Medical Knowledge.* Princeton: Princeton University Press; 1991.

21. Barnard D. Joining the healing community: Images and narratives to promote inter-professional professionalism. J Allied Health. 2015;44(4):244–248.

22. Charon R. Narrative medicine: The essential role of stories in medical education and communication. In: Fernandes I, Martins C, Reis A, Sanches Z, eds. *Creative Dialogues: Narrative and Medicine.* Newcastle-upon-Tyne: Cambridge Scholars Publishing, Lady Stephenson Library; 2015:95–111.

23. Kleinman A. The illness narratives: Suffering, healing, and the human condition. Acad Med. 2017;92(10):1406–1407.

24. Barnard D. A case of amyotrophic lateral sclerosis: A reprise and reply. Lit Med. 1992;11(1):133–146.

25. Kleinman A. *The Illness Narratives.* New York: Basic Books; 1988.

26. Frank AW. *At the Will of the Body: Reflections on Illness.* New York: Houghton Mifflin; 1992.

27. Frank AW. *The Wounded Storyteller: Body, Illness, and Ethics.* 2nd ed. Chicago: University of Chicago Press; 2013.

28. Hawkins J, Lindsay E. We listen but do we hear? The importance of patient stories. Br J Community Nurs. 2006;11(9):S6–14.

29. Byock I. *Dying Well: The Prospect for Growth at the End of Life.* New York: Riverhead; 1997.

30. Quill TE. *A Midwife Through the Dying Process: Stories of Healing and Hard Choices at the End of Life.* Baltimore: Johns Hopkins University Press; 1996.

31. Banks JT, Hawkins AH, eds. The art of the case history. Lit Med. 1992;11(1):1–182.

32. Boston P, Towers A, Barnard D. Embracing vulnerability: Risk and empathy in palliative care. J Palliat Care. 2001;17(4):248–253.

Suggestions for Further Reading

Buckman R. *How to Break Bad News.* Baltimore: Johns Hopkins University Press; 1992.

Byock I. *Dying Well: The Prospect for Growth at the End of Life.* New York: Riverhead; 1997.

Callanan M, Kelley P. *Final Gifts: Understanding the Special Needs, Awareness, and Communications of the Dying.* New York: Simon and Schuster; 2012.

Cassell EJ. The nature of suffering and the goals of medicine. *N Eng J Med.* 1982;306(11):639–645.

Cassell EJ. *The Nature of Suffering and the Goals of Medicine.* 2nd ed. New York: Oxford University Press; 2004.

Charon R. *Narrative Medicine: Honoring the Stories of Illness.* New York: Oxford University Press; 2006.

Cherny NI, Fallon MT, Kaasa S, Portenoy RK, Currow DC, eds. 2021. *Oxford Textbook of Palliative Medicine.* 6th ed. New York: Oxford University Press; 2021.

Chochinov HM, Breitbart W, eds. *Handbook of Psychiatry in Palliative Medicine.* 2nd ed. New York: Oxford University Press; 2009.

Crawley L, Payne R, Bolden J, et al. Palliative and end-of-life care in the African American community. *JAMA.* 2000;284(19):2518–2521.

Crawley L, Singer MK. Racial, cultural, and ethnic factors affecting the quality of end-of-life care in California. California HealthCare Foundation. 2007. https://www.chcf.org/wp-content/uploads/2017/12/PDF-CulturalFactorsEOL.pdf. Accessed August 10, 2022.

De Boulay S, Rankin M. *Cicely Saunders: The Founder of the Modern Hospice Movement.* London: SPCK Publishing; 2007.

Denholm DB. *The Caregiving Wife's Handbook: Caring for Your Seriously Ill Husband, Caring for Yourself.* Alameda, CA: Hunter House; 2012.

Didion J. *The Year of Magical Thinking.* New York: Knopf; 2005.

Elbaum A. Black lives in a pandemic: Implications of systemic injustice for end-of-life care. *Hastings Cent Rep.* 2020;50(3):58–60.

Ferrell B, Paice J, eds. *Oxford Textbook of Palliative Nursing.* 5th ed. New York: Oxford University Press; 2019.

Frankl VE. *Man's Search for Meaning.* New York: Washington Square Press; 1988.

Gawande A. *Being Mortal: Medicine and What Matters in the End.* New York: Metropolitan Books; 2014.

Hain R, Goldman A, Rapoport A, Meiring M, eds. *Oxford Textbook of Palliative Care for Children.* 3rd ed. New York: Oxford University Press; 2021.

Halifax J. *Being with Dying: Cultivating Compassion and Fearlessness in the Presence of Death.* Boston: Shambhala Publications; 2008.

Holloway K. *Passed On: African American Mourning Stories.* Durham, NC: Duke University Press; 2003.

Hooijer G, King D. The racialized pandemic: Wave one of COVID-19 and the reproduction of global north inequalities. The Cambridge Core. *Perspect. Politics.* August 11, 2021:1–21. https://doi.org/10.1017/S153759272100195X.

Hutchinson TA, ed. *Whole Person Care: A New Paradigm for the 21st Century.* New York: Springer International; 2011.

Hutchinson TA. *Whole Person Care: Transforming Healthcare.* New York: Springer International; 2017.

Kearney M. Palliative medicine: Just another speciality? *Palliat Med.* 1992;6:39–46.

Kearney M. *Mortally Wounded: Stories of Soul Pain, Death and Healing.* New York: Scribner; 1996.

Kuhl D. *What Dying People Want: Practical Wisdom for the End of Life.* Toronto: Anchor Canada; 2002.

Lewis CS. *A Grief Observed.* New York: Harper Collins; 1994.

Macdonald S, Herx L, Boyle A, eds. *Palliative Medicine: A Case Based Manual.* 4th ed. New York: Oxford University Press; 2021.

Mount B, Boston P, Cohen S. Healing connections: On moving from suffering to a sense of wellbeing. *J Pain Symptom Manag.* 2007;33(4):372–388.

Mount B. Healing, quality of life, and the need for a paradigm shift in health care. *J Palliat Care.* 2013;29(1):45–48.

Mount B. *Ten Thousand Crossroads: The Path as I Remember It.* Montreal and Kingston: McGill-Queens University Press; 2020.

Nuland SB. *How We Die: Reflections on Life's Final Chapter.* New York: Knopf; 1994.

Payne R, London D, Latson S, eds. *Key Topics on End-of-Life Care for African Americans: An Intellectual Discourse Derived from The Last Miles of the Way Home 2004 National Conference to Improve End-of-Life Care for African Americans.* Durham, NC: Duke Institute on Care at the End of Life; 2006. https://divinity.duke.edu/sites/divinity.duke.edu/files/documents/tmc/KTFULL.pdf.

Rosa WE, Ferrell BR, Applebaum AJ. The alleviation of suffering during the COVID-19 pandemic. *Palliat Support Care.* June 23, 2020:376–378. https://doi.org/10.1017/S1478951520000462.

Schiffman DD. *Coping with the Death of a Child: An Integrated Clinical Approach to Working with Bereaved Families.* New York: Routledge; 2020.

Simmons P. *Learning to Fall: The Blessings of an Imperfect Life.* New York: Bantam Books; 2002.

Thomas K, Lobo B, Detering K, eds. *Advance Care Planning in End-of-Life Care.* 2nd ed. Oxford: Oxford University Press; 2018.

Tolstoy L. *The Death of Ivan Ilych.* Trans. by Richard Pevear and Larissa Volokhonsky. New York: Vintage Books; 2010.

Webb NB. The child and death. In: Webb NB, ed. *Helping Bereaved Children: A Handbook for Practitioners.* New York: Guilford; 2010:3–19.

Youngner SJ, Arnold RM, eds. *The Oxford Handbook of Ethics at End of Life.* New York: Oxford University Press; 2016.

Index of Themes